Pitfalls in Diagnosis and Treatment of Shoulder Joint Diseases

Yu-jie Liu • Chang-ming Huang • Jing Xue
Editors

Pitfalls in Diagnosis and Treatment of Shoulder Joint Diseases

Springer

北京大学医学出版社
PUMP 1989

Editors
Yu-jie Liu
Orthopaedics
Chinese PLA General Hospital
Beijing, China

Chang-ming Huang
Orthopaedics
The 73 Group Army Hospital, Chenggong
Hospital Affiliated to Xiamen University
Xiamen, Fujian Province, China

Jing Xue
Orthopaedics
Air Force Medical Center of Chinese PLA
Beijing, China

ISBN 978-981-96-2474-4 ISBN 978-981-96-2472-0 (eBook)
https://doi.org/10.1007/978-981-96-2472-0

Jointly published with Peking University Medical Press
The print edition is not for sale in China (Mainland). Customers from China (Mainland) please order the print book from: Peking University Medical Press.

This Springer imprint is published by the registered company Springer Nature Singapore Pte Ltd.
The registered company address is: 152 Beach Road, #21-01/04 Gateway East, Singapore 189721, Singapore

Contents

Part I

Countermeasures for Cervical Diseases Misdiagnosed as Shoulder Joint Conditions: An Introduction and Summary

Jing Xue

Introduction

Neck and shoulder pain are common clinically, and sometimes the diagnosis of the condition that causes them is difficult to differentiate. In particular, cervical spinal cord disease causes symptoms of the shoulder joint, such as Keegan's disease, which is easily misdiagnosed as rotator cuff injury; Charcot joints caused by syringomyelia induce bone destruction of the shoulder joint, shoulder instability, and lift dysfunction; and neck injury-induced brachial plexus injury, which can lead to atrophy of muscles around the shoulder joint and weakness of shoulder lift. If the above conditions are not well diagnosed, it is very easy to misdiagnose or mistreat clinically. Doctors cannot only treat the head when there is a headache and the foot when there is a foot pain. This part will delve into the differential diagnosis of shoulder instability caused by syringomyelia, Keegan disease, and rotator cuff injury, as well as the issues of cervical injury-induced brachial plexus injury and shoulder joint diseases.

Summary

1. Shoulder pain is not always caused by diseases of the shoulder joint itself. Clinicians should improve their understanding of the shoulder symptoms induced by cervical spine diseases and should not only seek the cause from the shoulder joint itself. They should also avoid confusing cervical vertebra, spinal cord, and brachial plexus injuries with shoulder diseases.
2. Charcot's joint is the destruction of osteochondral cartilage of the shoulder joint caused by the denervation of the sensory neuron lesions in the spinal cord. For patients with sensorimotor separation, cervical syringomyelia should be highly suspected. Cervical spine MRI is of great value for its diagnosis. In addition, surgical treatment decisions should be carefully made for Charcot's joint.
3. Keegan's disease is caused by motor nerve compression of the cervical spine, which manifests as shoulder joint motor dysfunction, mainly characterized by supraspinatus and deltoid weakness, with no abnormal limb sensation, making it easy to be misdiagnosed as a rotator cuff injury. MRI shows compression of anterior motor nerve roots of the cervical

J. Xue (✉)
Orthopaedics, Air Force Medical Center of Chinese PLA, Beijing, China

spine or anterior horn of the spinal cord. Keegan's disease is a self-limiting disease, and most of them can be cured with correct conservative treatment, so don't rush to surgery.

4. Clinicians should not only pay attention to imaging examinations without examining patients but should inquire in detail about the patient's posture at the time of injury, symptoms after injury, and analyze the mechanism of injury and the process of post-injury diagnosis and treatment. Carefully perform visual inspection, palpation, percussion, measurement, and special examinations, paying attention to limb sensation, movement, muscle strength, and range of motion, and do not be confused by imaging. It is necessary to see through the appearance to perceive the essence, expand the thinking, eliminate the false, and retain the true. Through differential diagnosis, one can obtain the correct diagnosis.
5. Clinicians should be familiar with nerve and muscle anatomy and pay special attention to the examination of the spinal cord and brachial plexus for neck and shoulder injuries. Surgeons should strictly screen patients, do not arbitrarily expand the indications for surgery, and pay attention to conservative treatment and postoperative rehabilitation.

Syringomyelia-Induced Shoulder Instability

1

Yu-jie Liu and Jing Xue

Charcot arthropathy, also known as neuropathic arthropathy, is mostly due to diabetes, syringomyelia, spinal cord trauma, leprosy, chronic alcoholism, and other factors. Charcot arthritis often affects the shoulder joint, resulting in bone destruction, shoulder instability, and lifting dysfunction. Syringomyelia causes nerve dysfunction around the shoulder joint, which is a common cause of shoulder Shakk's arthritis [1], manifested by repeated shoulder dislocation and osteoarticular degeneration and destruction.

1.1 Overview of the Diagnosis and Treatment Process

The patient, a 39-year-old male, has had unexplained recurrent dislocations of the left shoulder joint for more than 10 years, and each dislocation can be reduced by himself. Ten days ago, the left shoulder joint was dislocated again, and the self-traction reduction was unsuccessful, so he came to the hospital. Physical examination: left shoulder abduction, forward flexion, dorsiflexion, internal rotation, and external rotation were all limited. The left elbow, wrist, and knuckles moved freely, muscle strength was normal, and the left upper limb had decreased temperature and pain sensation. The left shoulder joint presented with a square shoulder deformity (Fig. 1.1), accompanied by palpation of emptiness in the shoulder joint. The left biceps brachii muscle was more prominent than the contralateral side, presenting with a positive "Popeye sign" (Fig. 1.2), Dugas sign (Fig. 1.3), and Sulcus sign test (Fig. 1.4). X-ray showed a left shoulder dislocation with calcification visible on the lateral side (Fig. 1.5). Computed tomography (CT) showed a left humeral head dislocation downward and forward, with the anterior inferior edge of the glenoid embedded in the bone defect of the humeral head (Fig. 1.6). Magnetic resonance imaging (MRI) showed cluttered signals in left shoulder joint with rotator cuff and amounts of high signal in the joint. No signal of biceps longus tendon found in the intertubercular groove. The glenoid was embedded in the humeral head (Fig. 1.7).

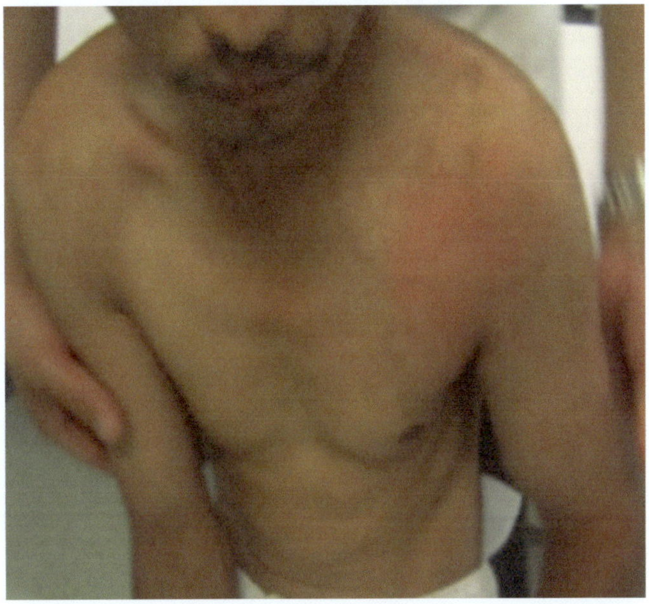

Fig. 1.1 The left shoulder showed a square shoulder, with a palpation of emptiness

According to the diagnosis of left shoulder dislocation and Hill-sach injury, manual reduction was successfully applied without anesthesia, and X-ray examination confirmed successful reduction. During the process of reduction, the patient had no pain or painful expression. After reduction, a shoulder sling was applied, and the left shoulder joint dislocated again the next day.

Y.-j. Liu
Orthopaedics, Chinese PLA General Hospital, Beijing, China

J. Xue (✉)
Orthopaedics, Air Force Medical Center of Chinese PLA, Beijing, China

Y.-j. Liu et al. (eds.), *Pitfalls in Diagnosis and Treatment of Shoulder Joint Diseases*,
https://doi.org/10.1007/978-981-96-2472-0_1

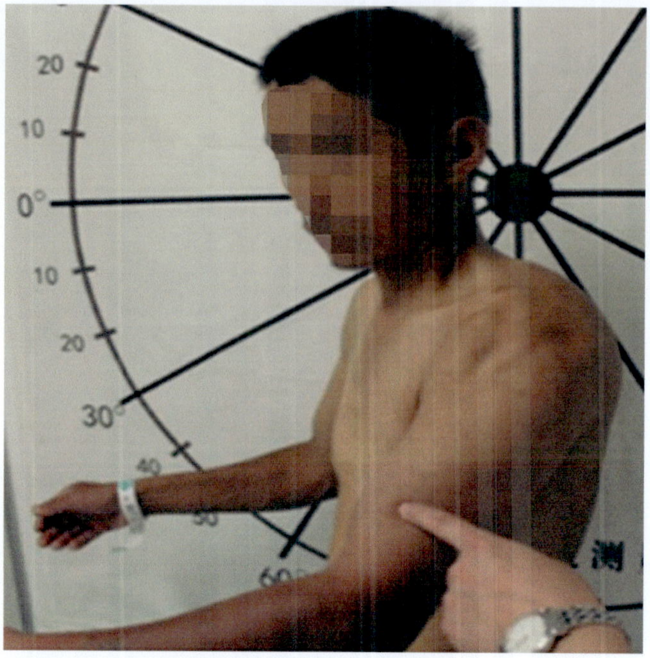

Fig. 1.2 Positive "Popeye sign" with left biceps brachii muscle

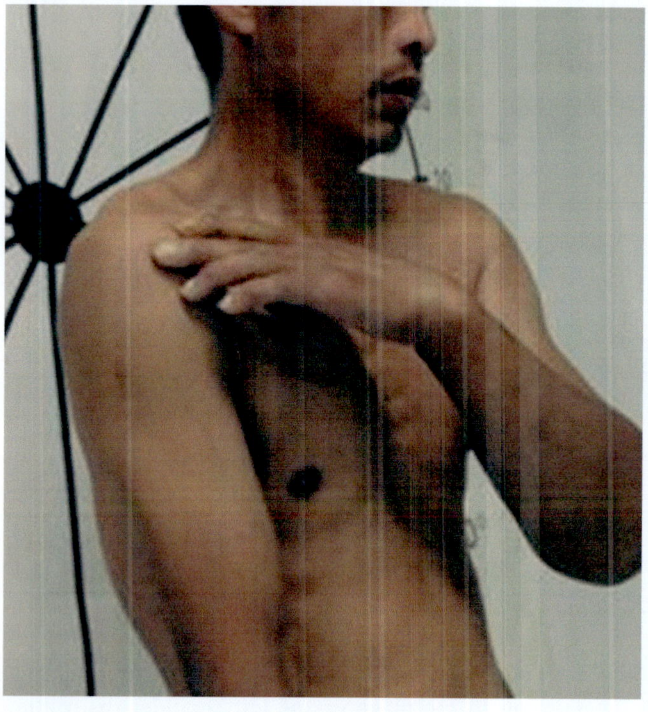

Fig. 1.3 Positive Dugas sign with left shoulder

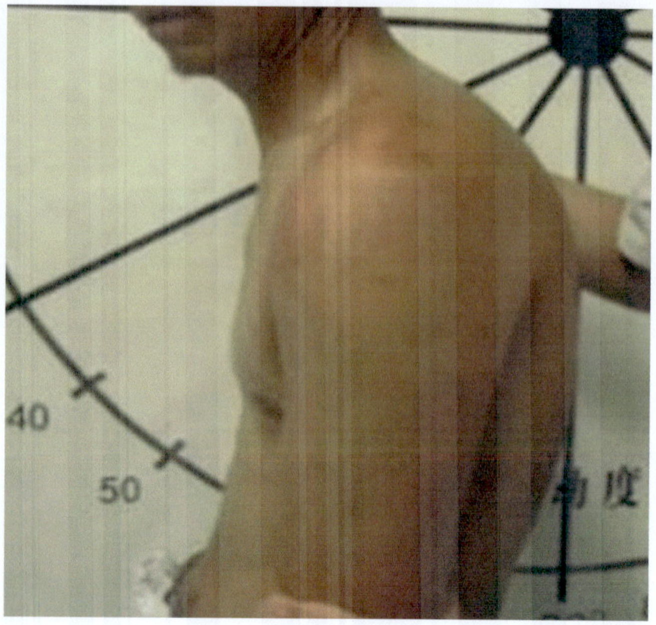

Fig. 1.4 Positive Sulcus sign test with left shoulder

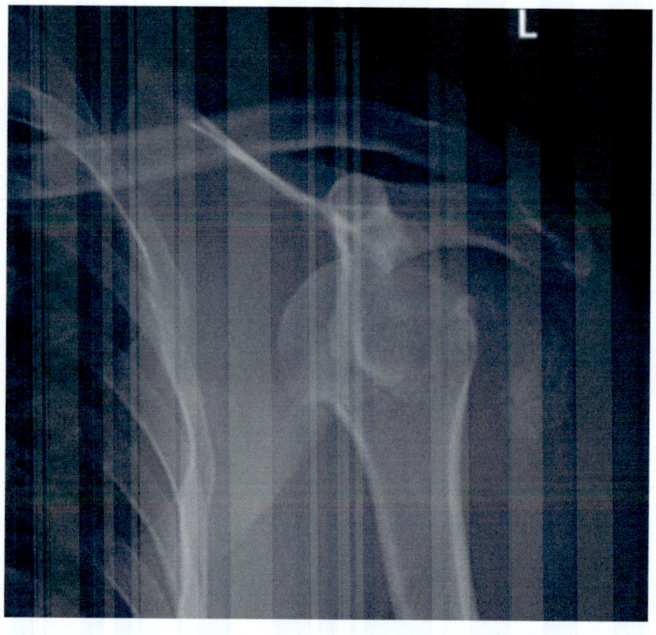

Fig. 1.5 The X-ray showed a dislocation of the left shoulder with soft tissue calcification

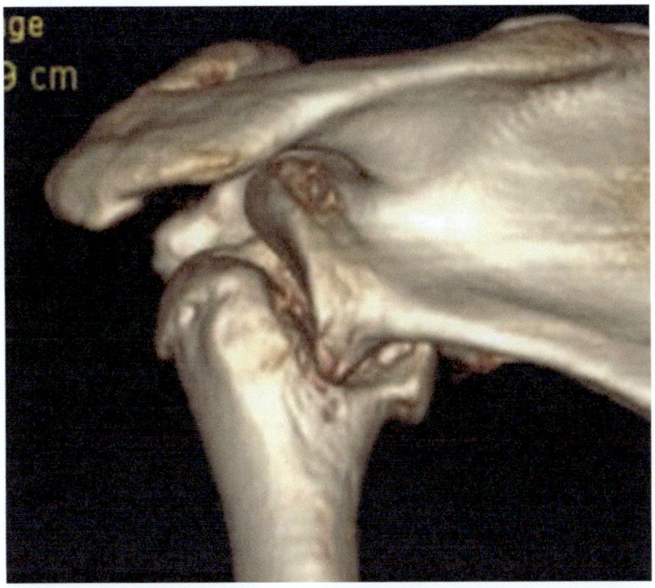

Fig. 1.6 3D reconstruction Computed tomography (CT) showed left humeral head dislocated downward and forward, with the anterior inferior edge of the glenoid embedded in the bone defect of the humeral head

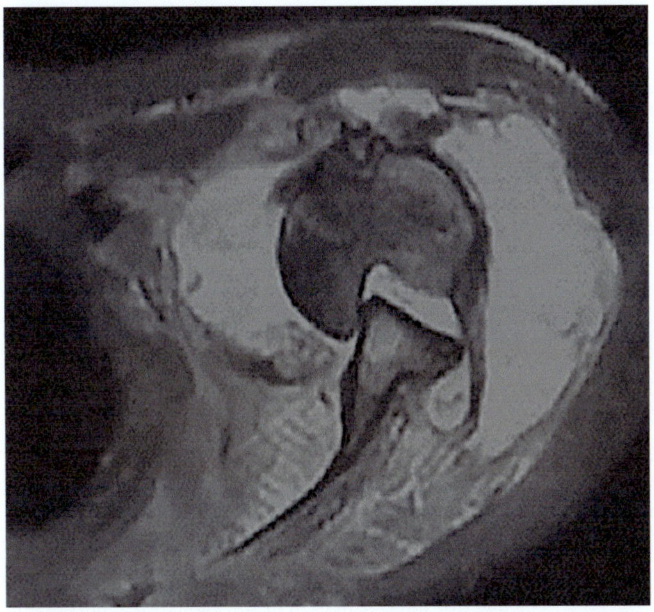

Fig. 1.7 Magnetic resonance imaging (MRI) showed cluttered signals in left shoulder joint with rotator cuff and amounts of high signal in the joint. No signal of biceps longus tendon found in the intertubercular groove. The glenoid was embedded in the humeral head

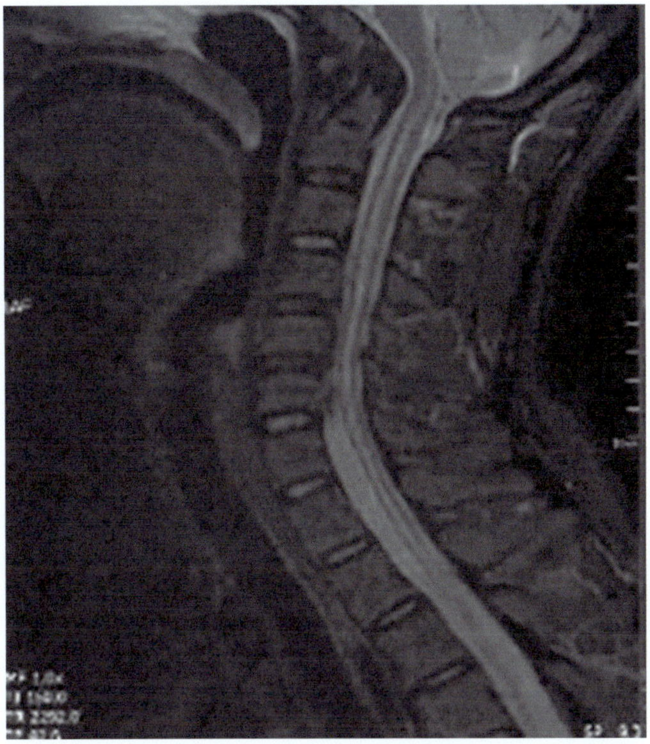

Fig. 1.8 MRI of the cervical spine showed abnormal signal at the C2-T2 level, low signal in T1 WI and high signal in T2 WI

MRI of the cervical spine showed abnormal signal at the C2-T2 level, low signal in T1 WI and high signal in T2 WI (Fig. 1.8). Electromyographic examination showed neurogenic injury in the bilateral common digital extensor, first interbony muscle, and abductor pollicis.

Arthroscopic exploration revealed hyperplasia, congestion, and edema of the synovial tissue in the shoulder joint (Fig. 1.9), tears of the supraspinatus tendon and subaspinatus tendon, and the joint cavity communicating with subacromial pouch (Fig. 1.10); rupture of long-head tendon of the biceps brachii (Fig. 1.11); large area damage to the humeral head and glenoid cartilage, with exposure of subchondral bone. The anterior inferior margin of the glenoid is embedded in the groove-like defect area of the humeral head, presenting a locked bite (Fig. 1.12). After debridement under arthroscopy, the dislocated humeral head was successfully relocated.

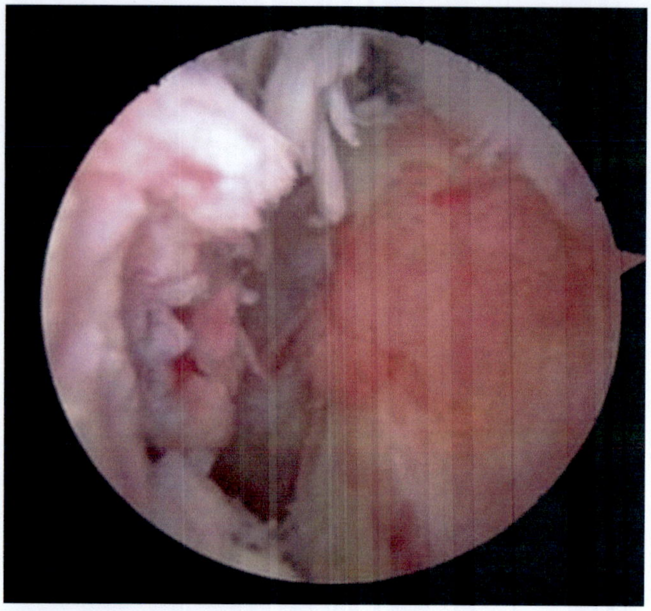

Fig. 1.9 The hyperplasia and edema of the synovial membrane of the shoulder joint cavity

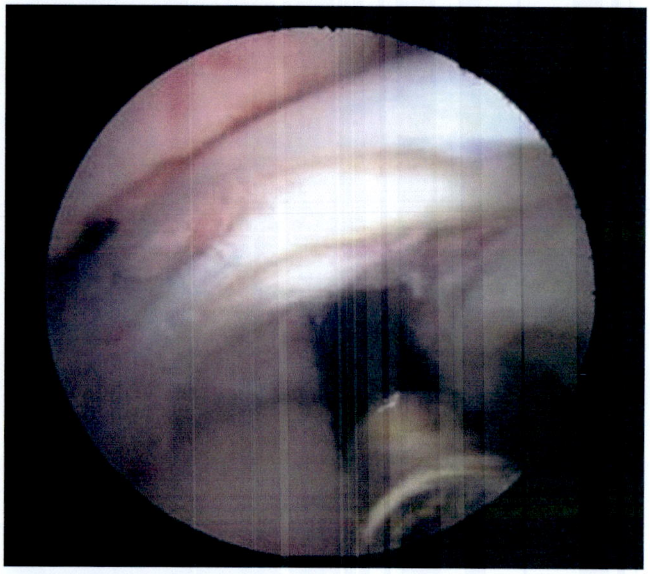

Fig. 1.10 Supraspinatus tendon injury with large area defect

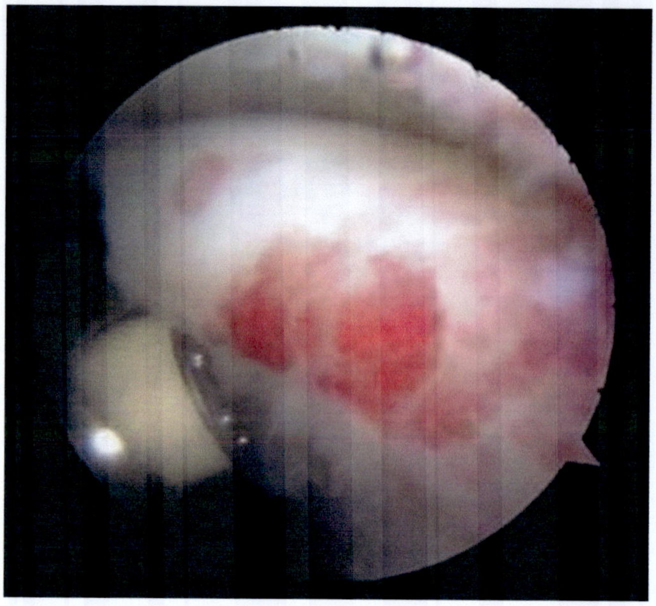

Fig. 1.11 Long-head tendon of the biceps brachii muscle ruptured and absent

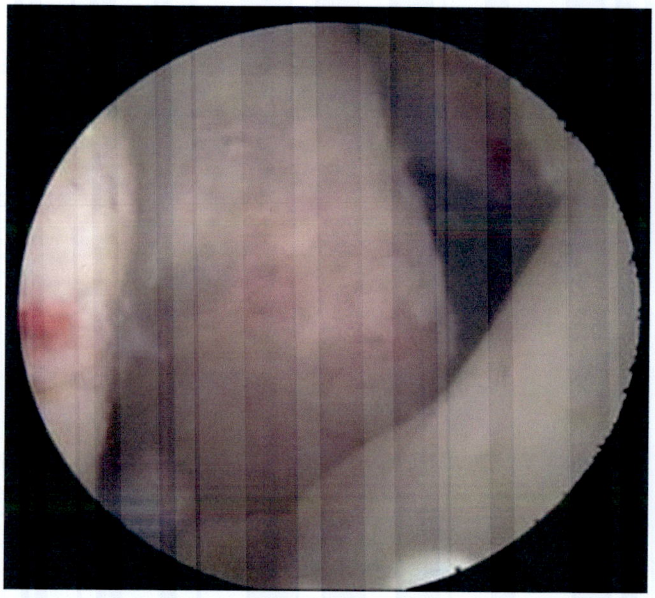

Fig. 1.12 The anterior inferior margin of the glenoid is embedded in the groove-like defect area of the humeral head, presenting a locked bite

1.2 Misconceptions in Diagnostic and Treatment of Shoulder Joint Injuries and Syringomyelia

Shoulder instability and irreparable huge rotator cuff injury are easier to diagnose according to routine physical examination and imaging examination. However, if the shoulder instability was caused by cervical disease, most inexperienced doctors rarely associate the cervical spinal cord and cervical plexus neuropathy with shoulder disease, and only seek the cause around the shoulder joint, which is the main reason for misdiagnosis or mistreatment. When the physical examination finds the separation of sensory and motor movement of the affected limb, cervical spinal cord disease should be suspected, and the cervical MRI examination is an important means to diagnosis. In this case, the cervical MRI showed an expansion of the central aqueduct of the cervical spinal cord (Fig. 1.8).

The central canal runs throughout the spinal cord, and obstruction of cerebrospinal fluid circulation can lead to syringomyelia formation [2]. Syringomyelia is a chronic, progressive spinal cord disease in which the central aqueduct in the spinal cord dilates tubularly, manifested by progressive expansion of the cystic cavity from the inside out and compression of spinal cord tissue, resulting in sensory, motor separation, and neurotrophic disorders, manifested by decreased pain and temperature sensation and normal deep sense [3]. Astrocytosis is the main pathological manifestation [4]. MRI is important for the diagnosis of syringomyelia, which manifests as segmental long T1 and T2 signaling cystic lesions of the spinal cord [5].

The "Charcot joint" was proposed by the French scholar Jean-Marie Charcot in 1868 and refers to destructive diseases of osteoarthritis caused by sensory abnormalities and neurotrophic disorders [2]. Syringomyelia is one of the main causes of Charcot joints, and lesions are more common in the cervical spinal cord and are neurotrophic disorders characterized by joint swelling and limited mobility [4]. Due to the lack of protective response of joints, joint cartilage wear and damage are serious, especially in long-term heavy labor workers. Charcot's arthritis, early X-rays show swollen soft tissues and dense bones. In advanced patients, there are varying degrees of bone resorption, destruction, intra-articular free bodies, osteophytes or new bone formation, joint dislocation and deformity, and periarticular structural destruction and pathological fractures.

There are not many reports in the literature on Charcot's shoulder arthritis. In 2018, Xin Wang counted reports of Charcot's arthritis published in Pubmed in 34 cases, of which 17 (50%) involved the shoulder joint [5]. In the same year, J. Hernigou also reported only 18 cases of Charcot's joint involvement in the shoulder in the English literature, accounting for 5% of all Charcot's arthritis [6].

Because Charcot's shoulder arthritis is relatively rare; insufficient clinical understanding is prone to missed diagnosis. For patients with recurrent shoulder dislocation without obvious cause of injury, temperature, pain, and touch sensations should be routinely examined during physical examination, and imaging of the cervical spine should be performed if necessary. Early detection and early treatment can effectively improve prognosis. Although Charcot's shoulder arthritis has very serious pathological changes on imaging and arthroscopy, the patient's pain symptoms and muscle strength disorders are not obvious, due to protective pain loss. The shoulder joint can be repeatedly dislocated, and the humeral head and the shoulder glenoid repeatedly collide, resulting in serious damage and bone defects of the humeral head and osteochondrage. Patients with Charcot's shoulder arthritis can reduce their shoulder dislocation on their own and should not be overtreated at the first time, mainly to maintain shoulder joint function. In the later stage, because the shoulder glenoid is embedded in the humeral head, occlusal twisting is difficult to reduce and requires surgical management.

Although patients with Charcot's knee osteoarthritis have been treated with rotary hinge knee replacement surgery, the short-term efficacy is good, but the long-term efficacy remains to be explored [7]. Charcot's shoulder arthritis has previously used shoulder fusion, hemishoulder replacement, and shoulder surface replacement, and its long-term efficacy has been unsatisfactory [1]. Many scholars believe that the key to treatment is to prevent the progression of the primary disease of cervical syringomyelopathy [3, 8]. Makihara et al. reported a patient with syringomyelia complicated by severe shoulder osteoarthritis who underwent spinal decompression surgery with a glenoid defect that continued to regenerate in the 3 years after surgery, and the range of motion of the shoulder joint almost returned to normal [9]. Matsuhashi et al. also reported that three patients who underwent humeral head replacement after spinal decompression surgery had 8 years of follow-up, and pain and range of motion improved, and no postoperative failure occurred [10]. Self-absorption of some spinal cord cavities has also been reported [11].

In summary, the treatment of Charcot's shoulder arthritis and dislocation caused by syringomyelia is premised on the diagnosis and treatment of syringomyelia by neurosurgery and the maintenance of joint function through conservative treatment. For occlusal shoulder dislocations that are difficult to reduce, arthroscopic surgical exploration and treatment is also a good treatment choice.

References

1. Snoddy MC, Lee DH, Kuhn JE. Charcot shoulder and elbow: a review of the literature and update on treatment. J Shoulder Elb Surg. 2017;26(3):544–52. https://doi.org/10.1016/j.jse.2016.10.015.
2. Kumar DR, Aslinia F, Yale SH, Mazza JJ. Jean-Martin Charcot: the father of neurology. Clin Med Res. 2011;9(1):46–9. https://doi.org/10.3121/cmr.2009.883.
3. Zheng G, Xia H. Research progress of pathogenesis and surgical management in syringomyelia. Chin J Spine Spinal Cord. 2015;25(4):374–8.
4. Sanders LJ. Jean-Martin Charcot (1825–1893). The man behind the joint disease. J Am Podiatr Med Assoc. 2002;92(7):375–80. https://doi.org/10.7547/87507315-92-7-375.
5. Wang X, Li Y, Gao J, Wang T, Li Z. Charcot arthropathy of the shoulder joint as a presenting feature of basilar impression with syringomyelia: a case report and literature review. Medicine (Baltimore). 2018;97(28):e11391. https://doi.org/10.1097/MD.0000000000011391.
6. Hernigou J, Boulares S, Delahaut O. Spontaneous posterior shoulder dislocation as the first symptom of a Charcot arthropathy. Acta Orthop Belg. 2018;84(1):73–7.
7. Zhuang ZK, Xu ZQ, Lin HH, et al. Rotating hinged total knee arthroplasty for end-stage Charcot's joint of the knee. Orthoped J China. 2022;30(3):277–80.
8. Zhou Y, Zhu L, Lin YX, Cheng HL. Charcot elbow joint as the initial symptom in Chiari malformation with syringomyelia. Chin Med J. 2015;128(24):3381–2. https://doi.org/10.4103/0366-6999.171466.
9. Makihara T, Onishi S, Wadano Y, Fujii K, Nagata H, Sakane M. Regrowth of the deteriorated glenoid in advanced Charcot shoulder after suboccipital decompression for syringomyelia: a case report. J Shoulder Elb Surg. 2015;24(8):e223–8. https://doi.org/10.1016/j.jse.2015.04.022.
10. Matsuhashi T, Nagahama K, Suenaga N, Oizumi N, Minami A. Midterm outcomes after humeral head replacement with rotator cuff repair in patients with syringomyelia shoulder neuroarthropathy: a report on three cases. J Shoulder Elb Surg. 2011;20(8):e8–15. https://doi.org/10.1016/j.jse.2011.04.032.
11. Zhang HQ, Chen LQ, Guo CF, Liu SH, Chen J, Luo J. Should syrinx be treated in patients with scoliosis complicated by syringomyelia without neurologic symptom. Orthoped J China. 2008;16(13):961–5.

Keegan's Disease Was Misdiagnosed as Rotator Cuff Injury

2

Chao Zheng, Ji Wu, and Jing Xue

2.1 Overview of Disease Diagnosis and Treatment

A 47-year-old female patient had a sudden sensation of right shoulder joint abduction and lifting weakness recently (Fig. 2.1). She presented to the hospital for treatment mainly because of the right shoulder combing difficulties, accompanied by local acid distension and mild pain. The symptoms gradually worsened. Since the onset of the disease, the patient has no symptoms in other limb joints and denies any history of trauma.

During the physical examination, it was observed that there was no significant atrophy of the right deltoid muscle, with a muscle strength grade of 2. The biceps muscle showed no signs of atrophy and was graded as 3. The strength of the triceps, subscapularis, pectoralis major, rhomboideus, teres major, teres minor, latissimus dorsi, forearm muscle group, and internal muscles of the hand were all graded 5. The affected side has no obstruction in deep sensation, shallow sensation, and pain perception. The lift test, bear hug test, and swallow-tail sign were all positive, while the lift off test and shrug test were negative. The passive movement of the shoulder joint was not limited. The biceps reflex was reduced, and the bilateral Huffman sign and long bundle sign were negative. The examination of the cranial nerve and the rest of the limb nervous system revealed no abnormalities.

The imaging examination demonstrated that the cervical spine radiographs in sagittal position displayed no physiological lordosis. The cervical MRI disclosed mild compression of the dural sac at C4–6 (Fig. 2.2), along with partial disruption of cerebrospinal fluid flow. Axial T2-weighted images showed right side disc herniation at the C4–5 segments, accompanied by significant compression of the right ventral motor nerve root at C5 (Fig. 2.3).

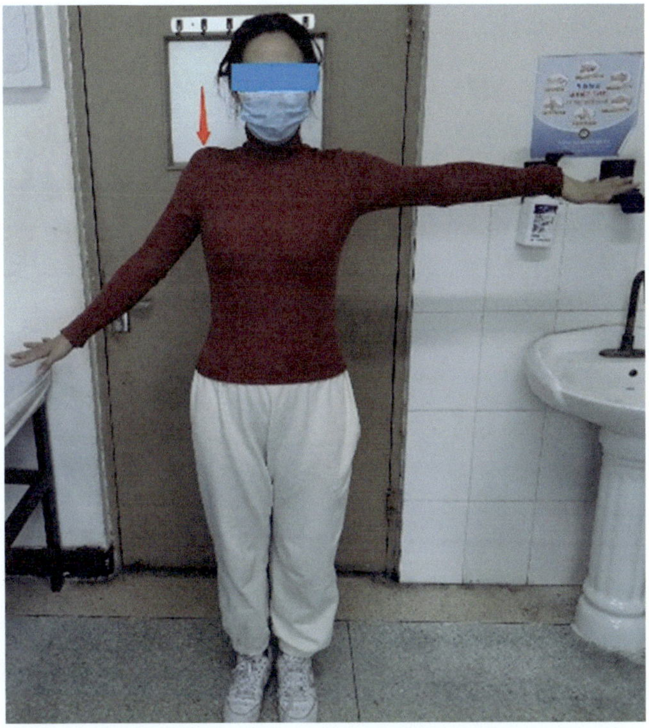

Fig. 2.1 Right shoulder joint abduction and lift weakness

Based on the patient's clinical manifestations symptoms, physical examination results, and imaging findings, the patient was diagnosed with Keegan's disease. A conservative treatment plan was developed including restricting neck movement with a neck brace, administering neuronutrition, dehydration, hormones, and other medications, implementing rehabilitation physiotherapy, and conducting strict follow-up observations of the patient's condition. After 1 week of treatment, the patient's shoulder abduction and lift function began to gradually improve. This treatment regimen was maintained to reinforce its effects, and the shoulder abduction and lift function normalized 1 month later (Fig. 2.4).

C. Zheng (✉)
Air Force Medical Center, Beijing, China

J. Wu · J. Xue
Orthopaedics, Air Force Medical Center of Chinese PLA, Beijing, China

Y.-j. Liu et al. (eds.), *Pitfalls in Diagnosis and Treatment of Shoulder Joint Diseases*, https://doi.org/10.1007/978-981-96-2472-0_2

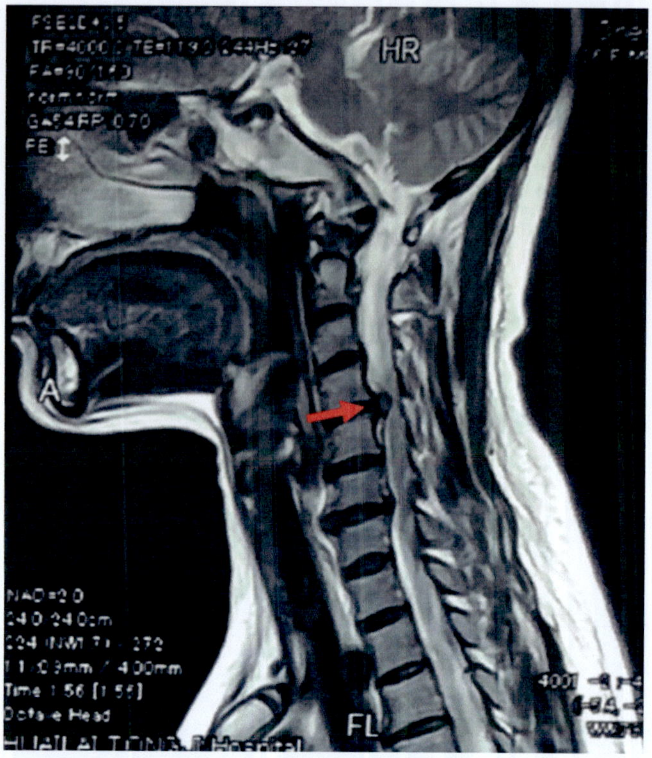

Fig. 2.2 The sagittal T2-weighted MRI images of the cervical spine demonstrated compression of the dural sac from C4–6

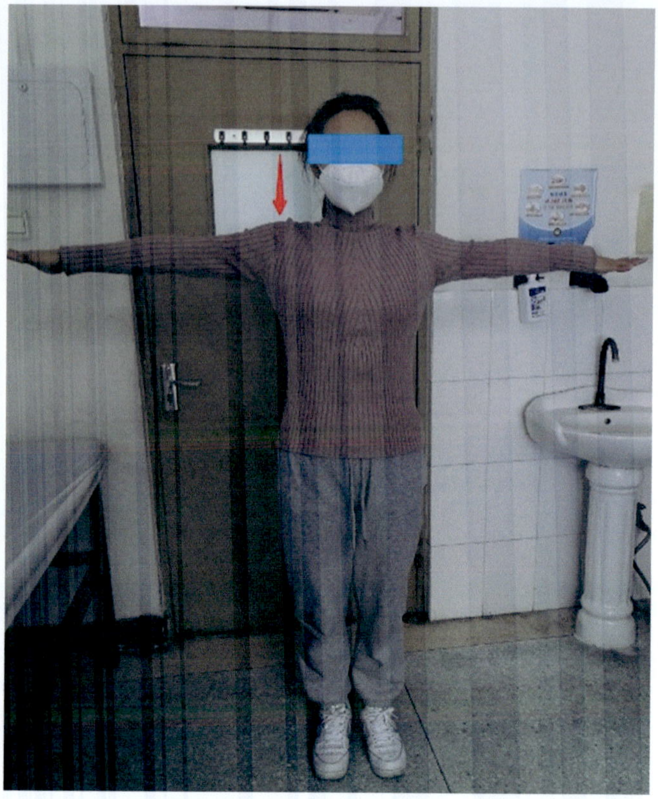

Fig. 2.4 One month following conservative treatment, the right shoulder joint's abduction and lift function normalized

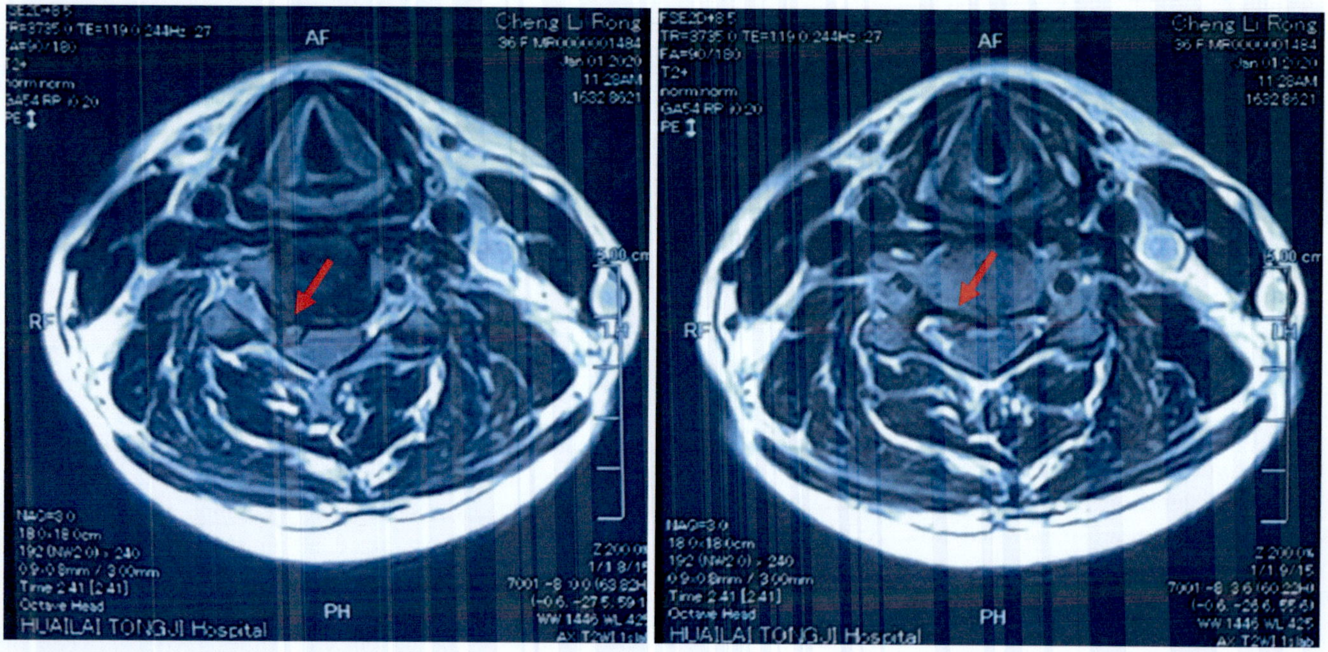

Fig. 2.3 Axial T2-weighted MRI images of the cervical spine demonstrated a right-sided disc herniation from C4–5, resulting in significant compression of the right ventral motor nerve root

2.2 Why Does Keegan's Disease Result in Only Shoulder Joint Dysfunction?

Keegan's disease is a rare disease [1] characterized by a high propensity for misdiagnosis and mistreatment. The illness is typified by a weakening of the deltoid and biceps muscles, accompanied by an inability of the shoulder joint to abduct and lift actively, without any manifestations of paresthesia or spinal cord damage. This disease often has no obvious history of trauma and characterized by rapid onset and swift progression. The imaging manifestation is typical selective compression of the cervical ventral motor nerve root or anterior horn of the spinal cord [1]. Electrophysiological examination shows neurogenic damage to the deltoid and biceps brachii muscles.

Due to the damage of selective ventral motor nerve roots at the C5 and 6 segments or selective anterior spinal horn, the abduction function of the affected shoulder joint innervated by these nerves can be easily impaired [1]. However, in clinical practice, middle-aged and elderly patients with shoulder abduction and lift dysfunction often receive treatment in the sports medicine department. Physicians may misdiagnose a rotator cuff injury based on the abnormal signals of such an injury depicted by magnetic resonance imaging (MRI), or even resort to premature surgical intervention.

The author has frequently encountered some patients with the shoulder joint abduction dysfunction in the clinic. Professional physical examination and related imaging examination were performed on the patients at the first diagnosis. After careful differential diagnosis, Keegan's disease was confirmed. Patients are cured by early and correct treatment.

The differential diagnosis of Keegan's disease is difficult. Rotator cuff injury mainly involves the supraspinatus muscle, while Keegan's disease mainly affects the deltoid and biceps muscles. The biceps atrophy and weakness are the key to distinguish rotator cuff injury [2]. When middle-aged and elderly people suffer from Keegan's disease, most of them are also accompanied by imaging changes such as rotator cuff degeneration injury. The probability of misdiagnosis as rotator cuff injury is as high as 40% [2], and some even perform wrong surgical operations according to shoulder joint disease treatment.

Diagnosis and differential diagnosis should be conducted through a joint consultation among spinal surgery, neurology, sports medicine, and other multidisciplinary experts. Electrophysiological examination may be necessary. Clinicians must possess not only specialized skills but also strong spinal clinical knowledge and multidisciplinary experience in imaging. This is crucial to avoid misdiagnosis or missed treatment opportunities. The electrophysiological examination of Keegan's disease revealed motor potential, polyphasic and giant potential, and even denervated potential in the deltoid and biceps muscles. However, the specific parameters of the examination were not completely consistent from different reports [3].

In the event of damage to the ventral cervical motor nerve root or the corresponding segmental selective spinal cord anterior horn, the emergence of corresponding segmental motor dysfunction is observed, which is characterized by dissociative upper limb motor disorder. Based on the distinct sites, this condition can be categorized into three subtypes: proximal type (classic Keegan's disease), distal type, and mixed type. If the ventral motor root of C4 is impaired, abnormalities in phrenic nerve function might also occur. The fundamental pathological mechanism underlying the various types is the failure of the ventral motor nerve roots of the cervical nerve to enter the dural canal or the selective compression of the motor neurons in the anterior horn of the spinal cord. Meanwhile, the dorsal sensory roots and the anterior and posterior columns of the spinal cord remain unaltered, thus leading to the absence of abnormal manifestations in other parts of the limbs [1].

An American study on microanatomy of 128 C3-T1 nerve roots discovered that C5 nerve roots exhibit minimal angulation with the spinal cord, possess a short stroke, and were easily compressed by the adjacent vertebral artery. In conjunction with the constraints imposed by the dentate ligament, the nerve root tension is elevated, the available movement space is limited, and the blood supply is inadequate. The hypertrophy of the uncinate vertebral joint may lead to compression of the anterior branch motor nerve roots, particularly the C5 motor nerve roots [4]. This can result in a reduction of cervical lordosis, narrowing of the cervical canal, and multi-segmental degeneration. The dentate ligaments hinder the retreat space of nerve roots and compress the "weak area" of the ventral motor nerve root of C5 or the anterior horn of the spinal cord, causing motor dysfunction without sensory impairment or spinal cord damage [1]. In cases where selective compression of the anterior horn of the spinal cord is impaired, the "snake eye" sign may be observed in the T2-weighted image. The characteristic "fried egg sign" in the anterior horn of the spinal cord can be detected via myelographic CT scan, indicating pathological changes in that region [2, 4]. Some researchers have also noted that the potassium channel conduction of motor axons is diminished, and the vulnerability of motor axons is heightened, which might also contribute to the disease's susceptibility to injury.

The Keegan's disease may self-recovery without any intervention [2, 5]. In clinical practice, the author has observed that patients with Keegan's disease experiencing simple motor nerve root compression often recover spontaneously and completely during the early stages following timely conservative treatment. Therefore, it is crucial to avoid rushing into surgical intervention. After 4–6 weeks or more of active and appropriate conservative treatment, the majority of patients can gradually regain their health. Should there be no signs of improvement, cervical surgery can be considered if necessary.

In conclusion, the main clinical manifestations of Keegan's disease are shoulder joint active abduction movement disorder, with no sensory and limb abnormalities. Imaging revealed compression of the C5 or C6 anterior motor nerve roots or the anterior horn of the spinal cord. In patients with shoulder symptoms, Keegan's disease should not be mistaken for rotator cuff injury for surgical treatment.

2.3 Key Points of Diagnosis and Treatment

Keegan's disease is a rare condition characterized by self-recovery, primarily caused by damage to the C5 and C6 segments of the ventral motor root or anterior horn motor neurons, leading to impaired shoulder joint abduction and lift functions. When patients with Keegan's disease exhibit abnormal rotator cuff signals on imaging for the first time, it may be misdiagnosed as a rotator cuff injury, resulting in inappropriate treatment, including shoulder joint surgery. Rotator cuff injuries primarily involve the supraspinatus muscle, whereas Keegan's disease primarily affects the deltoid and biceps muscles. The key distinction between the two conditions lies in the biceps atrophy and weakness. Electrophysiological and MRI examinations should be performed. Clinicians should possess a multidisciplinary understanding of spinal surgery, neurology, sports medicine, and other related fields to ensure accurate diagnosis and avoid misdiagnoses. Multidisciplinary consultations may be necessary for diagnosis and differential diagnosis when required.

References

1. Keegan JJ. The cause of dissociated motor loss extremity with cervical spondylosis:a cause report. J Neurosurg. 1965;23(5):528–36.
2. Iwata E, Shigematsu H, Inoue K, et al. Biceps-related physical findings are useful to prevent misdiagnosis of cervical spondylotic amyotrophy as a rotator cuff tear. Asia Spine J. 2018;12(1):69–73.
3. Luo WQ, Li YY, Xu QL, et al. Cervical spondylotic amyotrophy: a systematic review. Eur Spine J. 2019;28:2293–301.
4. Alleyne CH, Cawley CM, Barrow DL, et al. Microsurgical anatomy of the dorsal cervical nerve roots and the cervical dorsal root ganglion/ventral root complexes. Surg Neurol. 1998;50(3):213–811.
5. Shinomiya K, Komori H, Matsuoka N, et al. Neuroradiologic and electrophysiologic assessment of cervical spondylotic amyotrophy. Spine. 1994;19(1):21–5.

Brachial Plexus Injury Was Misdiagnosed as Rotator Cuff Injury

3

Yu-jie Liu and Chun-bao Li

3.1 Case Report

The patient was a 19-year-old male soldier. While participating in a military training exercise, he experienced a dislocation and strain in his left shoulder (Fig. 3.1). The manual reduction procedure lasted for a period of 3 months. The individual resumed combat training but subsequently reported increasing numbness and pain below the left shoulder joint, along with difficulty in applying force when lifting objects. An MRI examination of the shoulder joint revealed abnormal signal at the attachment site of the supraspinatus muscle of the left shoulder to the greater tuberosity of the humerus (Fig. 3.2). The patient was admitted to the hospital with rotator cuff injury and was scheduled for surgical treatment.

Following admission, the patient was consistently queried regarding his medical history. In addition to the previously noted shoulder dislocation, it was observed that during combat training 1 week prior, the patient's head and neck were inadvertently immobilized under the armpit of the opposing individual (Fig. 3.3). Subsequently, the patient presented with symptoms including pain and weakness in the left shoulder joint, numbness and discomfort in the shoulder skin, gradual atrophy of the surrounding shoulder muscles, and trembling weakness during shoulder lifting activities.

Physical examination:

It was observed that the left deltoid and pectoralis major muscles exhibited signs of atrophy (Fig. 3.4), while the supraspinatus, infraspinatus, biceps, and triceps brachii muscles displayed significant atrophy (Fig. 3.5).

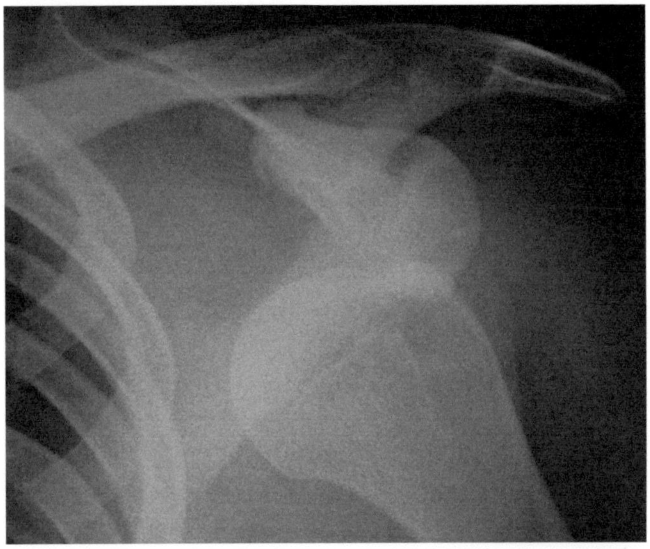

Fig. 3.1 Anterior dislocation of the left shoulder

Weakness in shoulder abduction and lifting was noted, accompanied by muscle tremors. No apparent abnormalities were detected in the forearm flexor carpal muscles, extensor carpal muscles, or internal hand muscles. Decreased skin sensation was observed in the subacromial deltoid region (Fig. 3.6), while normal skin sensation was present in the palm and back of the forearm. Additionally, a positive Tinel's sign was elicited in the neck during examination. The MRI examination indicated indistinct signals in the left brachial plexus root sleeve (Fig. 3.7), while electromyography demonstrated an injury to the left upper brachial plexus meridian.

The patient received a diagnosis of upper brachial plexus injury through clinical examination and experienced gradual relief of pain symptoms following treatment with acupuncture, rehabilitation, physiotherapy, and neurotrophic drugs. After 3 months, the patient reported normal shoulder function, with improvements in muscle atrophy of the supraspinatus, infraspinatus, deltoid, and biceps brachii muscles, and a recovery of muscle strength to grade 4.

Y.-j. Liu
Orthopaedics, Chinese PLA General Hospital, Beijing, China

C.-b. Li (✉)
Department of Orthopedics, The Fourth Medical Center, Chinese PLA General Hospital, Beijing, China

Y.-j. Liu et al. (eds.), *Pitfalls in Diagnosis and Treatment of Shoulder Joint Diseases*,
https://doi.org/10.1007/978-981-96-2472-0_3

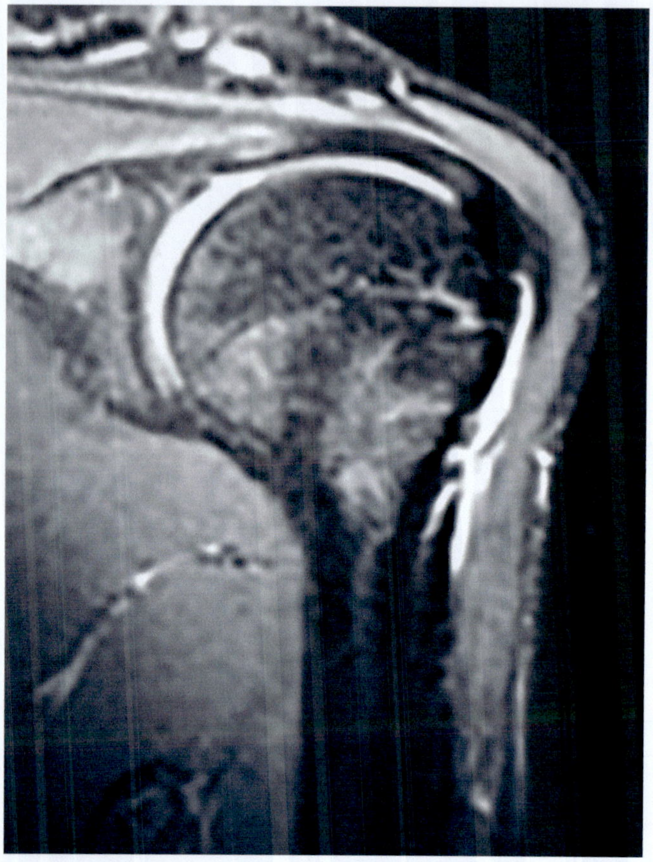

Fig. 3.2 MRI of the left shoulder showed abnormally low signal intensity at the attachment of the supraspinatus tendon

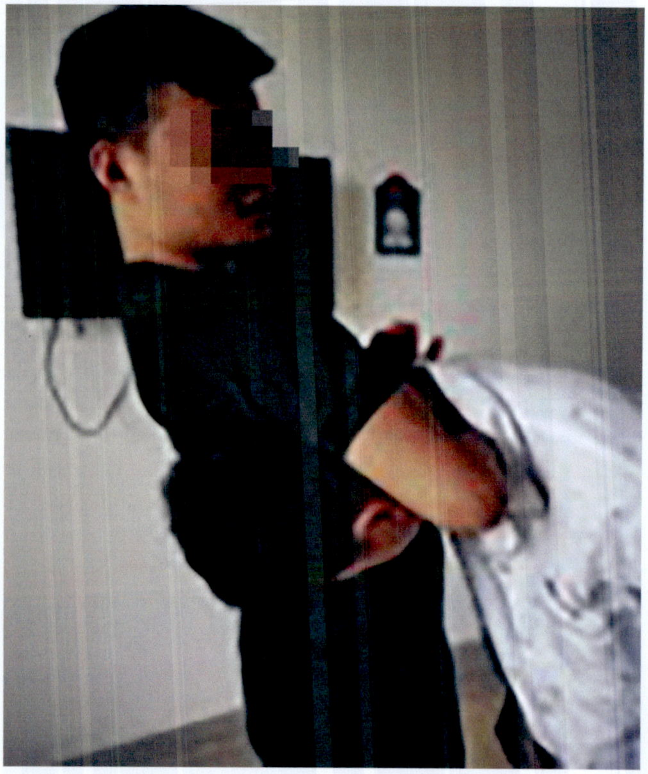

Fig. 3.3 The head and neck of the patient was clamped during the combat training

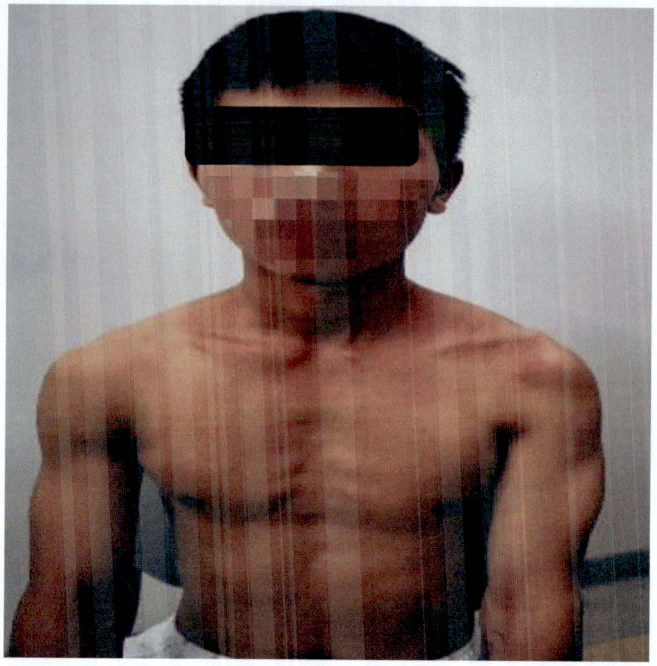

Fig. 3.4 Atrophy occurred in the left deltoid and pectoralis major muscles

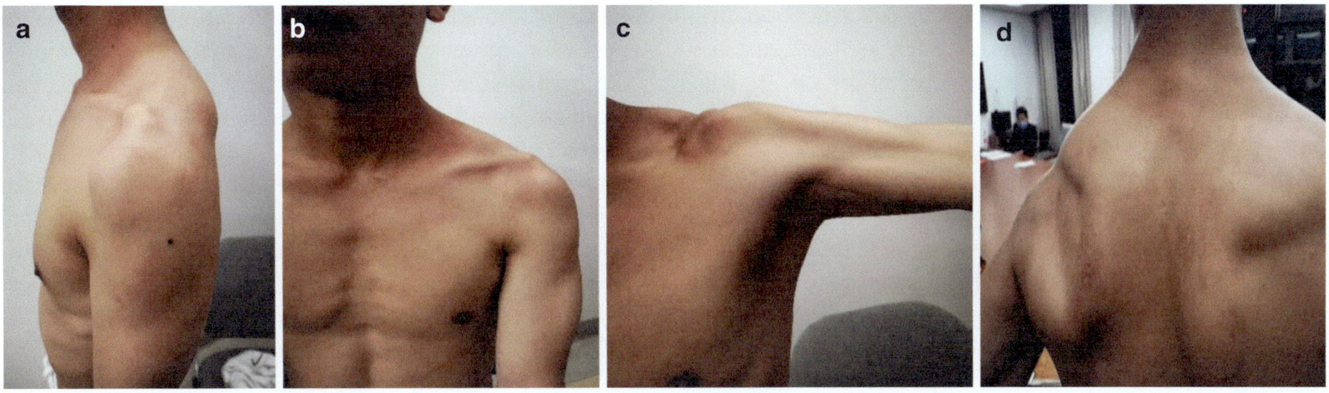

Fig. 3.5 Atrophy occurred in the infraspinatus (**a**), supraspinatus (**b**), biceps brachii (**c**), and triceps brachii (**d**) muscles

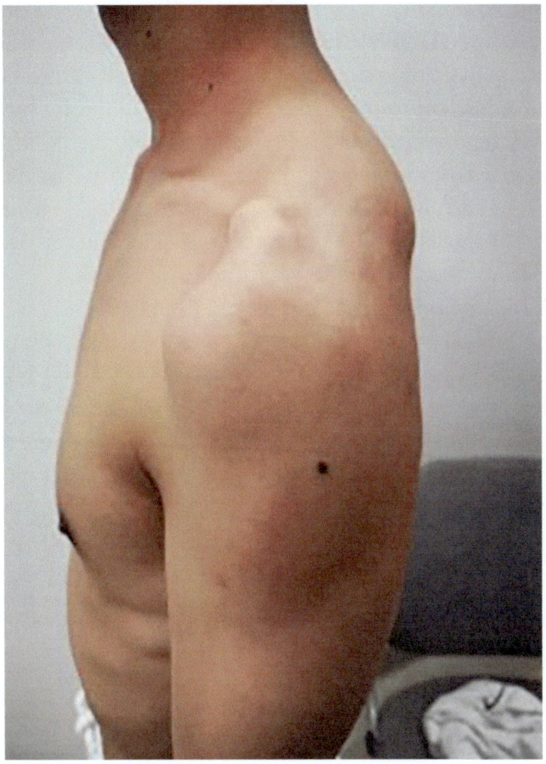

Fig. 3.6 Area of hypoesthesia in the skin of the shoulder joint

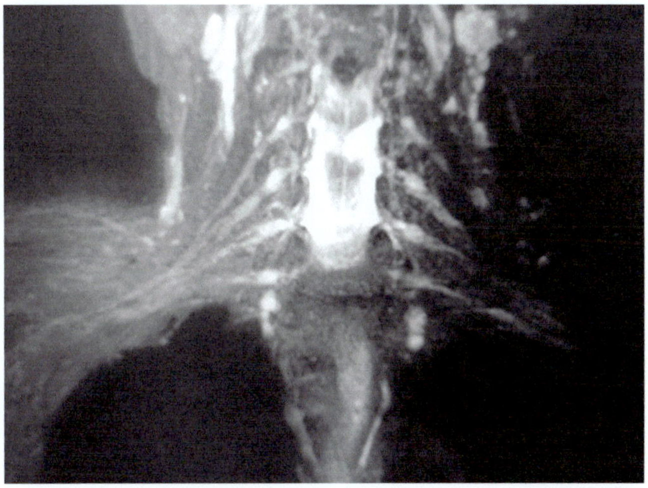

Fig. 3.7 MRI of the cervical spine showed that the signal of the left brachial plexus nerve root sleeve was not obvious

3.2 Misunderstanding of Diagnosis and Treatment

Fractures and dislocations of cervical vertebrae, circular vertebrae, and axis are frequently observed in wrestling, boxing, sanda, and other sports. Shoulder joint fractures and dislocations are prevalent in grappling. Nevertheless, brachial plexus injuries resulting from neck and shoulder traction or separation injuries are frequently overlooked. Lower brachial plexus injuries typically stem from unilateral suspension and traction of the upper limb, presenting as impaired thumb extension, finger extension, wrist extension, hand grasping, and hand muscle atrophy. The paper pinch test yields positive results in these cases.

Upper brachial plexus injuries can occur as a result of neck–shoulder separation injuries, such as those sustained during grappling training. This type of injury occurs when the patient's head and neck become trapped in the opponent's armpit, leading to a pulling and separating force on the neck and shoulder. Clinical manifestations typically include pain in the affected neck and shoulder, as well as atrophy of the upper arm and deltoid muscles. MRI imaging of the shoulder joint may reveal low signal changes at the attachment site of the greater tuberosity of the supraspinatus muscle, there was no signal of rotator cuff tear, and the underlying pathological changes should not be overlooked for obvious radiographic changes.

3.3 Summary

1. Shoulder pain may not always be attributed to shoulder joint pathology. Clinicians should enhance their comprehension of shoulder joint symptoms stemming from cervical spondylosis, rather than solely focusing on shoulder joint etiology, and should differentiate between injuries of the cervical spine, spinal cord, and brachial plexus and shoulder joint diseases.
2. Charcot joint arises from sensory neuron dysfunction of the spinal cord, leading to bone and soft tissue destruction in the shoulder joint. In cases of sensory and motor dissociation, clinicians should consider cervical syringomyelia as a potential diagnosis. MRI of the cervical spine is a valuable diagnostic tool for identifying Charcot joint induced by syringomyelia, and caution should be exercised in selecting surgical treatment options.
3. Keegan's disease, caused by cervical motor nerve compression, presents with motor dysfunction in the shoulder joint, particularly weakness in the supraspinatus and deltoid muscles, without abnormal limb sensation, leading to potential misdiagnosis as a rotator cuff injury. MRI images typically reveal compression of the cervical anterior motor nerve roots or the anterior horn of the spinal cord. Keegan's disease is considered a self-limited condition, and most patients can be cured with correct conservative treatment, and surgery is not necessary.
4. Clinicians are advised to thoroughly assess patients by inquiring about the nature of the injury, symptoms experienced post-injury, and analyzing the mechanism of injury, as well as the subsequent diagnosis and treatment process, rather than solely relying on imaging. It is imperative to conduct a comprehensive physical examination, including visual observation, palpation, percussion, measurements, and specialized tests, to accurately assess limb sensation, movement, muscle strength, and joint range of motion, in order to avoid misinterpretation of imaging results. Additionally, clinicians should strive to discern the underlying cause of symptoms, engage in critical thinking, distinguish between genuine and misleading findings, and formulate an accurate diagnosis.
5. Clinicians need to have a thorough understanding of the anatomical structures of nerves and muscles, with particular emphasis on assessing the spinal cord and brachial plexus in cases of neck and shoulder injuries. Surgeons must exercise caution in expanding surgical indications, prioritize conservative treatment options, and emphasize postoperative rehabilitation.

Part II

Complications of Rotator Cuff Surgery: A Guide and Summary

Chang-ming Huang

Guides

Why do suture anchors fail in rotator cuff repair? Why do anchors pull out? Why do anchors cause damage to the articular cartilage of the shoulder joint? Why do absorbable anchors fracture? These are the hotspots and difficulties in arthroscopic surgical repair and reconstruction for massive rotator cuff injuries. When performing rotator cuff injury repair and reconstruction, whether to take into account and avoid and solve this series of problems brought by anchor fixation should be highly concerned.

This part focuses on exploring how to conduct a comprehensive evaluation before surgery for rotator cuff injury, select surgical indications, prevent re-tearing after rotator cuff injury repair surgery, use edge suture technology, and use long head tendon transposition technology of biceps brachii and treatment strategies for irreparable large rotator cuff injury.

Summary

Careful preoperative evaluation of the patient's overall condition, quality of rotator cuff tissue, muscle atrophy and fat infiltration, size of rotator cuff injury, and degree of tendon contracture is of great significance for correctly formulating treatment plans.

Imaging examinations are used to assess the size of rotator cuff injuries, the degree of muscle atrophy and retraction, the grade of fat infiltration, and the upward displacement of the humeral head, so that the correct treatment plan can be selected based on the specific condition of the patient.

Special attention should be paid to the imaging changes of the humeral tuberosity bone in the shoulder joint before surgery. Bone grafting is recommended for cysts with a diameter of 5–10 mm or more. It is not advisable to use multiple anchor screws to fill and fix the cysts. Osteoporosis and cystic changes, as well as the selection of anchor diameter, are the main reasons for anchor fixation failure.

Pay attention to the osteophytic hyperplasia of the humeral tuberosity in the shoulder joint, grind the osteophytic hyperplasia of the humeral tuberosity, preserve the bone cortex, and do not remove too much to avoid reducing the strength of anchor fixation.

Anchor nail implantation should pay attention to matching the diameter of the nail hole with the anchor nail. If the nail path is too thick, the anchor nail is easy to pull out; if the nail

C. Huang (✉)
Department of Orthopedics, The 73rd Group Army Hospital,
Chenggong Hospital Affiliated to Xiamen University, Xiamen, China

path is too thin or too shallow, it is difficult to implant the anchor nail; if the nail tail is exposed, it is prone to shoulder peak impact.

When implanting anchor bolts, attention should be paid to the angle of the anchor bolts to prevent them from accidentally entering the joint surface of the humeral head; double row stitching technology pays attention to the distance and angle of the inner and outer row anchor bolts to avoid interference between the anchor bolts.

Suture bridge technique should pay attention to the distance, angle, and suture tension of the internal and external anchor bolts to avoid interference between the anchor bolts and excessive suture tension, which may lead to cutting fractures.

Once the anchor is pulled out, timely surgical treatment is necessary to avoid adverse effects caused by anchor migration.

The incidence of re-tear after giant rotator cuff repair surgery is high. The use of technique of marginal convergence of rotator cuff tissue and transposition of the long head tendon of the biceps brachii muscle can help reduce the tension of rotator cuff tissue and prevent re-tearing after rotator cuff suture surgery.

For the treatment of irreparable rotator cuff injuries, appropriate surgical methods should be selected based on the patient's age, degree of injury, living needs, skills mastered by the doctor, socio-economic situation, and other factors.

Complications and Countermeasures of Rotator Cuff Injury Treated with Anchor Fixation

4

Yu-jie Liu, Chang-ming Huang, and Yang-pan Fu

4.1 Overview of Disease Diagnosis and Treatment

The patient was a 69-year-old male. His pain in the right shoulder joint with limited mobility for over 2 years has been relieved after massage, physical therapy, and closed treatment according to shoulder periarthritis. Half a year ago, after moving a heavy object (20 kg), the pain in the right shoulder joint worsened, and lifting and rotating activities were restricted, affecting work, life, and sleep. A shoulder joint X-ray examination was performed at a local hospital, which showed osteophyte hyperplasia and osteoporosis in the humeral tuberosity of the right shoulder joint, with a hooked shoulder peak (Fig. 4.1). MRI shows right rotator cuff tear with synovitis (Fig. 4.2).

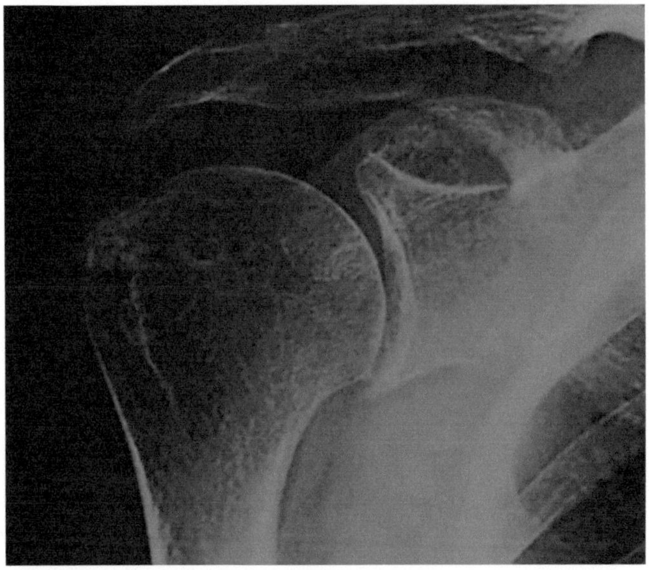

Fig. 4.1 Right shoulder joint AP X-ray image

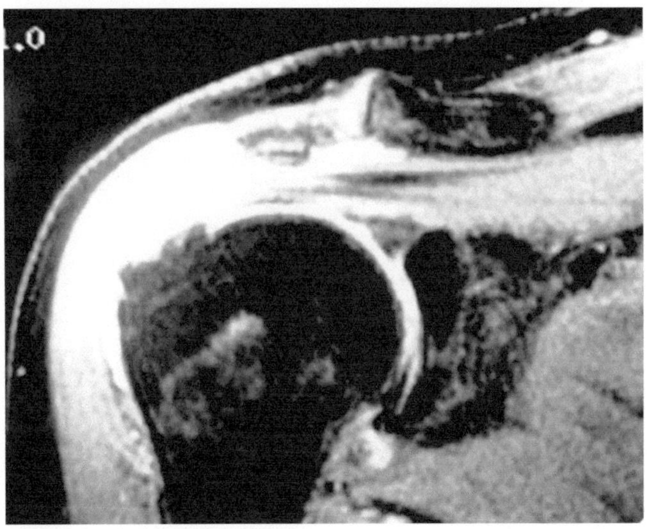

Fig. 4.2 T2 coronal MRI images of right shoulder joint with lipid pressure

Physical examination showed atrophy of the deltoid, supraspinatus, and infraspinatus muscles of the right shoulder joint, limited abduction and adduction of the shoulder joint (Fig. 4.3), maximum abduction of 30° (Fig. 4.4), anterior flexion and posterior extension of 45°–0–15°, shoulder tenderness, shoulder impact induced test (Neer sign) (+), and shoulder joint impact test (+).

After completing preoperative examination, arthroscopic exploration and cleaning of the right shoulder and repair of rotator cuff injury were performed under general anesthesia. During the operation, rotator cuff tear and humeral tuberosity osteophyte hyperplasia were found (Fig. 4.5). Arthroscopic grinding of hypertrophic osteophytes (Fig. 4.6) reveals severe osteoporosis in the greater tuberosity of the humerus (Fig. 4.7). Two metal anchor screws with a diameter of 4.5 mm were implanted into the greater tuberosity of the humerus (Fig. 4.8), and the torn rotator cuff tissue was

Y.-j. Liu
Orthopaedics, Chinese PLA General Hospital, Beijing, China

C.-m. Huang (✉) · Y.-p. Fu
Department of Orthopedics, The 73rd Group Army Hospital, Chenggong Hospital Affiliated to Xiamen University, Xiamen, China

Y.-j. Liu et al. (eds.), *Pitfalls in Diagnosis and Treatment of Shoulder Joint Diseases*,
https://doi.org/10.1007/978-981-96-2472-0_4

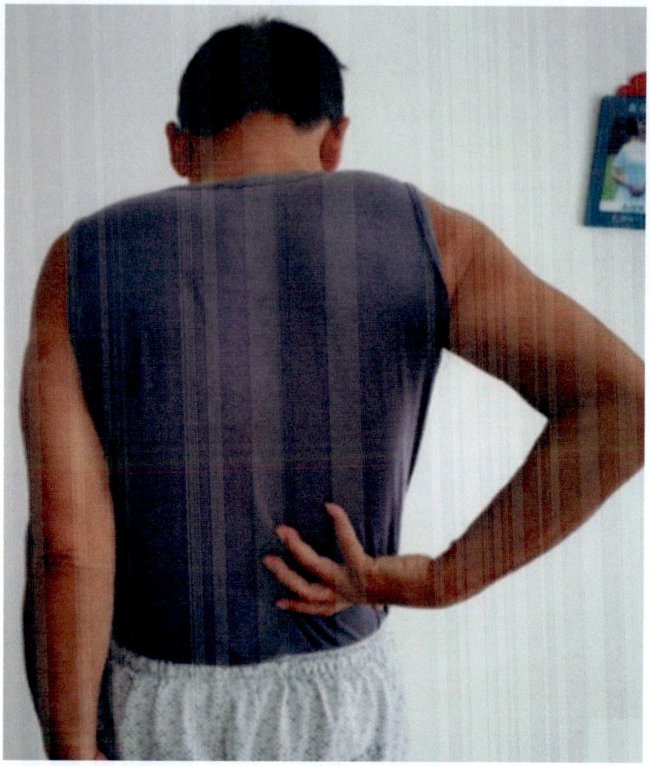

Fig. 4.3 Restricted movement of the right shoulder joint

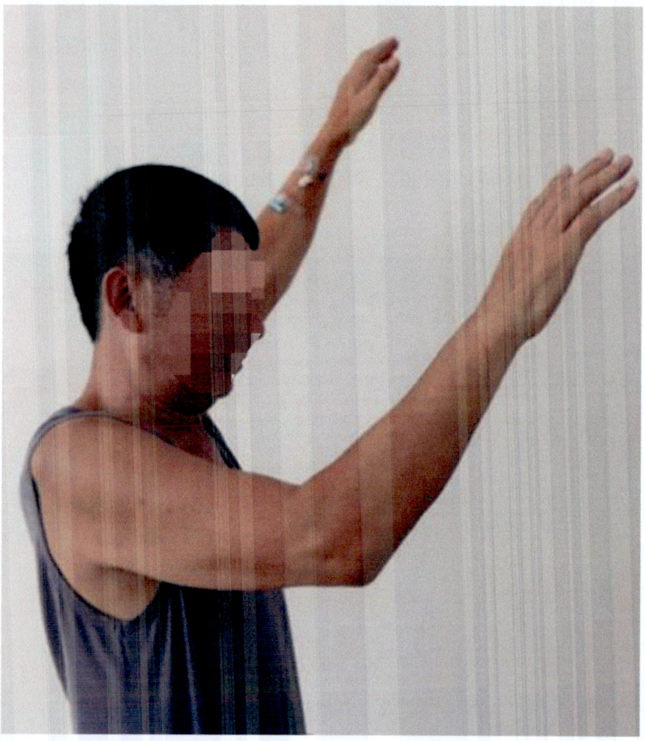

Fig. 4.4 Restricted right shoulder joint abduction and lifting activity

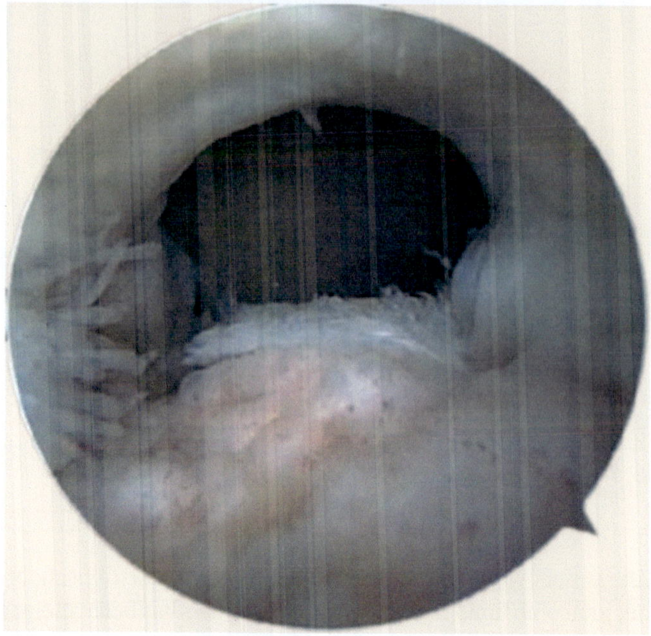

Fig. 4.5 Arthroscopic exploration shows rotator cuff tear and humeral tuberosity osteophyte hyperplasia

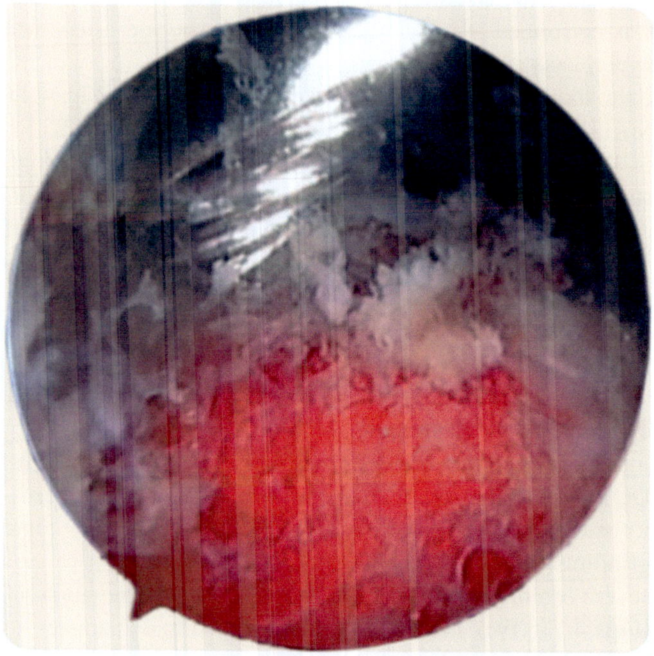

Fig. 4.6 Arthroscopic grinding of osteophytes with hyperplasia of the greater tuberosity of the humerus, severe subcortical osteoporosis

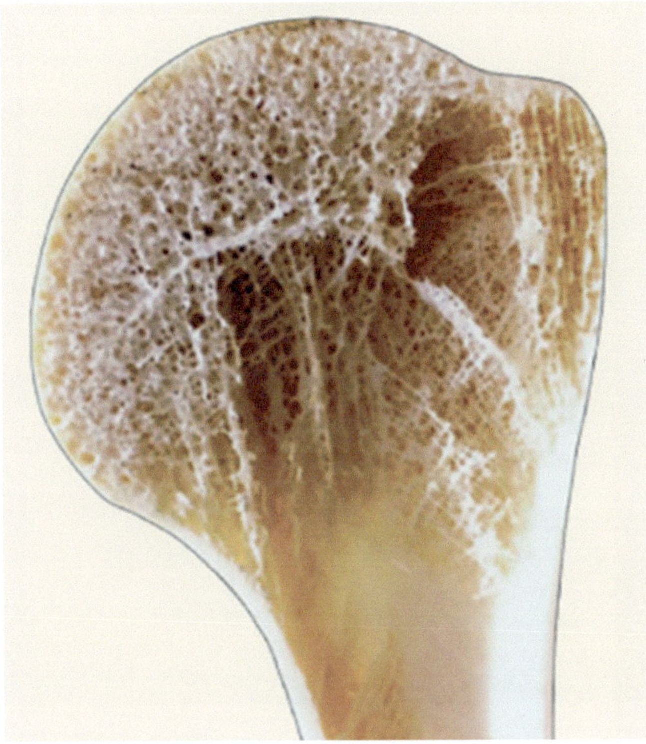

Fig. 4.7 Osteoporosis specimen of humeral head

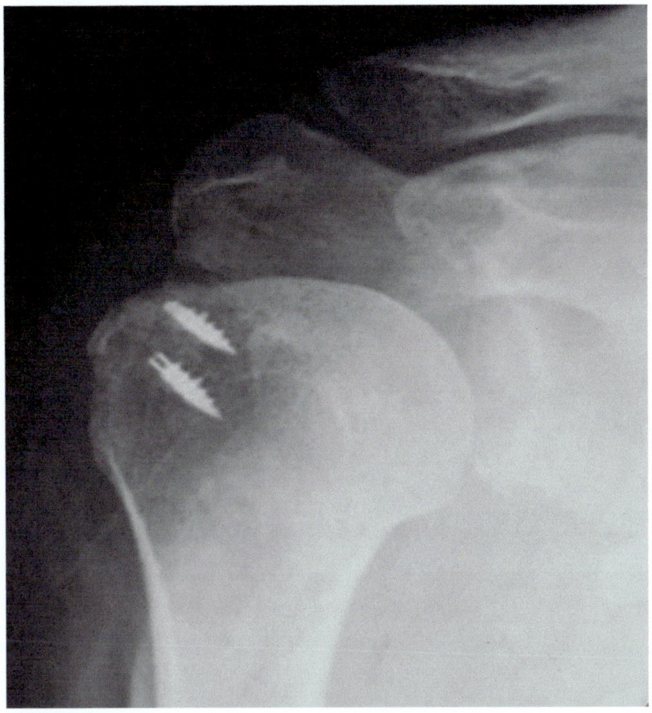

Fig. 4.9 X-ray examination shows the placement of anchor screws in the site of osteoporotic cystic transformation

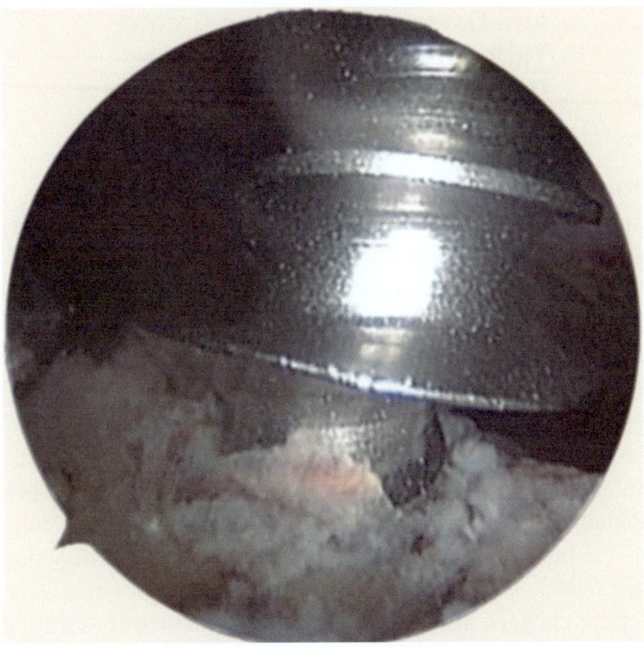

Fig. 4.8 Grinding area for anchor nail implantation in osteophytes

sutured to investigate whether the rotator cuff was well sutured. Postoperative X-ray of the shoulder joint showed that the anchor nail was located at the site of cystic transformation of the greater tuberosity of the humerus (Fig. 4.9). One month after surgery, a follow-up X-ray was taken at the outpatient clinic, and it was found that an anchor nail was pulled out from the greater tuberosity of the humerus (Fig. 4.10). Arthroscopic exploration revealed that the anchor was located in the subacromial space (Fig. 4.11). The anchor was removed, and a bone-rich area was selected for re-implantation, then the rotator cuff was sutured and repaired. Postoperative care included the use of shoulder brace protection and functional rehabilitation training according to rehabilitation procedures.

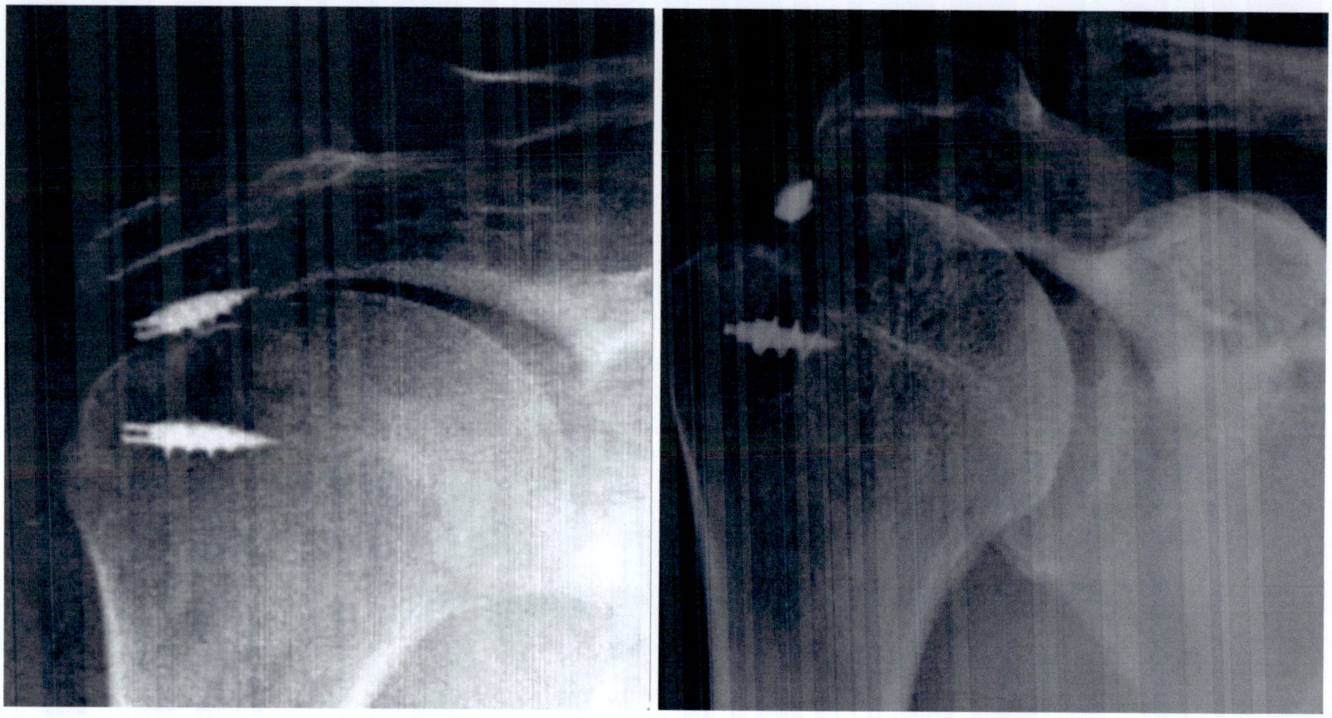

Fig. 4.10 X-ray examination shows (1 month after surgery) that the metal anchor is pulled out from the osteoporotic area of the humeral head

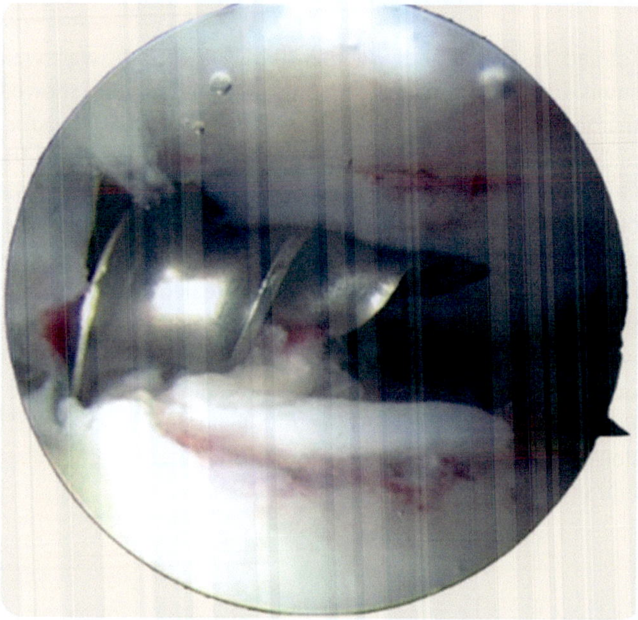

Fig. 4.11 Arthroscopic exploration reveals that the extracted metal anchor is located in the subacromial space of the shoulder peak

4.2 Cystic Degeneration and Osteoporosis of the Greater Tuberosity of the Humerus Are Important Causes of Anchor Screw Extraction

The incidence rate of rotator cuff injury in the elderly is higher, and conservative treatment is often used in the early stage. Due to old age, long disease course, and limited shoulder joint mobility, secondary shoulder joint adhesion, muscle wasting atrophy, and osteoporosis occur. Preoperative X-ray examination (Fig. 4.12) and CT examination (Fig. 4.13) were used. If X-ray examination reveals cystic changes in the greater tuberosity of the humerus, it should be highly suspected of rotator cuff injury. MRI has important diagnostic value for rotator cuff injury and cystic changes (Fig. 4.14). Patients with cystic transformation of the greater tuberosity of the humerus accompanied by shoulder joint dysfunction and muscle atrophy are more likely to have rotator cuff tears. Cystic changes at the insertion point of the rotator cuff are one of the factors contributing to the low healing rate and high failure rate after rotator cuff repair surgery.

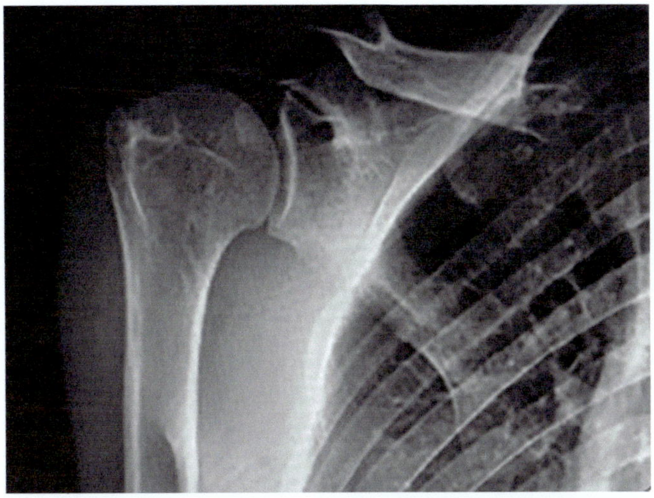

Fig. 4.12 X-ray examination shows low-density shadows of the greater tuberosity of the humerus

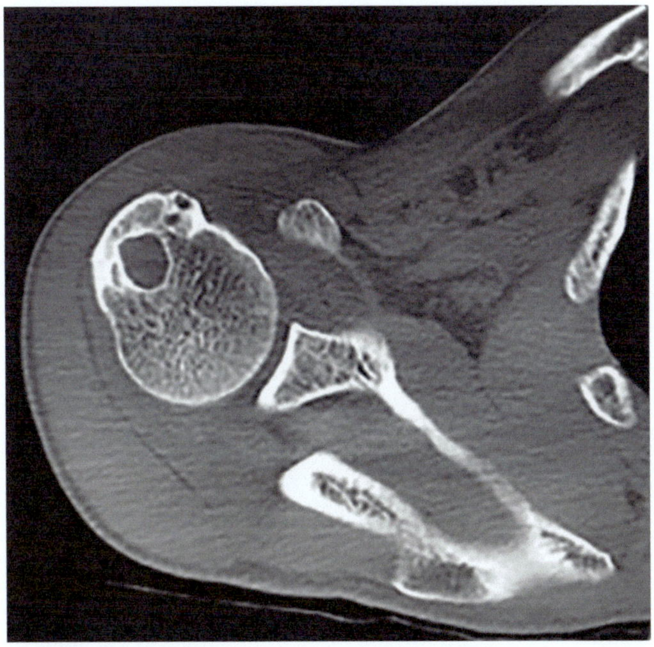

Fig. 4.13 CT findings of cystic changes in the greater tuberosity of the humerus

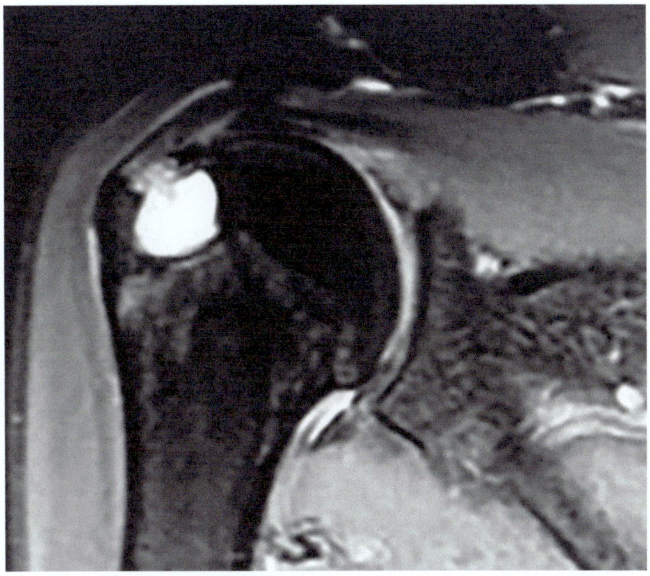

Fig. 4.14 MRI showing cystic changes at the attachment of the supraspinatus tendon of the greater tuberosity of the humerus with rotator cuff tear

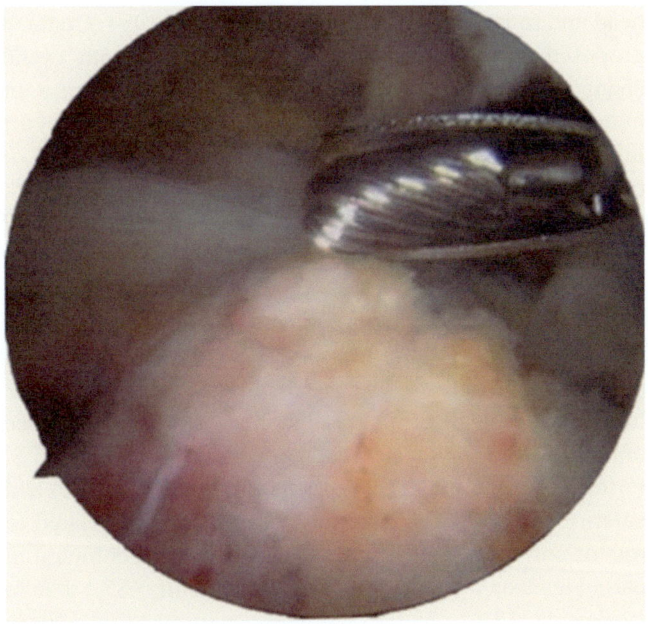

Fig. 4.15 Humerus tuberosity osteophyte

In recent years, the surgical technique of rotator cuff repair has been widely popularized. When choosing a treatment plan, special attention must be paid to the treatment of humeral tuberosity osteophyte (Fig. 4.15) and osteoporosis. When grinding osteophytes, it is important to preserve sufficient bone cortex (Fig. 4.16). Do not excessively grind cortical bone and overcorrect it, because the anti-extraction force of cancellous bone is lower than that of cortical bone, which can easily lead to anchor nail extraction. According to literature reports, after the anchor is removed, it can migrate freely to the lungs, subclavian bone, and adjacent to the spine [1]. Therefore, once the anchor is found to be pulled out, timely measures should be taken for early surgery to prevent the anchor from migrating and wandering to important tissues and organs.

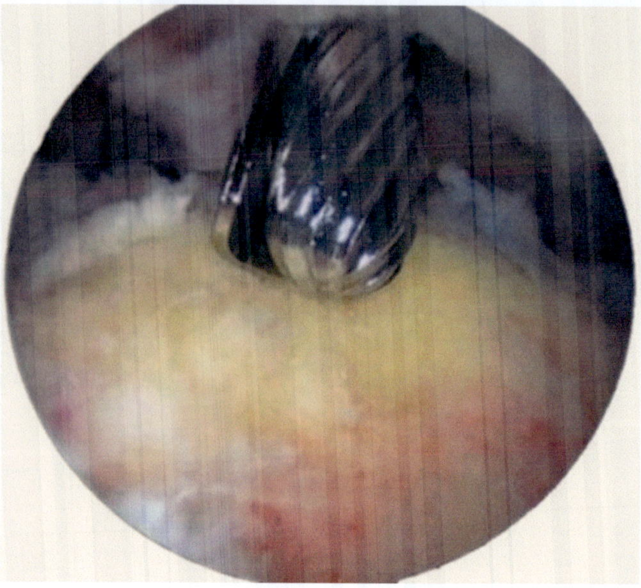

Fig. 4.16 Grinding of humeral tuberosity osteophyte while preserving cortical bone

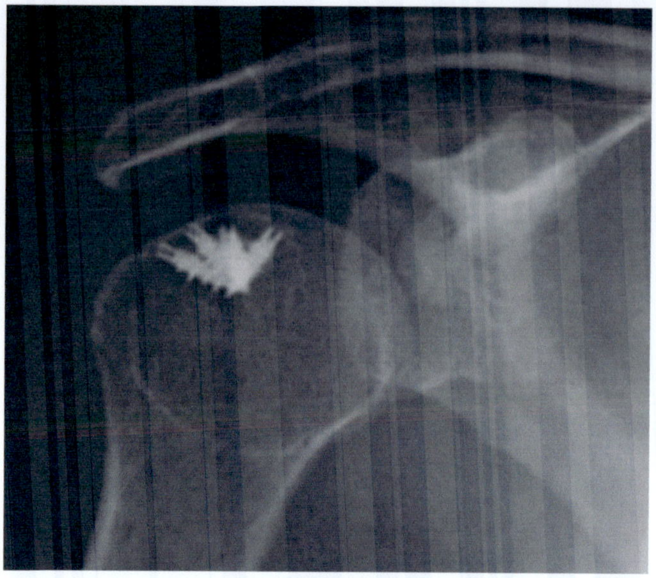

Fig. 4.17 Multiple metal anchor screws filled in the cystic loosening area of the greater tuberosity of the humerus

The relationship between cystic changes in the humeral head and rotator cuff tears is not yet clear. In 1934, Codman proposed that rotator cuff tear is associated with cystic changes in the humeral head, especially in the case of humeral tuberosity cysts [2]. The incidence of rotator cuff injury combined with bone cysts accounts for 1/2 to 4/5 of rotator cuff injuries. Is the humeral tuberosity bone cyst related to age or rotator cuff tear or degeneration? Postoperative humeral tuberosity cyst may be related to the reaction of suture anchor screw to rotator cuff injury. In 2007, Fritz et al. [3] retrospectively studied 238 cases of shoulder arthroscopy or open surgery, with an average age of 43 years. Among them, 50.8% had normal rotator cuff, 5.5% had tendinitis, and 43.7% had rotator cuff tear. The incidence of bone cysts in the greater tuberosity of the humerus is 66%. Posterior cyst of greater tuberosity of humerus (56.7%) and anterior cyst (22.7%). Anterior cysts are closely related to rotator cuff disease, and anterior cysts are more common in partial tears on the joint side of the rotator cuff (48%) than in cystic side (13%).

When the diameter of the humeral tuberosity cyst is greater than 5 mm, it is recommended to use bone grafting for treatment. Autologous bone, allogeneic bone, artificial bone, etc. can be commonly used. In 2005, Burkhart et al. [4] reported a group of cases of rotator cuff injury and humeral tuberosity cyst. Under arthroscopy, allogeneic bone was used to compress and graft bone, obtaining a sturdy bone bed. Single row anchor screws were used for fixation, and the clinical effect was satisfactory. In 2007, Kim et al. [5] reported arthroscopic removal of bone cysts with bone grafting (autologous and allogeneic bone) and double row reconstruction of the rotator cuff insertion point. In 2012, Levy et al. [6] used whole allograft bone and double row anchor bolts. Bone transplantation has good bone induction and bone conduction effects. The giant cyst of the greater tuberosity of the humerus with rotator cuff tear requires thorough scraping of the tissue inside the cyst, bone grafting to seal the cyst area, and firm fixation and reconstruction of the rotator cuff for reliable results. Anchor nail implantation points must avoid areas of osteoporosis and cystic changes. If the cystic cavity is accidentally entered, it is not advisable to hastily close it by simply using multiple anchor screws to fill the cystic area (Fig. 4.17). If necessary, select a site with better bone under X-ray fluoroscopy and re-implant anchor bolts or use a double row fixation method (Fig. 4.18).

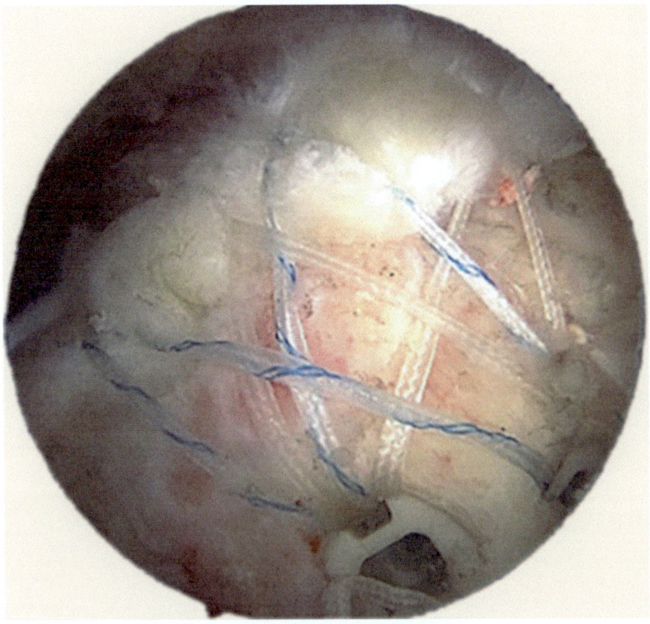

Fig. 4.18 Double row fixation technique for reconstructing the rotator cuff, with external anchor screws implanted at the normal greater tuberosity of the humerus

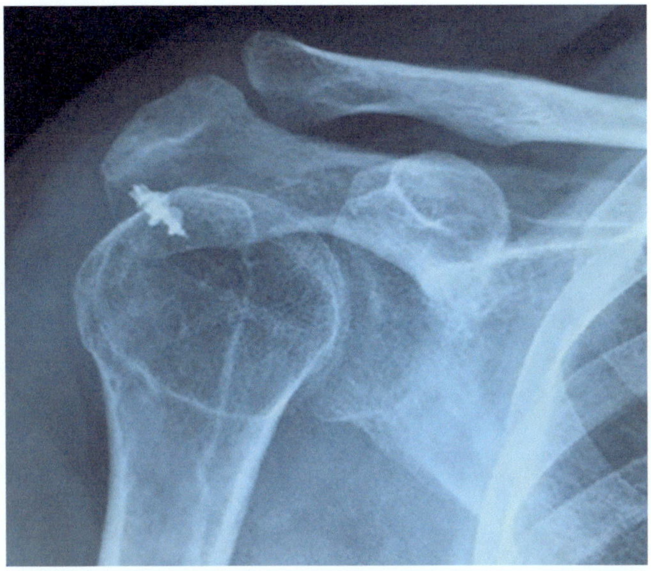

Fig. 4.19 The tail end of the anchor nail is too long and exposed outside the bone, causing impact with the shoulder peak

4.3 Issues to Pay Attention to When Implanting Anchor Bolts

Before the anchor implantation, it is necessary to pay attention to the matching of the diameter of the anchor and the nail path. If the nail path is too thin or shallow, the nail implantation will be difficult, and the nail tail will be exposed outside the cortical bone (Fig. 4.19), resulting in impact and wear with the acromial peak. Intertubercular sulcus anchor implantation should pay special attention to the implantation angle of the anchor. A hole opener should be prefabricated and then screwed into the anchor, otherwise the anchor will slide under the cartilage and cause fixation failure (Fig. 4.20).

For patients with osteoporosis in the shoulder joint, the depth of insertion of the metal anchor into the greater tuberosity of the humerus should be controlled. If the anchor is inserted too deeply, it will penetrate the cartilage of the humeral head, causing wear of the shoulder glenoid cartilage (Fig. 4.21) and leading to severe osteoarthritis.

If suture bridge fixation technology is used, the distance and angle between the inner and outer row anchor screws and the tension of the suture should be adjusted (Fig. 4.22) to prevent the suture from being too tight and causing humeral tuberosity cutting fracture. The inclination angle of the outer anchor bolts is too large, which can interfere with the stability of the inner anchor bolts. When the anchor is implanted in the outer row, pay attention to expanding the hole with a reamer matching the diameter of the anchor, otherwise the anchor will be crushed (Fig. 4.23) or broken (Fig. 4.24) during implantation. At the same time, the distance of the outer row anchors should be appropriate, and it is not reliable to be too close, otherwise it is easy to fracture the bone between the anchors (Fig. 4.25) or fracture of the greater tubercle of humerus (Fig. 4.26).

Rotator cuff injury is accompanied by severe osteoporosis, and anchor bolts are prone to extraction. Therefore, the allogeneic biological bone anchor designed by the author (Fig. 4.27) was used for the repair and reconstruction of rotator cuff injuries (Fig. 4.28), which has anti-cutting and anti-pull-out effects and achieved good therapeutic effects (Fig. 4.29).

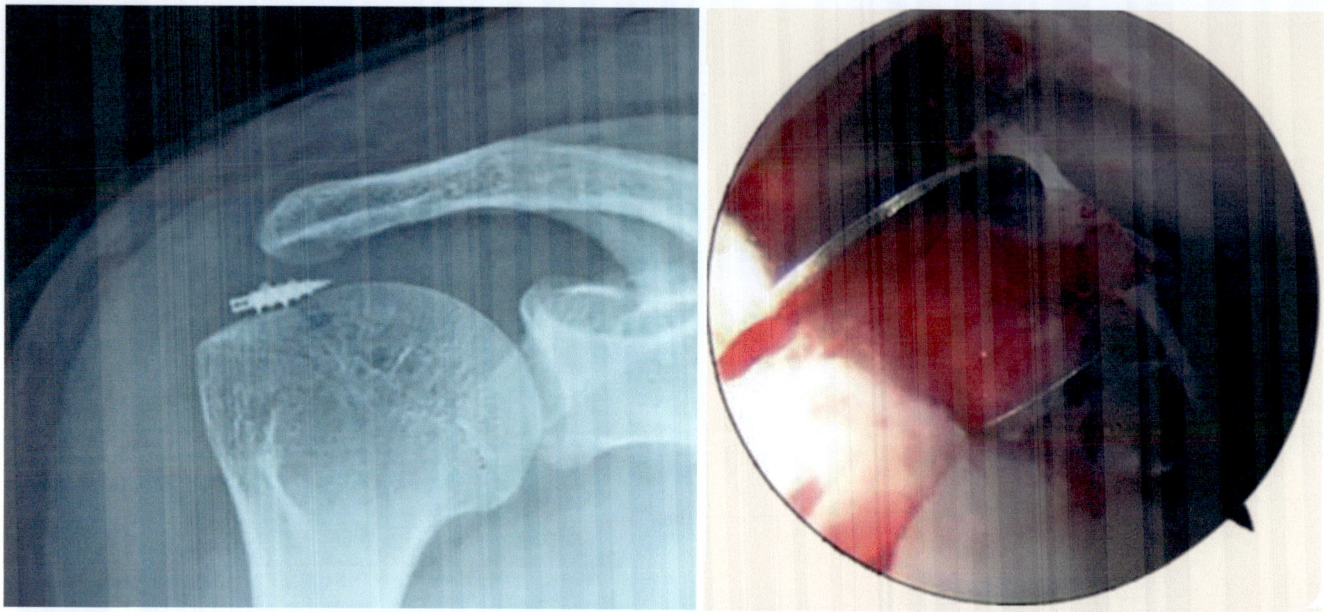

Fig. 4.20 Incorrect angle and position of anchor screw implantation, anchor screw implanted under the cartilage of the humeral head

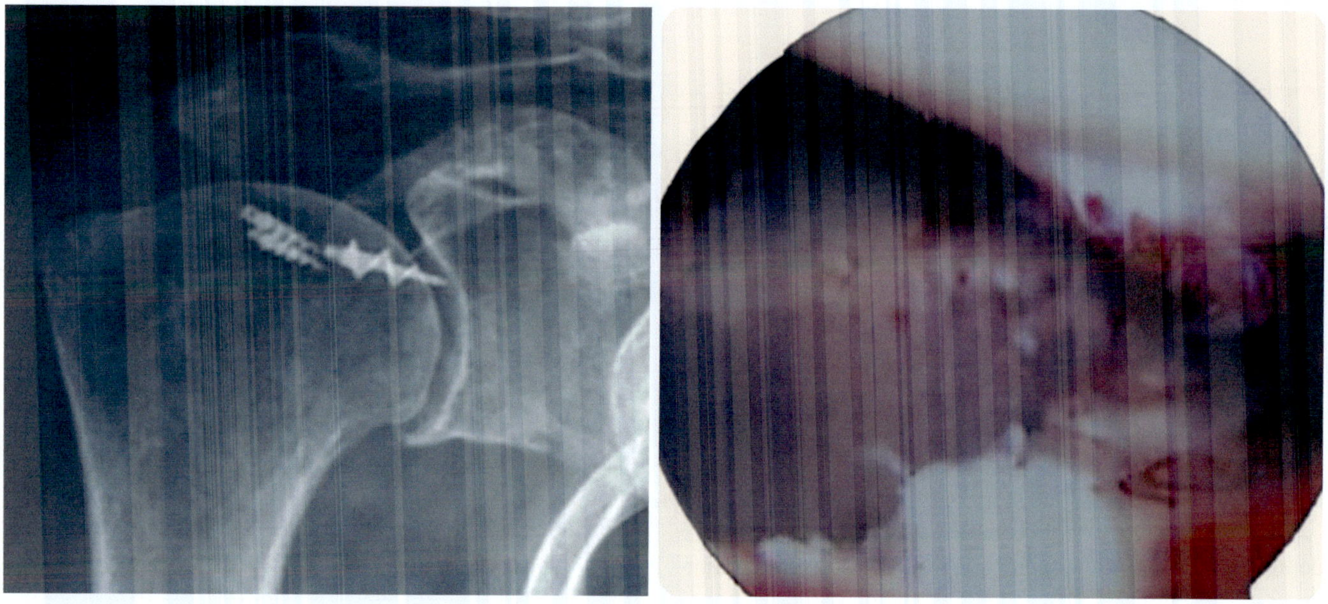

Fig. 4.21 Metal anchor penetrating the humeral head, causing damage to the glenoid cartilage

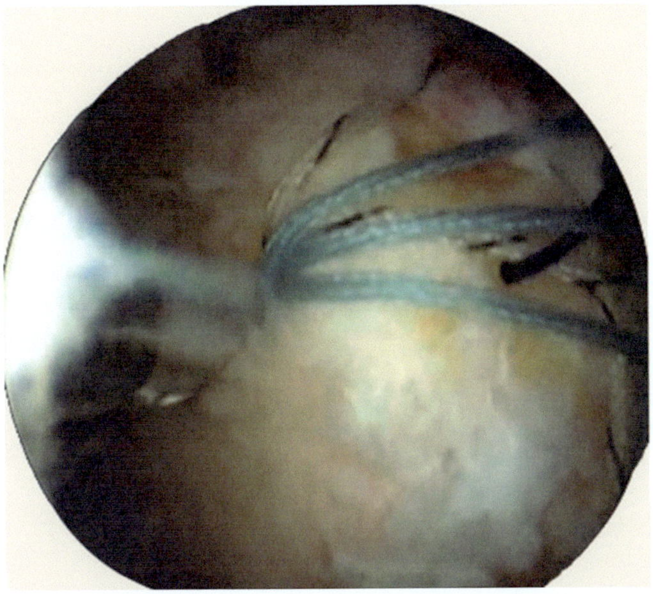

Fig. 4.22 Double row anchor nail suture bridge fixation technique, paying attention to suture tension to prevent cutting fractures

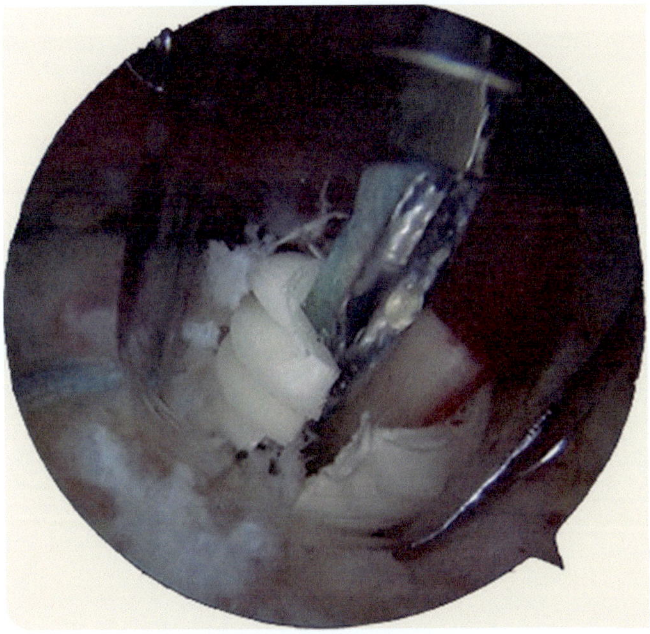

Fig. 4.23 Crush outer row anchor bolts

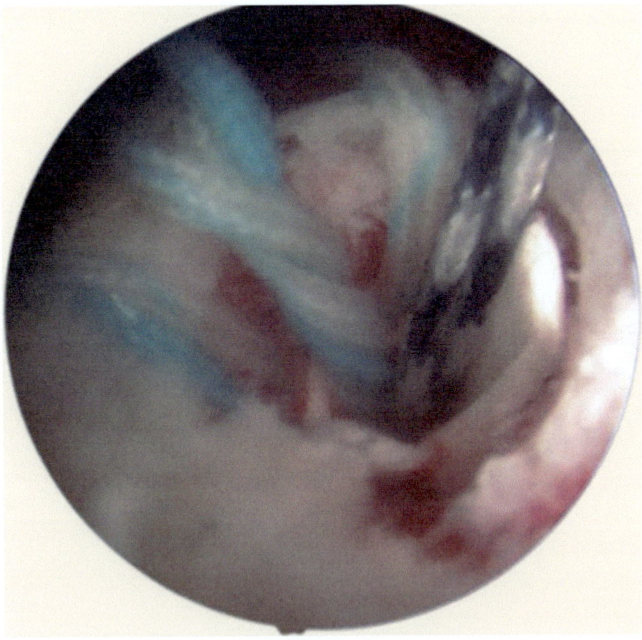

Fig. 4.24 Broken outer row anchor bolts

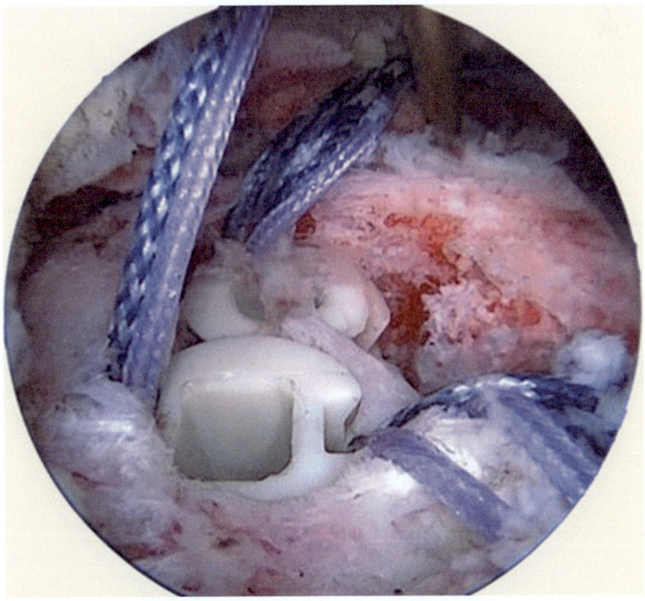

Fig. 4.25 Bone fracture between external anchor screws

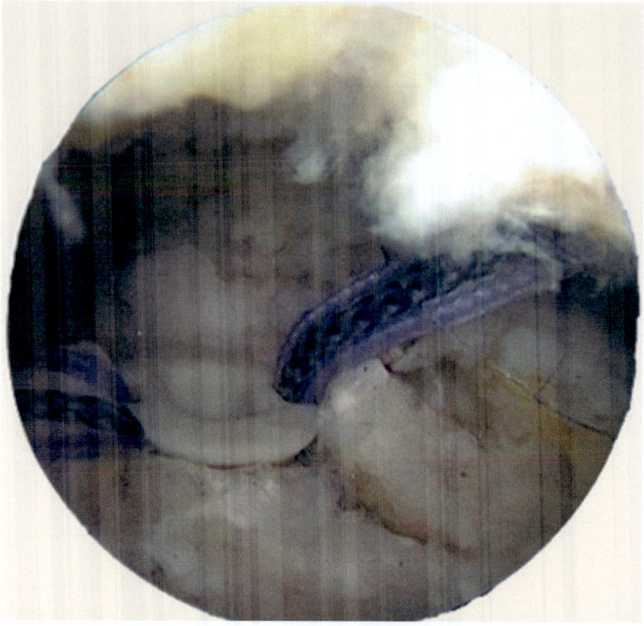

Fig. 4.26 Fracture of the greater tuberosity of the humerus after external anchor screw implantation

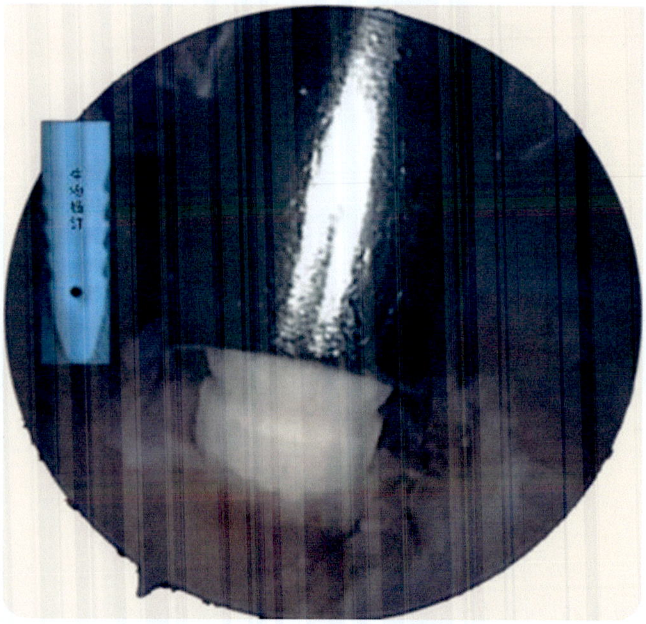

Fig. 4.27 Allogeneic biological bone anchor nail inserted into the greater tuberosity of the humerus

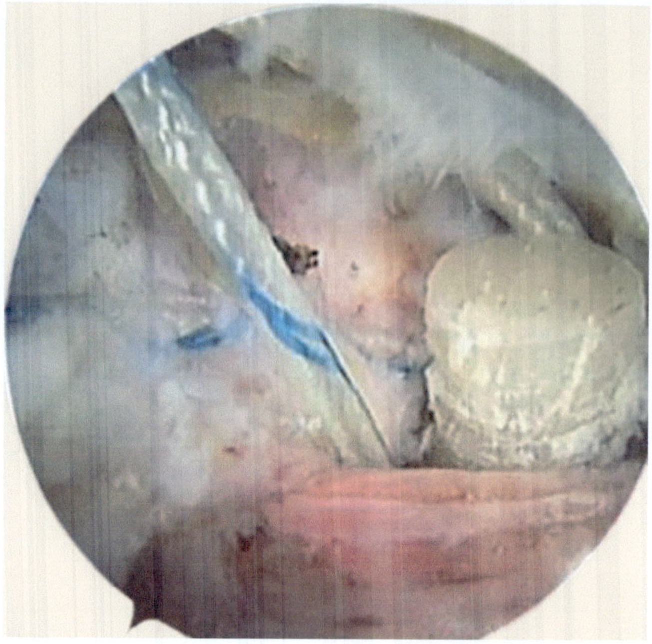

Fig. 4.28 Biological bone anchor fixation for repairing rotator cuff injury

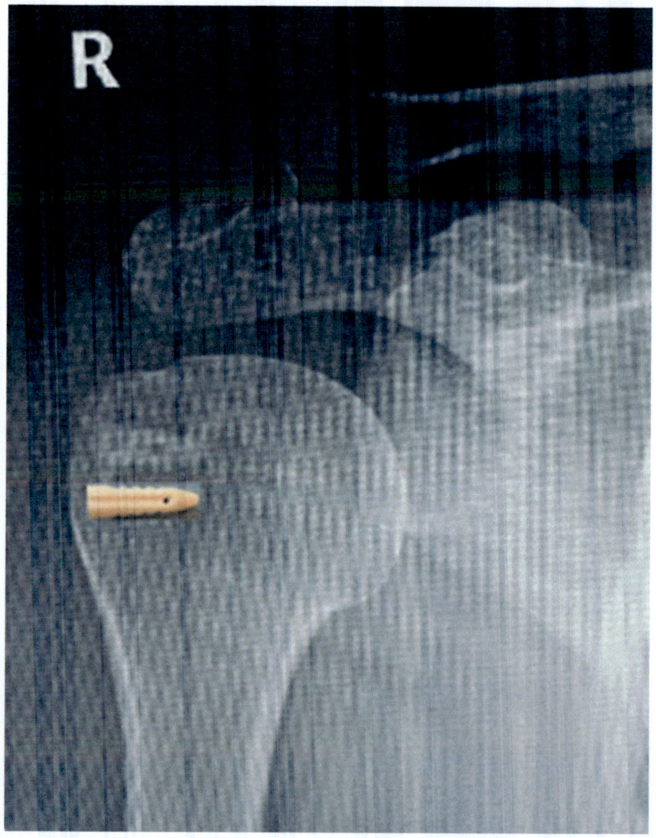

Fig. 4.29 X-ray examination shows the humeral tuberosity bone anchor after surgery for rotator cuff injury

References

1. Lyons FA, Rockwood CA. Migration of pin used in operations on the shoulder. J Bone Joint Surg. 1990;72A:1262–7.
2. Codman EA. The shoulder: rupture of the supraspinatus tendon and other lesions in or about the subacromial bursa. Malabar: Krieger Pub Co; 1934.
3. Fritz LB, Ouellette HA, O'Hanley TA, et al. Cystic changes at supraspinatus and infraspinatus tendon insertion sites: association with age and rotator cuff disorders in 238 patients. Radiology. 2007;244(1):239–348.
4. Burkhart SS, Klein JR. Arthroscopic repair of rotator cuff tears associated with large bone cysts of the proximal humerus: compaction bone grafting technique. Arthroscopy. 2005;21(7):900–1.
5. Kim KC, Rhee KJ, Shin HD, et al. Arthroscopic fixation for displaced greater tuberosity fracture using the suture-bridge technique. Arthroscopy (2008) 24(1):120.
6. Levy DM, Moen TC, Ahmad CS. Bone grafting of humeral head cystic defects during rotator cuff repair. Am J Orthop (Belle Mead NJ). 2012;41(2):92–4.

5 The Neglected Problems and Countermeasures of Massive Rotator Cuff Injury

Chang-ming Huang, Yu-jie Liu, and Yang-pan Fu

5.1 Introduction

The treatment of massive rotator cuff tears remains a clinical challenge, as it not only presents high surgical difficulty and poor prognosis but also significantly increases the rate of retearing after repair. The main manifestations of irreparable rotator cuff tears are shoulder joint pain, weakness, and pseudoparalysis. Imaging examination can evaluate the size of rotator cuff injury, muscle atrophy, degree of muscle contraction, grading of fat infiltration, and humeral head displacement. The correct treatment plan should be selected based on the patient's condition. For elderly patients, if the shoulder joint function is basically good, arthroscopic debridement, biceps tendon release, amputation, or tendon fixation surgery can be considered, while repairing part of the rotator cuff; For patients with irreparable massive rotator cuff tears accompanied by pseudoparalysis, patch techniques, superior capsule reconstruction, and transposition of the long head tendon of the biceps brachii muscle, or reverse total shoulder replacement surgery may be considered. For young patients, the main focus is on restoring rotator cuff muscle strength, and transfer surgery to the latissimus dorsi tendon and pectoralis major muscle can be used. For individuals with intact subscapularis muscle, latissimus dorsi muscle transfer can improve lateral rotation and partial lift function [1]. For simple irreparable tears of the subscapularis muscle, transfer of the pectoralis major tendon can help patients recover internal rotation of the shoulder joint. For irreparable ipsilateral supraspinatus muscle tears, this method may be ineffective [2].

C.-m. Huang (✉) · Y.-p. Fu
Department of Orthopedics, The 73rd Group Army Hospital, Chenggong Hospital Affiliated to Xiamen University, Xiamen, China

Y.-j. Liu
Orthopaedics, Chinese PLA General Hospital, Beijing, China

5.2 Overview of Disease Diagnosis and Treatment

The patient is a 68-year-old male with pain in the right shoulder joint accompanied by limited abduction and lifting activity for more than 5 years, which affects night time sleep and normal life. Physical examination showed significant atrophy of the supraspinatus, infraspinatus, and deltoid muscles. Shoulder joint active forward flexion and upward lift 70° (Fig. 5.1), abduction and external rotation 20°, passive forward flexion and upward lift 180° (Fig. 5.2), and lateral external rotation 50°. Neer sign (+), Jobe test (+) (Fig. 5.3), Lag sign (+), Belly press test (+) (Fig. 5.4), Lift off test (+) (Fig. 5.5), Hawkins sign (+) (Fig. 5.6), Speed test (−), and O'Brien test (−). Imaging examination: X-ray examination shows greater tuberosity of the humerus and osteophyte of

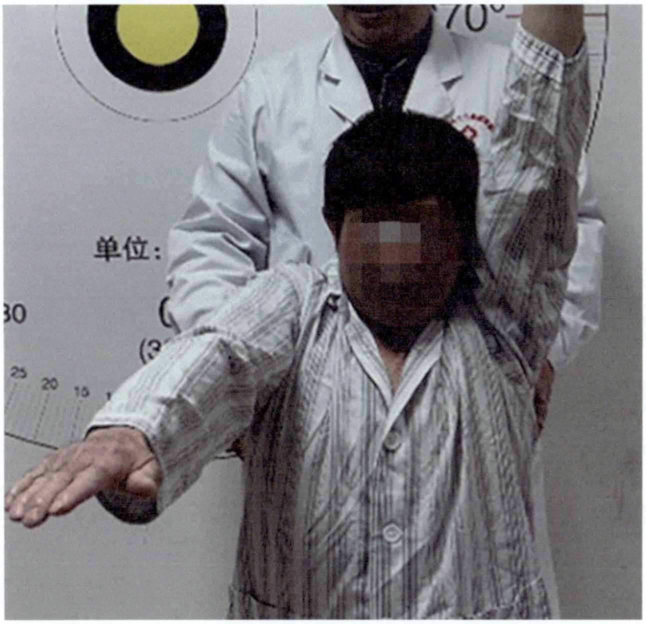

Fig. 5.1 Active flexion and lifting of the right shoulder joint at 70° (R)

Y.-j. Liu et al. (eds.), *Pitfalls in Diagnosis and Treatment of Shoulder Joint Diseases*, https://doi.org/10.1007/978-981-96-2472-0_5

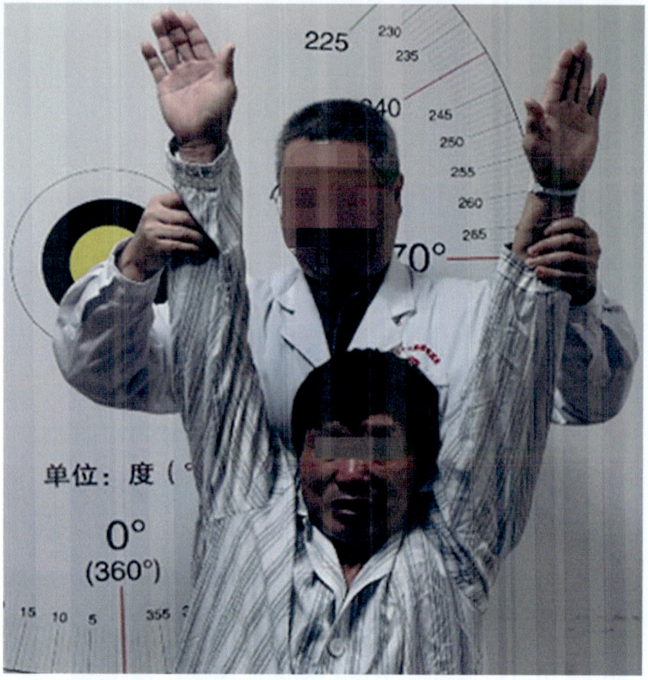

Fig. 5.2 Passive flexion and lifting of the right shoulder joint 180°

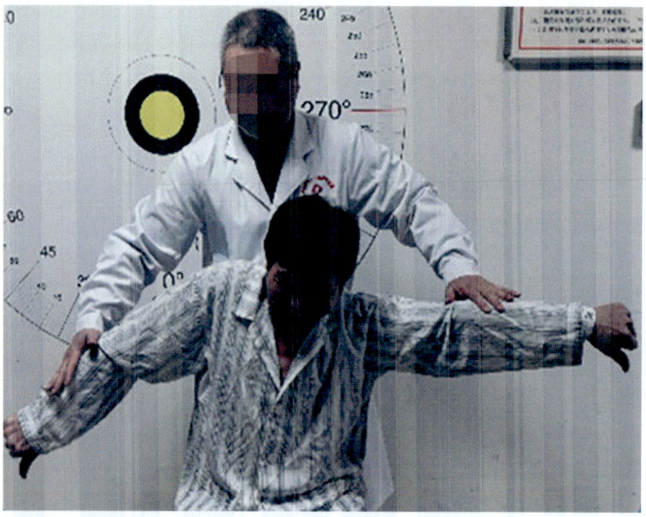

Fig. 5.3 Jobe test (+)(R)

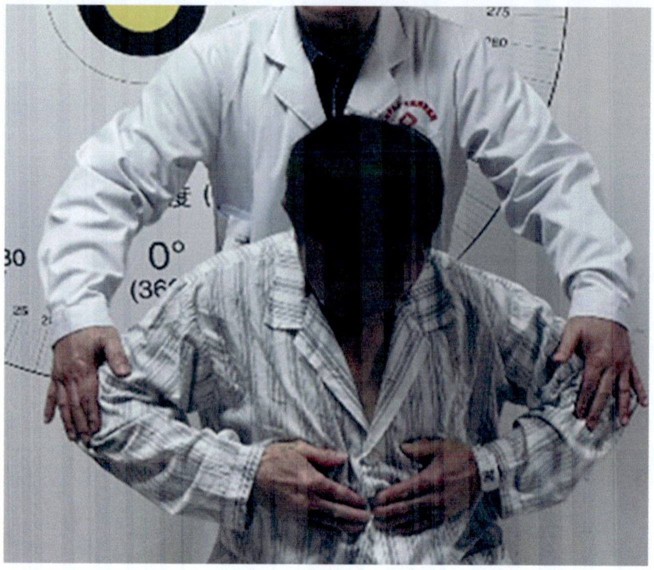

Fig. 5.4 Right shoulder belly press test (+)

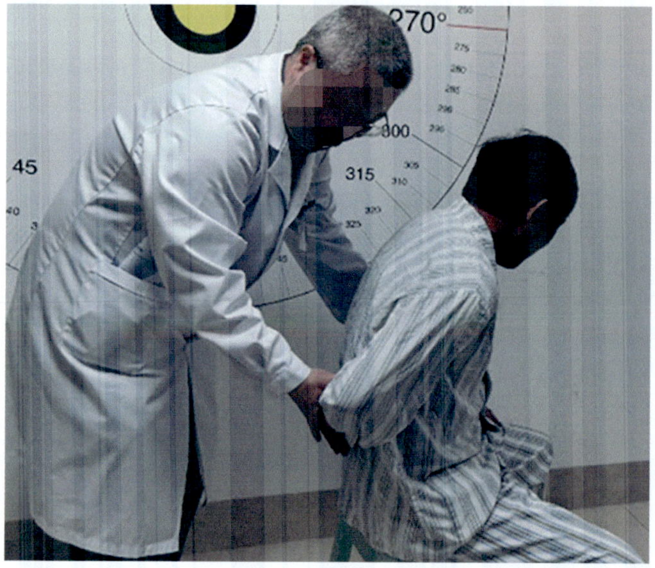

Fig. 5.5 Right shoulder lift off test (+)

the acromion, narrowing of the glenoid humeral joint space (Fig. 5.7), and CT shows upward displacement of the humeral head (Fig. 5.8). MRI shows a huge tear in the rotator cuff (Fig. 5.9) and fatty tissue in the supraspinatus muscle (Fig. 5.10).

Under general anesthesia, arthroscopic exploration revealed a massive tear in the right rotator cuff (Fig. 5.11), and the severed end of the supraspinatus tendon retracted to the edge of the shoulder glenoid (Fig. 5.12). The humeral tuberosity and acromion osteophyte are hypertrophic, and

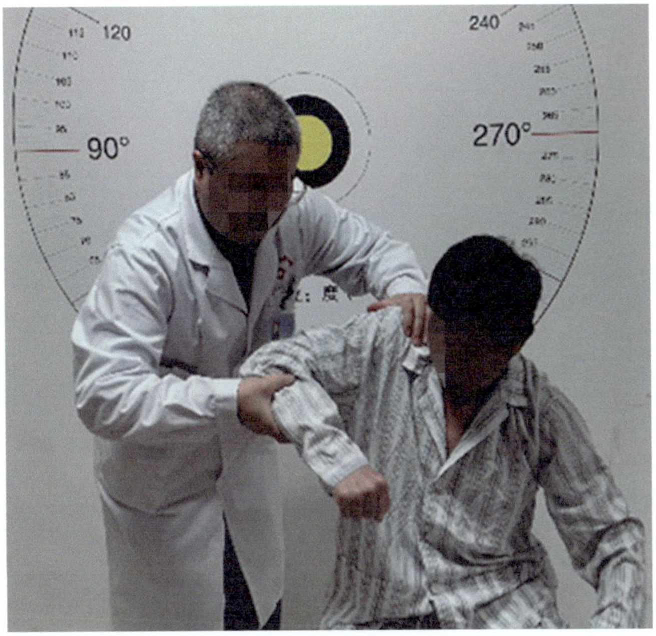

Fig. 5.6 Hawkins sign of right shoulder (+)

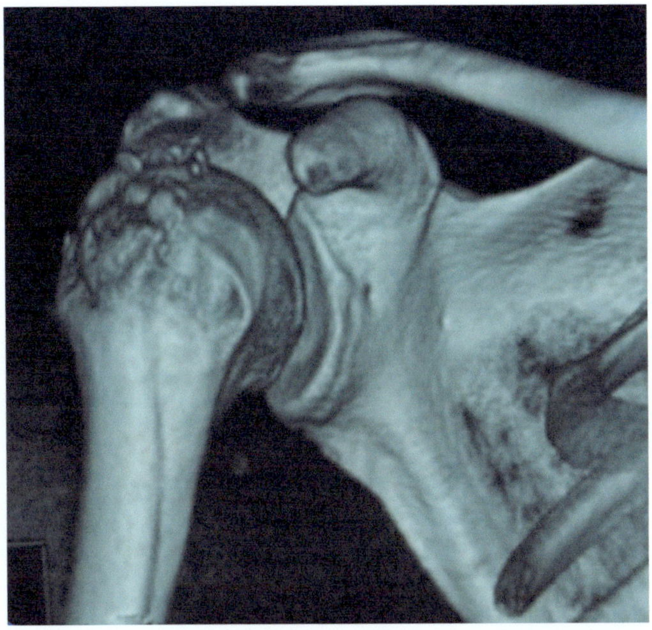

Fig. 5.8 CT three-dimensional reconstruction examination of the right shoulder joint shows upward displacement of the humeral head

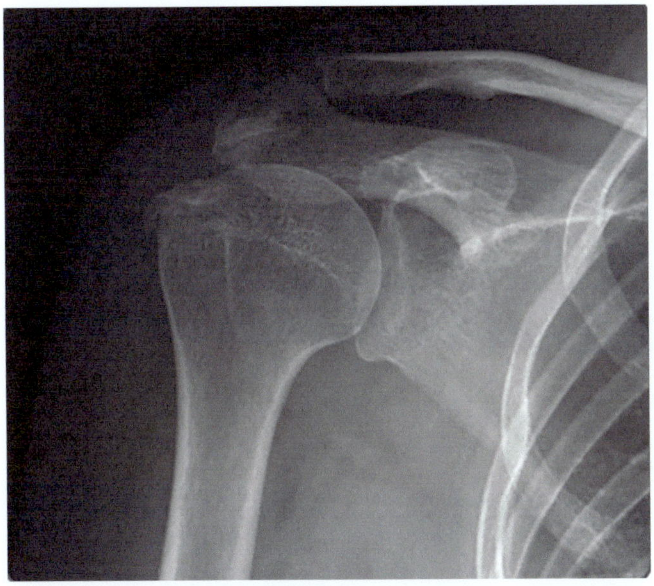

Fig. 5.7 X-ray examination of the right shoulder joint in an anteroposterior position shows bone hyperplasia in the greater tuberosity of the humerus and narrowing of the glenoid humeral joint space

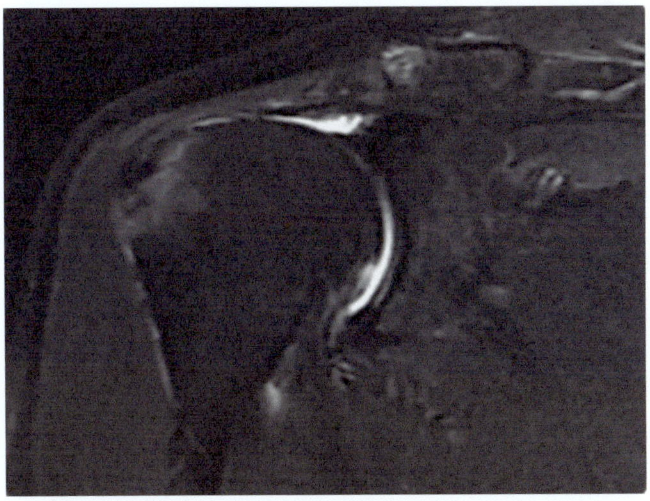

Fig. 5.9 Coronal PD fat suppression sequence on MRI of the right shoulder joint showing massive rotator cuff tear

acromioplasty is performed by grinding the osteophyte. The contracted rotator cuff tissue was released, and 4.5-mm diameter absorbable anchor was used for double row fixation in the foot print area of the humeral tuberosity rotator cuff. Due to poor quality of rotator cuff tissue, the torn rotator cuff was reluctantly closed after release (Fig. 5.13). After surgery, the shoulder joint was immobilized with a sling for routine functional rehabilitation training. Half a year after surgery, the right shoulder joint still suffered from pain and limited active movement. MRI examination revealed retear in the rotator cuff (Fig. 5.14).

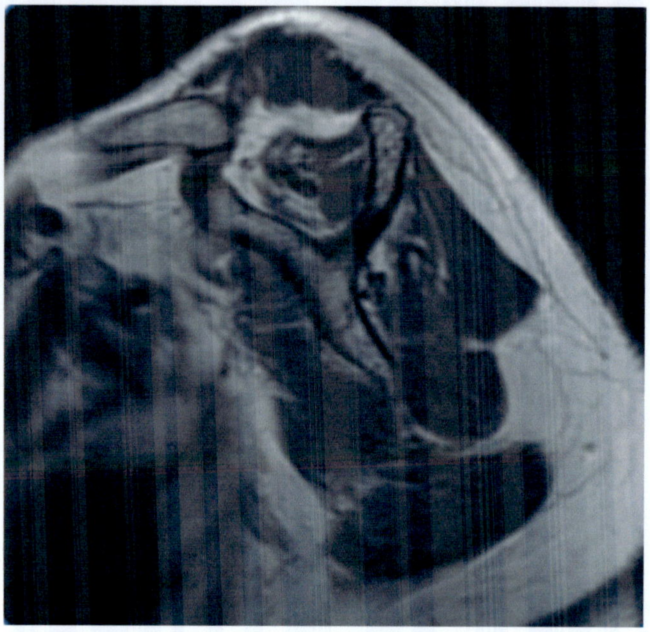

Fig. 5.10 MRI oblique sagittal T1 sequence of the right shoulder joint shows grade II fat infiltration, where the supraspinatus muscle is more abundant than fat

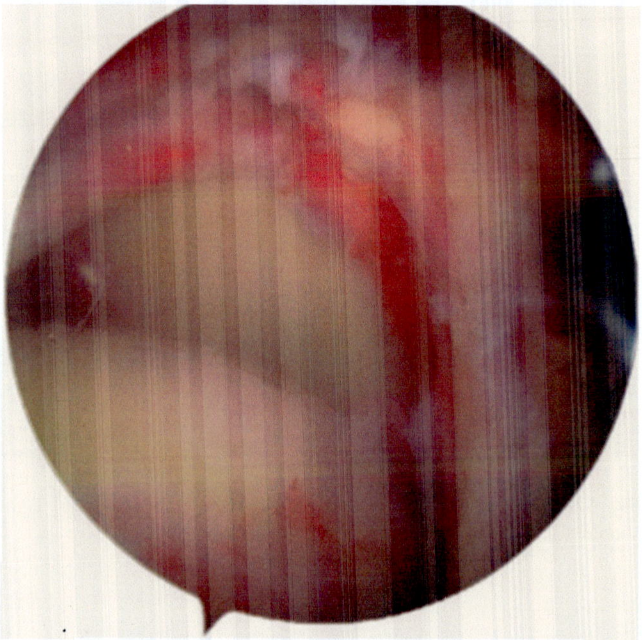

Fig. 5.11 Giant tear on right rotator cuff

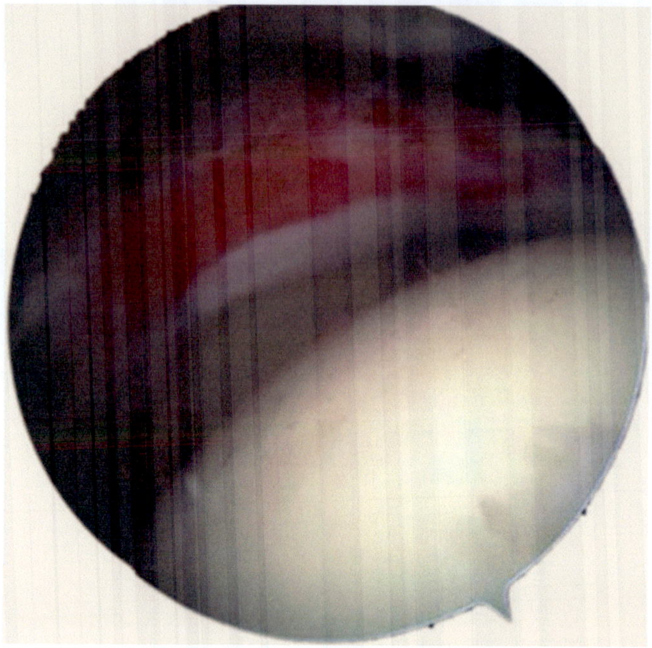

Fig. 5.12 The severed end of the supraspinatus tendon retracts to the edge of the shoulder glenoid

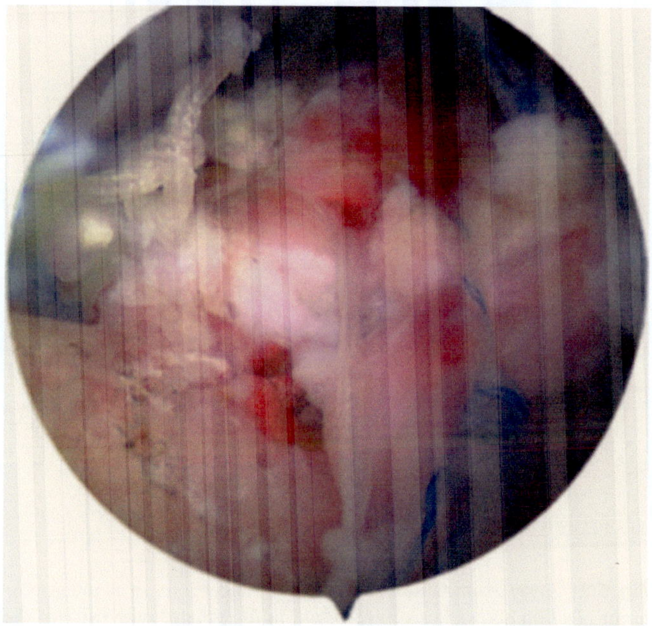

Fig. 5.13 Sutured rotator cuff tear, closed tear

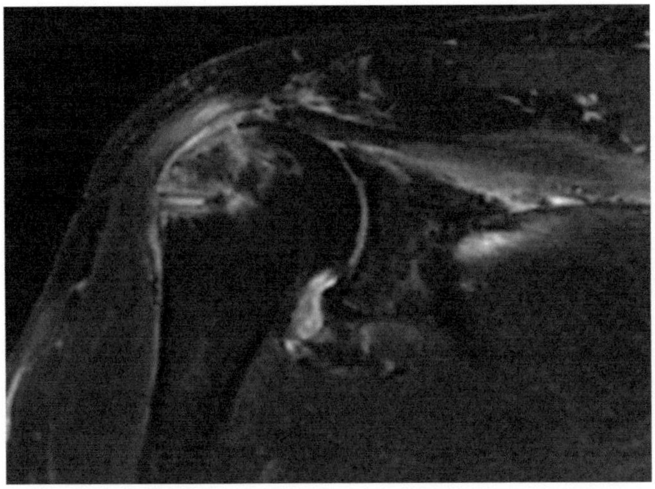

Fig. 5.14 Postoperative right shoulder joint MRI coronal PD fat suppression sequence showing recurrent rotator cuff tear

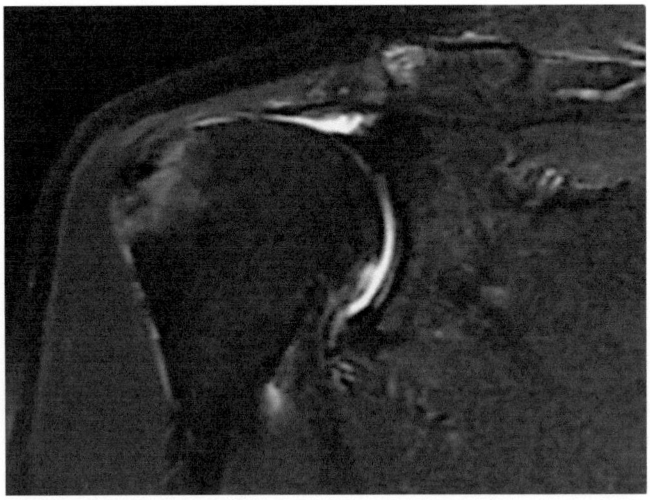

Fig. 5.15 MRI coronal PD fat suppression sequence of right rotator cuff third degree injury showing rotator cuff retraction to shoulder glenoid

5.3 Comprehensive Preoperative Assessment of the Patient's Condition Is an Important Measure

Preoperative evaluation of the patient's overall condition, including age, occupation, symptoms, signs, underlying disease, degree of rotator cuff injury, imaging examination, and if necessary, electromyography examination can help determine the presence of pseudoparalysis and axillary nerve injury, which is crucial for selecting surgical indications.

5.3.1 Imaging Evaluation of the Morphology of the Acromion and the Quality of Bone in the Greater Tuberosity of the Humerus

Bigliani [3] classifies the acromion into three types: Type I, flat shoulder peak; Type II, arc-shaped shoulder peak; Type III, hooked shoulder peak. Preoperative X-ray examination can determine the presence of rotator cuff joint disease. Hamada [4] classification is commonly used to classify the acromion into five types: Type I, with a distance between the acromion and the humeral head greater than 6 mm; Type II, with a distance of ≤5 mm between the shoulder peak and the humeral head; Type III, with a distance of ≤5 mm between the acromion and the humeral head, and a clubbing like change below the acromion; Type IV, divided into two subtypes A and B, with a distance of ≤5 mm between the shoulder peak and the humeral head. Type A is characterized by glenohumeral arthritis, narrow glenohumeral joint space, no clubbing or acetabulization. Type B is glenoid humeral arthritis, with narrow glenoid humeral joint space accompanied by clubbing and acetabulization. It also exhibits V-shaped, narrowing of the glenoid humeral joint space with pestle-like transformation, and collapse of the humeral head.

5.3.2 Evaluating the Quality of Rotator Cuff Is Helpful for Making Decisions on Surgical Plans for Rotator Cuff Surgery

The quality of rotator cuff is related to postoperative efficacy. North American scholars believe that rotator cuff injury is greater than 5 cm, while European scholars believe that complete injury to two or more tendons is a massive rotator cuff injury. Patte [5] classified rotator cuff injury into three degrees based on the degree of retraction in oblique coronal MRI: first degree, with mild retraction of the rotator cuff; second degree, the rotator cuff retracts to the level of the humeral head; third degree, the shoulder sleeves retract to the level of the shoulder glenoid (Fig. 5.15). Shoulder cuff muscle strength below grade 3, humeral head displacement, tendon retraction to shoulder glenoid level, and severe muscle atrophy are irreparable injuries.

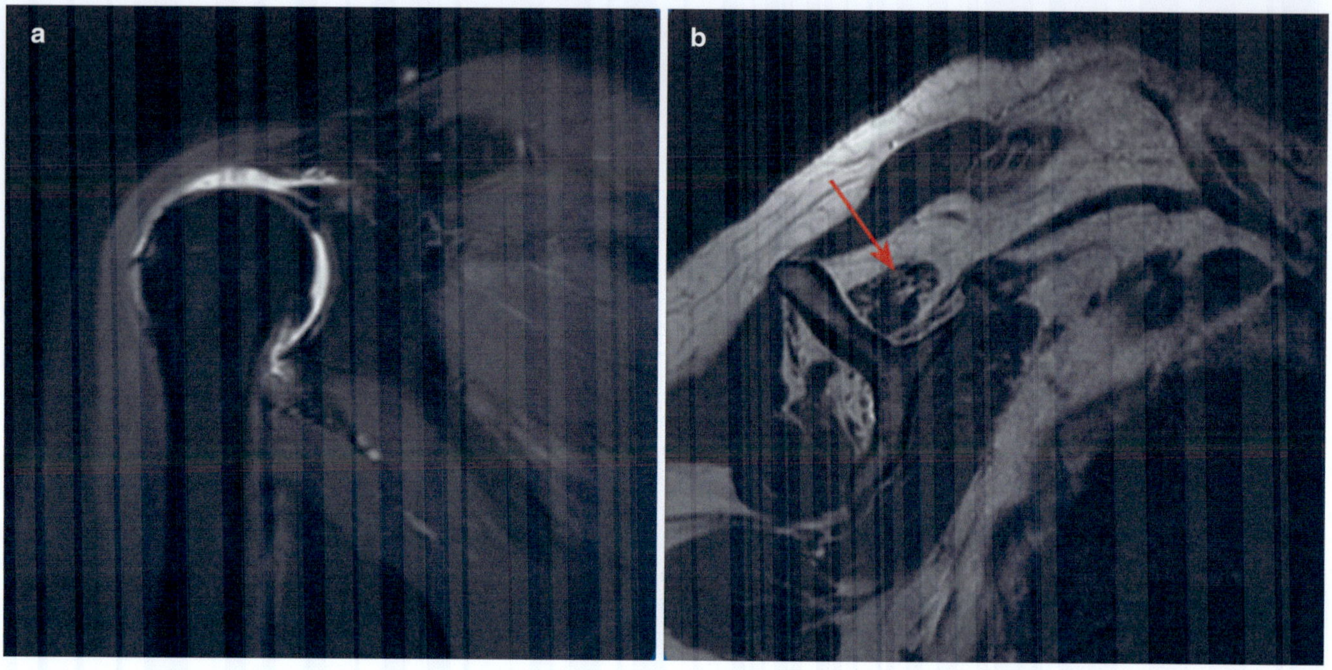

Fig. 5.16 MRI image of right shoulder joint (**a**) Diagonal coronal view shows a huge rotator cuff injury on the right shoulder; (**b**) T1 oblique sagittal view shows atrophy and fat infiltration in the rotator cuff supraspinatus muscle (red arrow)

The MRI examination of the shoulder joint selected oblique coronal, oblique sagittal, axial, and T1 oblique sagittal positions to evaluate changes such as rotator cuff muscle fat infiltration, muscle atrophy (Fig. 5.16), rotator cuff injury size, degree of retraction, and humeral head displacement. Goutellier [6] classified fat infiltration into five levels. Level 0: Normal muscle without fat infiltration; Level I: A small amount of intramuscular fat; Level II: Muscle is more than fat; Level III: Muscle is equal to fat; Level IV: Fat is more than muscle. Warner et al. [7] classified muscle atrophy into four degrees: normal, mild, moderate, and severe. Thomazeau et al. [8, 9] classified supraspinatus muscle atrophy into three degrees using MRI oblique sagittal imaging. Degree I: Muscle cross-sectional area ≥60%; Grade II, muscle cross-sectional area ≥40% and <60%; Grade III, muscle cross-sectional area <40%.

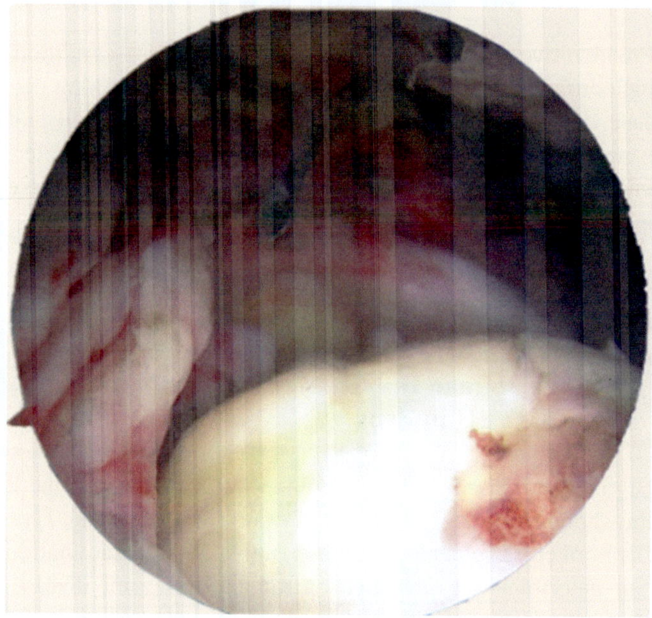

Fig. 5.17 Giant injury to the right rotator cuff

5.4 Reasons for Postoperative Retear

According to literature reports, the incidence of retear after repair surgery for massive rotator cuff injuries can reach up to 40%. The course of giant rotator cuff injury in elderly patients can last for several years, and the shoulder joint cannot move normally for a long time, leading to adhesions, osteoporosis, muscle atrophy, and severe rotator cuff muscle steatosis. Therefore, it is crucial to choose the appropriate surgical indication, especially for rotator cuff contracture with fatty infiltration after injury (Fig. 5.17). Although rotator cuff loosening and forced suturing were performed during surgery (Fig. 5.18), the rotator cuff tissue is fragile, the tensile strength is reduced, incorrect braking methods and functional training are not standardized in the early postoperative stage, and the limbs are difficult to withstand tensile strength after surgery, all of which are the reasons for postoperative retear.

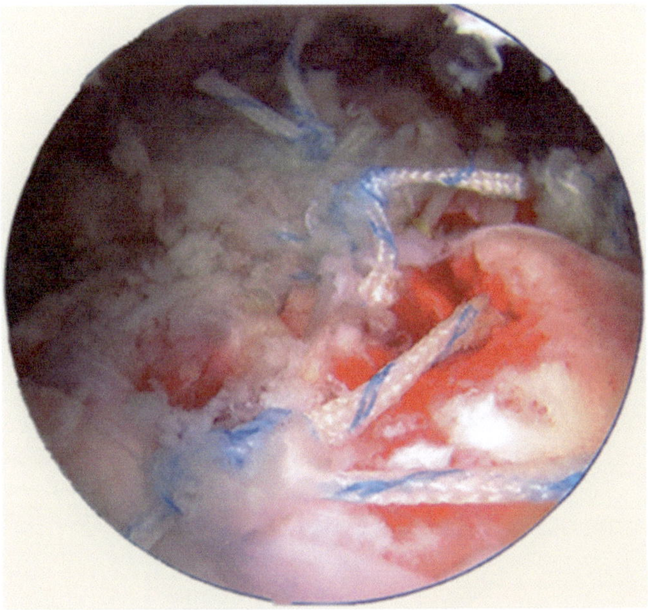

Fig. 5.18 Suturing of rotator cuff after internal movement of release

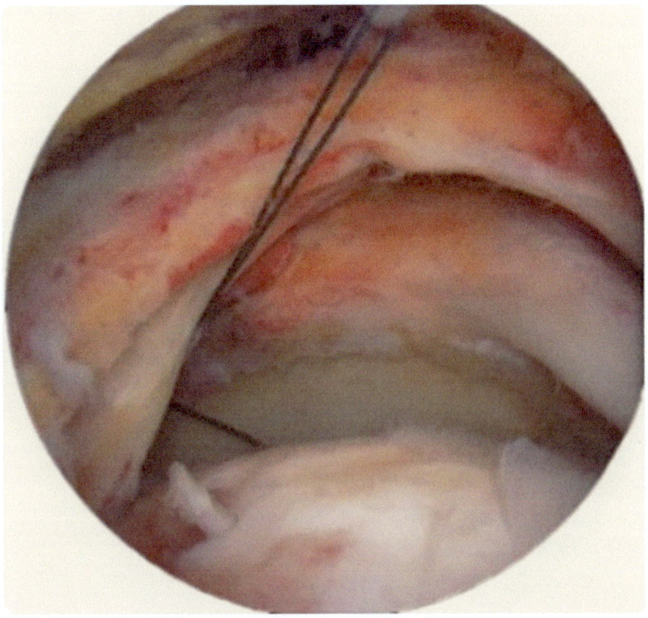

Fig. 5.19 Giant rotator cuff tear in a U-shape

5.5 Massive Rotator Cuff Injury with Technique of Marginal Convergence

Evaluating the quality of residual rotator cuff tendons under arthroscopy and selecting appropriate suture repair methods is beneficial for the treatment of rotator cuff injuries.

The purpose of partially repairing the tendon is to rebuild the stable fulcrum and coupling of the glenoid humeral joint and improve shoulder joint function. Burkhart et al. [10] believed that if partial repair of the rotator cuff is performed using the rotator cuff marginal convergence technique, the biomechanical balance of the shoulder joint can be restored. In the case of a large tear in the rotator cuff, the stress after forced suturing is mainly concentrated on the suture edge and anchor, which will cause anchor removal or rotator cuff retearing. Excessive tension in the shoulder sleeves can easily lead to early surgical failure [11]. The location and quantity of anchor bolts should be arranged according to the severity of rotator cuff injury and the tension of the rotator cuff. If the contraction tension of the rotator cuff is too high after injury, appropriate release of the rotator cuff can be performed first, and then marginal convergence can be performed to turn the "U" shaped rotator cuff wound (Fig. 5.19) into a "V" shape (Fig. 5.20) through edge to edge stitching, and finally the V-shaped shape can be transformed into a T-shaped shape. The articular cartilage at the inner edge of the greater tuberosity of the humerus should be cleaned (Fig. 5.21), suture anchor screws are implanted (Fig. 5.22), the rotator cuff is sutured and fixed at the greater tuberosity of the humerus (Fig. 5.23). To facilitate tendon healing, the subtuberoidal bone can be treated with microfracture. The injury of the huge rotator cuff was repaired by marginal convergence, and the anchor was moved inboard to the inner margin of the greater tubercle of humerus (Fig. 5.24).

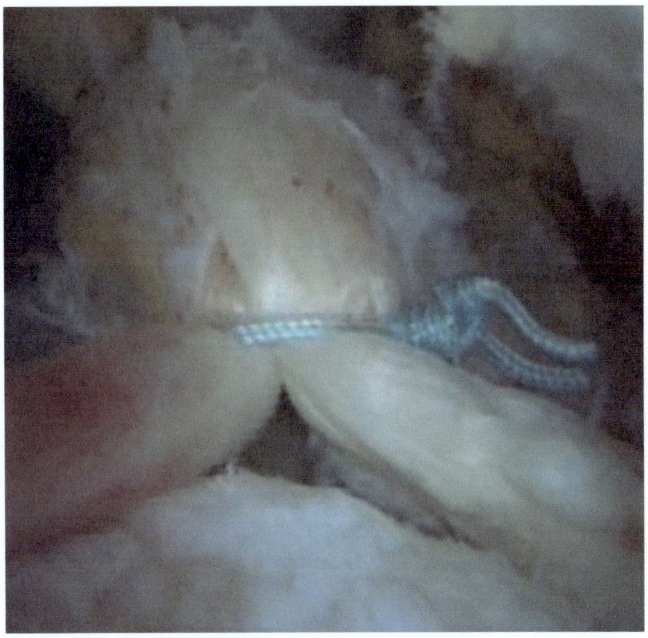

Fig. 5.20 The U-shaped is sutured side to side to form a V-shape

Based on anatomical and biomechanical research, it has been found that in order to maximize the holding strength of anchor screws, the angle of anchor screw implantation

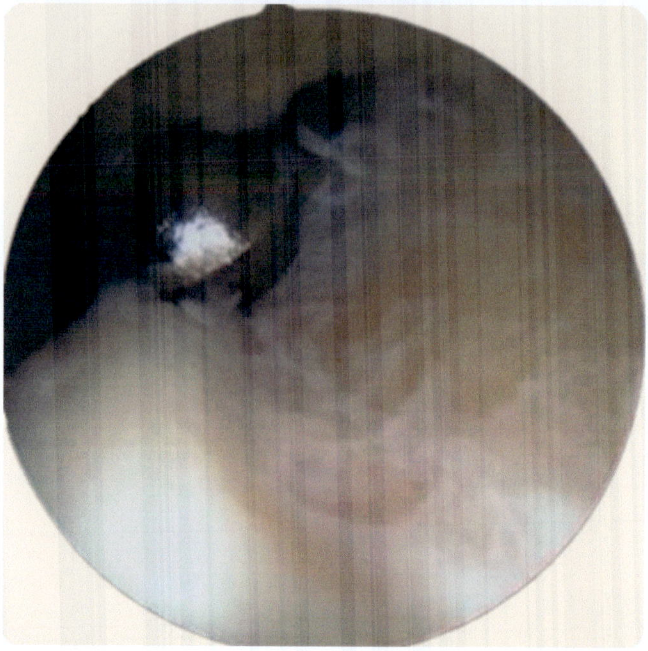

Fig. 5.21 Removing the articular cartilage at the inner edge of the greater tuberosity of the humerus as the anchor screw insertion point

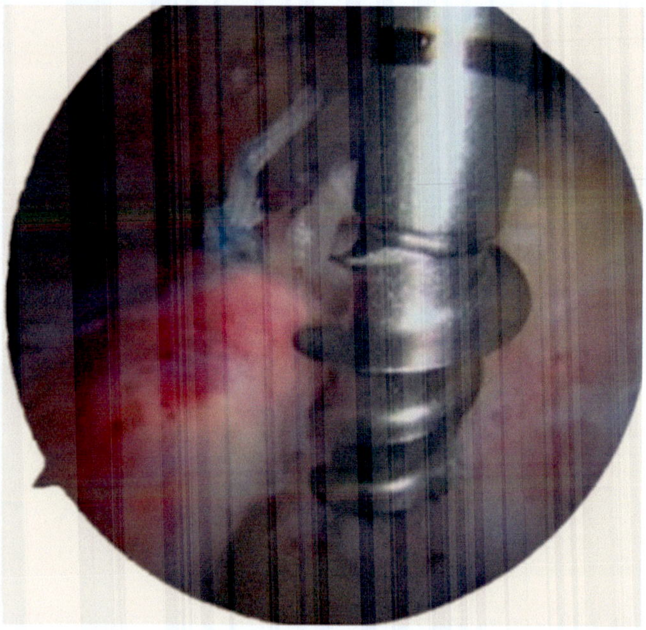

Fig. 5.22 Suturing and fixing the rotator cuff at the greater tuberosity of the humerus

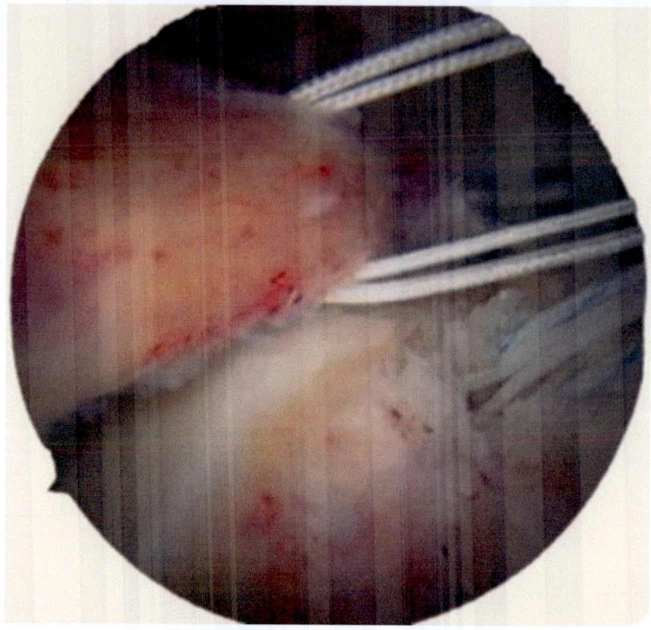

Fig. 5.23 Suture fixation of the rotator cuff edge at the inner edge of the greater tuberosity of the humerus

should be perpendicular to the suture angle. Therefore, the angle of anchor screw implantation should be less than 45 ° from the direction of the rotator cuff, and the anchor screw implantation point should be located behind the greater tuberosity of the humerus, with high bone density near the cartilage edge, which can achieve greater grip strength. The anterior lateral bone density is relatively low, and there is a possibility of anchor loosening during anchor implantation here.

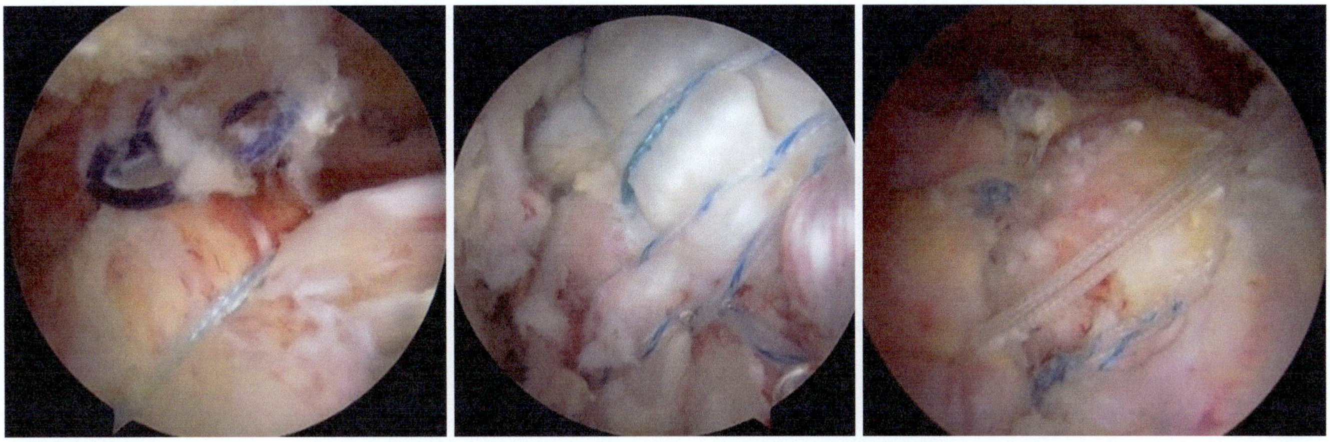

Fig. 5.24 Large rotator cuff marginal convergence, anchor fixed at the greater tuberosity of the humerus

5.6 Biceps Tendon Transposition and Enhanced Fixation (Chinese Way)

At present, many scholars believe that the long head tendon of the biceps brachii muscle may be the cause of pain in patients with rotator cuff injury. There is still controversy over whether to cut or reuse the long head tendon of the biceps brachii muscle in the repair of giant rotator cuff. In 2005, Walch et al. [12] performed a total of 307 patients with rotator cuff injury who underwent long head tendon resection of the biceps brachii muscle. The postoperative shoulder joint pain significantly improved.

Some scholars fixed the long head tendon of the biceps directly in the intertubercular sulcus, and some scholars fixed the long head tendon of the biceps after backward and external transposition. Many scholars have adopted the method of transposition of the long head tendon of the biceps after amputation, and the distal and proximal ends of the long head tendon were fixed with anchors. This will not increase the tension of the biceps long tendon too much, reduce pain and limited elbow extension, or cause the anchor to pull out due to increased tension. The translocation and fixation of the biceps tendon without amputation avoids the fixation of the two severed ends after the amputation of the tendon, which increases the amount of consumables, and more importantly, prevents the fixation failure caused by suture ligation or interfacial nail fixation of the severed ends of the tendon, necrosis, or tendon slip.

Scholars at home and abroad have achieved good therapeutic effects by transposing and fixing the biceps brachii tendon while dealing with huge rotator cuff injuries. French scholars Boutsiadis et al. [13] used the technique of cutting, transferring, and fixing the long head tendon of the biceps brachii muscle developed by Chinese scholar Professor Chen Shiyi to strengthen the repair of the rotator cuff, achieving good results. They referred to this surgical method as "Chinese Way." The long head tendon of the biceps tendon was not severed during the operation, and the long head tendon was transposed backward and laterally with sutures (Fig. 5.25). Anchor fixation was performed at a new position on the lateral side of the greater tuberosity of the humerus (Fig. 5.26). The advantage of this method is that it utilizes the force coupling change and pressure on the humeral head after the transposition of the biceps tendon, enhancing the tensile strength of the rotator cuff. Due to the arthroscopic synovial cleaning and relief of the intertubercular groove on the biceps brachii tendon, postoperative pain was relieved.

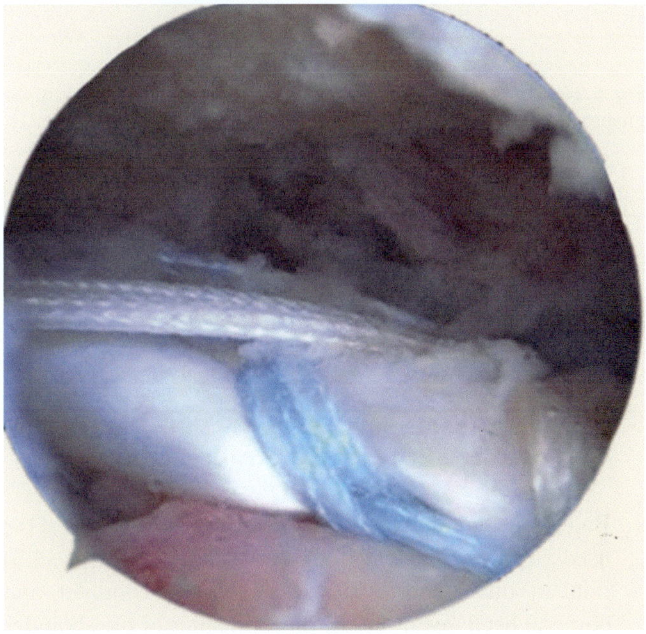

Fig. 5.25 Suture traction for release and transposition of biceps brachii tendon

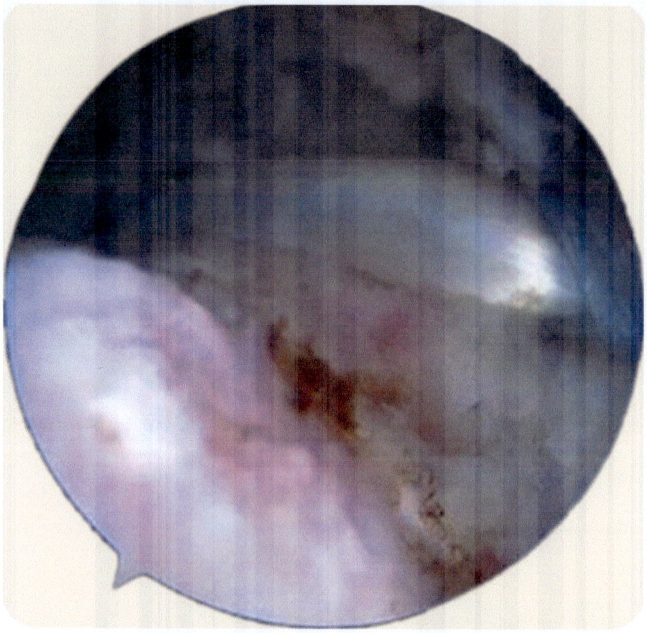

Fig. 5.26 Transfer of the biceps brachii tendon to the lateral side of the greater tuberosity of the humerus

The transposition of the long head tendon of the biceps brachii muscle can partially reconstruct the upper joint capsule and seal the defect of the massive rotator cuff tear, reducing the rate of postoperative retear.

5.7 Countermeasures for Irreparable Massive Rotator Cuff Injuries

1. Balloon technique: Israeli scholars Savarese et al. [14] used a biodegradable balloon pad technique (InSpace) to implant under arthroscopy between the shoulder and humeral head, restoring the biomechanics of the shoulder joint. The technique is simple and less invasive and can be used as a method to delay the reverse shoulder arthroplasty.
2. Superior capsule reconstruction technique: Ishihara et al. [15] studied the biomechanical characteristics of the shoulder joint capsule on the passive stability of the glenoid humeral joint using the reconstruction technique of the superior joint capsule. The tear of the superior joint capsule increases the displacement of the humeral head in front and below. The purpose of reconstructing the superior joint capsule is to restore the static stable structure of the shoulder joint. Mihata et al. [16] studied the efficacy of arthroscopic superior joint capsule reconstruction in the treatment of irreparable rotator cuff tears. The average active elevation and external rotation significantly increased after surgery, which helps prevent osteoarthritis or rotator cuff muscle atrophy and can restore shoulder joint stability and function. The reconstruction of the superior joint capsule and the bridging technique of the rotator cuff tissue have good therapeutic effects.
3. Reverse shoulder joint replacement: This surgery is commonly used in patients with irreparable rotator cuff tears. For patients with pseudoparalysis of the shoulder joint and active shoulder abduction <90°, it can improve shoulder joint range of motion, alleviate pain, and improve postoperative scores [17].

In summary, the incidence of retear after giant rotator cuff repair surgery is high. The use of marginal convergence of rotator cuff tissue and transposition of the long head tendon of the biceps brachii muscle can help reduce the tension of rotator cuff tissue and prevent retear after rotator cuff suture surgery. For the treatment of irreparable rotator cuff injuries, appropriate surgical methods should be selected based on the patient's age, degree of injury, living needs, skills mastered by the doctor, socioeconomic situation, and other factors.

References

1. Gerber C, Vinh TS, Hertel R, et al. Latissimus dorsi transfer for the treatment of massive tears of the rotator cuff. A preliminary report. Clin Orthop Relat Res. 1988;232:51–61.
2. Galatz LM, Connor PM, Calfee RP, et al. Pectoralis major transfer for anterior-superior subluxation in massive rotator cuff insufficiency. J Shoulder Elb Surg. 2003;12(1):1–5.
3. Bigliani LU, Cordasco FA, Mcllveen SJ, et al. Operative repair of massive rotator cuff tears: long-term results. J Shoulder Elb Surg. 1992;1(3):120–30.
4. Hamada K, Fukuda H, Mikasa M, et al. Roentgenographic findings in massive rotator cuff tears. A long-term observation[J]. Clin Orthop Relat Res. 1990;254:92–6.
5. Patte D. Classification of rotator cuff lesions. Clin Orthop Relat Res. 1990;254:81–6.
6. Goutallier D, Postel JM, Bernageau J, et al. Fatty infiltration of disrupted rotator cuff muscles. Rev Rhum Engl Ed. 1995;62(6):415–22.
7. Warner JP, Higgins L, Parsons IV, et al. Diagnosis and treatment of anterosuperior rotator cuff tears. J Shoulder Elb Surg. 2001;10(1):37–46.
8. Thomazeau H, Boukobza E, Morcet N, et al. Prediction of rotator cuff repair results by magnetic resonance imaging. Clin Orthop Relat Res. 1997;344:275–83.
9. Thomazeau H, Rolland Y, Lucas C, et al. Atrophy of the supraspinatus belly, assessment by MRI in 55 patients with rotator cuff pathology. Acta Orthop Scand. 1996;67(3):264–8.
10. Burkhart SS, Athanasiou KA, Wirth MA. Margin convergence:a method of reducing strain in massive rotator cuff tears. Arthroscopy. 1996;12(3):335–8.
11. Burkhart SS, Johnson TC, Wirth MA, et al. Cyclic loading of transosseous rotator cuff repairs: tension overload as a possible cause of failure. Arthroscopy. 1997;13(2):172–6.

12. Walch G, Edwards TB, Boulahia A, et al. Arthroscopic tenotomy of the long head of the biceps in the treatment of rotator cuff tears: clinical and radiographic results of 307 cases. J Shoulder Elb Surg. 2005;14(3):238–46.
13. Boutsiadis A, Chen SY, Jian CY, et al. Long head of the biceps as a suitable available local tissue autograft for superior capsular reconstruction: "the Chinese way". Arthrosc Tech. 2017;6(5):1559–66.
14. Savarese E, Romeo R. New solution for massive, irreparable rotator cuff tears: the subacromial "biodegradable spacer". Arthrosc Tech. 2012;1(1):e69–74.
15. Ishihara Y, Mihata T, Tamboli M, et al. Role of the superior shoulder capsule in passive stability of the glenohumeral joint. J Shoulder Elb Surg. 2014;23(5):642–8.
16. Mihata T, Lee TQ, Watanabe C, et al. Clinical results of arthroscopic superior capsule reconstruction for irreparable rotator cuff tears. Arthroscopy. 2013;29(3):459–70.
17. Wall B, Nové-Josserand L, O'Connor DP, et al. Reverse total shoulder arthroplasty: a review of results according to etiology. J Bone Joint Surg Am. 2007;89(7):1476–85.

Part III

Complications and Countermeasures in Shoulder Instability Anchor Fixation: An Introduction and Summary

Jing Xue

Introduction

This part focuses on the diagnosis and treatment of shoulder instability caused by glenolabral articular disruption (GLAD). It discusses complications associated with different suture anchor fixations, such as metal anchor protrusion, leading to secondary osteoarthritis of the glenohumeral joint. Factors contributing to failure and strategies for absorbable anchor and PEEK anchor fragmentation are also addressed. The development of bioabsorbable bone anchors for stabilizing and repairing shoulder instability is expected to become a future hotspot. The reasons behind post-Latarjet surgery screw breakage and nonunion of coracoid grafts are analyzed in detail. Additionally, technical key points and precautions for scapular spine and iliac bone grafting in the treatment of glenoid bony defects are elaborated.

Summary

1. GLAD injury is a rare etiology of shoulder instability, and arthroscopic exploration plays a pivotal role in both diagnosis and treatment. Surgical intervention primarily entails repairing labral tears and performing local microfracture surgery following cartilage fragment removal.
2. Inadequate surgical technique during the labral anchor repair procedure commonly contributes to failure and postoperative complications. The utilization of allograft bone anchors, devised by the author, offers facile substitution and promotes bony healing within the affected area, rendering it an optimal choice for revision surgery subsequent to unsuccessful labral anchor procedures.
3. Postoperative failure of the Latarjet procedure due to broken screws or nonunion of coracoid graft is not uncommon. Employing scapular spine as a graft material effectively addresses bone defects associated with Bankart lesions. The utilization of allogeneic cortical bone transverse nail presents a convenient and feasible approach for the fixation and repair of bony Bankart lesions, resulting in successful healing at both the bone graft and recipient site. The iliac bone graft is a straightforward, secure, and efficient technique for reconstructing glenoid bone defects.

J. Xue (✉)
Orthopaedics, Air Force Medical Center of Chinese PLA, Beijing, China

6 Shoulder Instability - Anteroinferior Labrum Injury

Lei Zhang

6.1 Clinical Evaluation and Diagnosis

6.1.1 Case 1

The patient is a 40-year-old woman who presented with pain in the right shoulder. She was pulled out of a swimming pool with direct, forceful traction on her right arm 1 month ago. She felt pain right after and persisted for a month.

Physical Examination Full range of motion in the right shoulder. Neer sign (+), the External Rotation Resistance Strength test (-), Hawkins sign(+).

Imaging The X-ray of the right shoulder joint showed no apparent abnormalities (Fig. 6.1). MRI of the shoulder joint revealed an anterior labrum injury with associated cyst formation (Fig. 6.2).

Intraoperative Findings Right shoulder labral tear with GLAD lesion observed (Fig. 6.3). After debridement of the cartilage fragments, two suture anchors were implanted in the glenoid to repair the labral injury (Fig. 6.4). Microfracture surgery was performed on the chondral lesion site of the glenoid (Fig. 6.5), forming a Fibrin clot in the defect (Fig. 6.6).

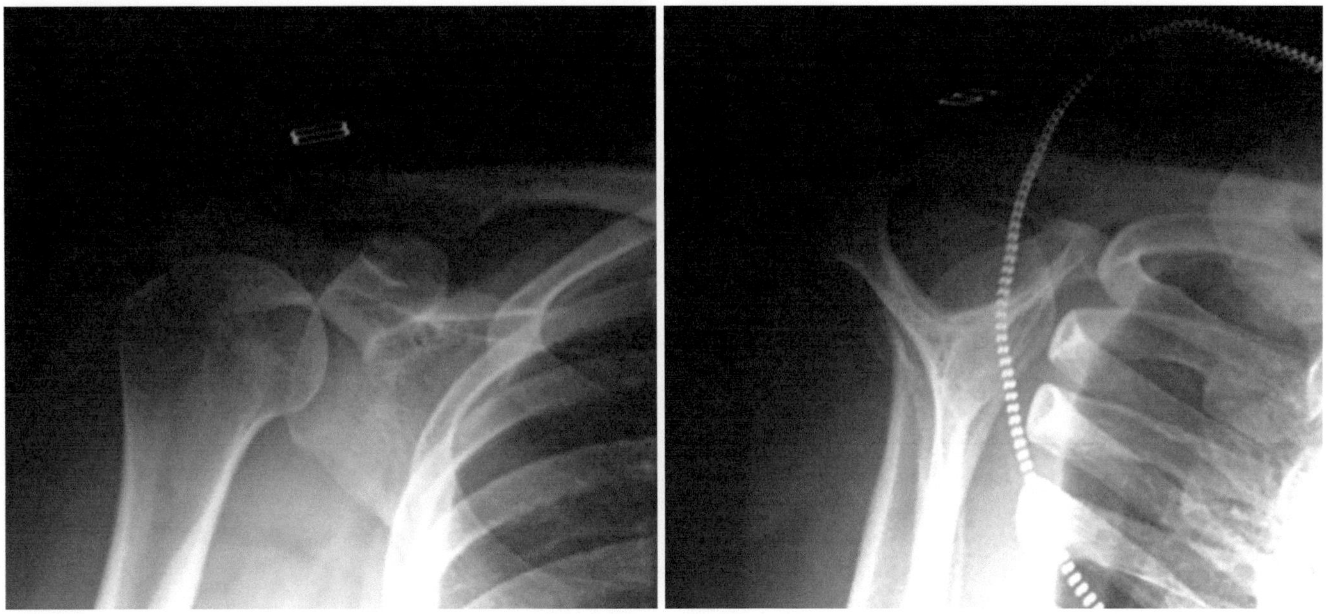

Fig. 6.1 The X-ray of the right shoulder joint showed no apparent abnormalities

L. Zhang (✉)
Wangjing Hospital, China Academy of Chinese Medical Sciences, Beijing, China

Y.-j. Liu et al. (eds.), *Pitfalls in Diagnosis and Treatment of Shoulder Joint Diseases*,
https://doi.org/10.1007/978-981-96-2472-0_6

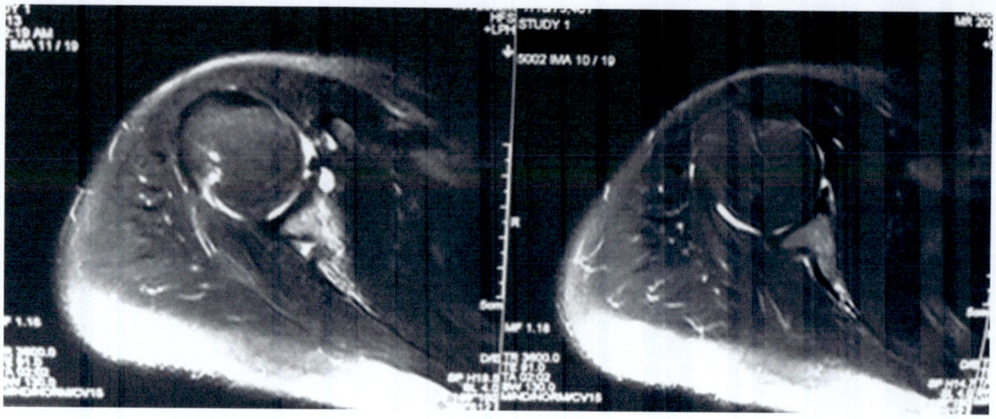

Fig. 6.2 MRI of the shoulder joint revealed an anterior labrum injury with associated cyst formation

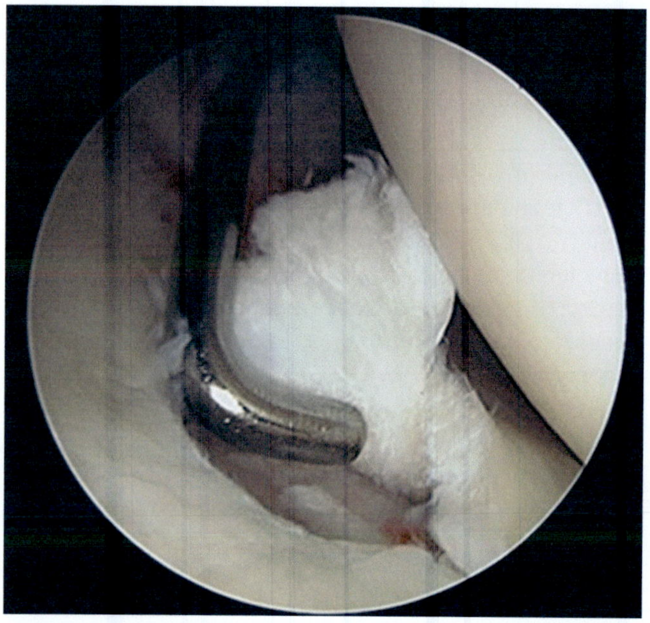

Fig. 6.3 Right shoulder labral tear with GLAD lesion observed

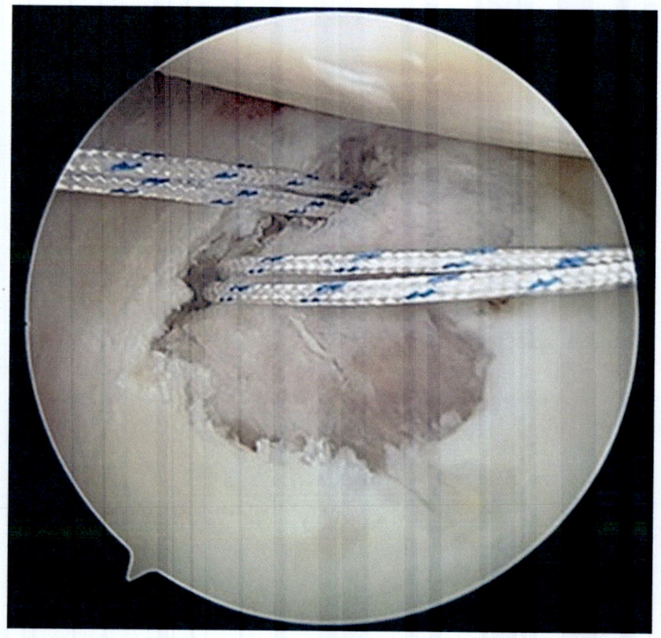

Fig. 6.4 Two suture anchors were implanted in the glenoid to repair the labral injury

6.1.2 Case 2

The patient is a 68-year-old with no history of trauma. He has been experiencing right shoulder pain for 2 months and conservative treatment for "peri arthritis" for 1 and a half months, with no significant improvement.

Physical Examination A significantly decreased range of motion of abduction 70°, forwarding flexion 80°, 0° external rotation 30°, 0° internal rotation 30°. Neer sign (+), the external rotation resistance strength test (+), Hawkins sign (+).

Imaging X-ray shows a Type II acromion (Bigliani classification) (Fig. 6.7). MRI reveals high-signal areas in the subchondral bone of the greater tubercle of the humerus and anteroinferior part of the glenoid (Fig. 6.8), with a preliminary diagnosis of GLAD injury.

Intraoperative Findings Arthroscopy was performed and revealed a GLAD injury (Fig. 6.9) and a tear of the glenoid (Fig. 6.10). After debridement of the cartilage lesion, a Bankart repair (Fig. 6.11) and microfracture surgery for the glenoid cartilage injury were performed.

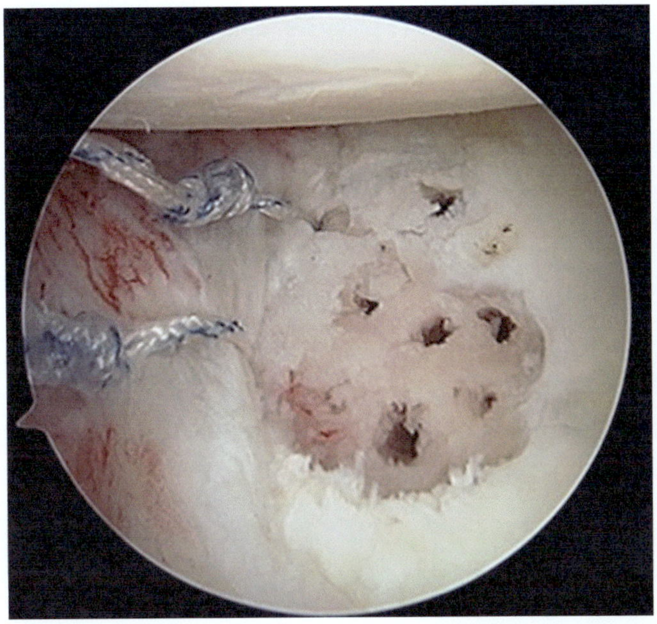

Fig. 6.5 Microfracture surgery was performed on the chondral lesion site of the glenoid

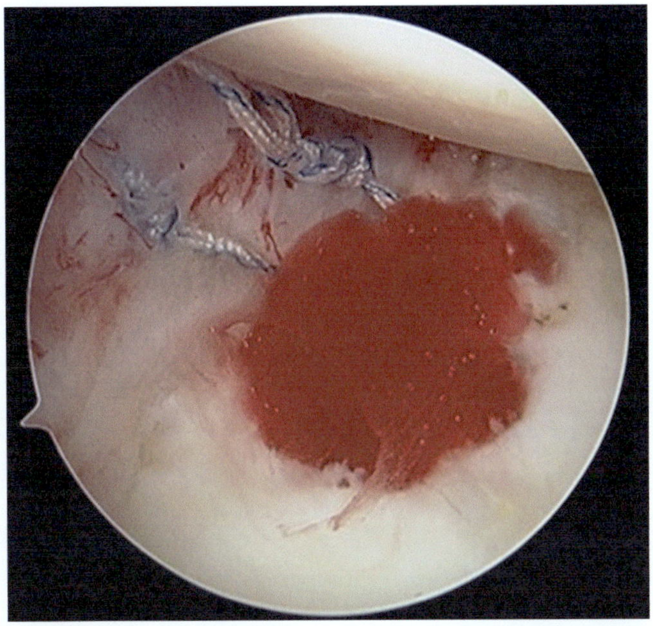

Fig. 6.6 Fibrin clot in the defect

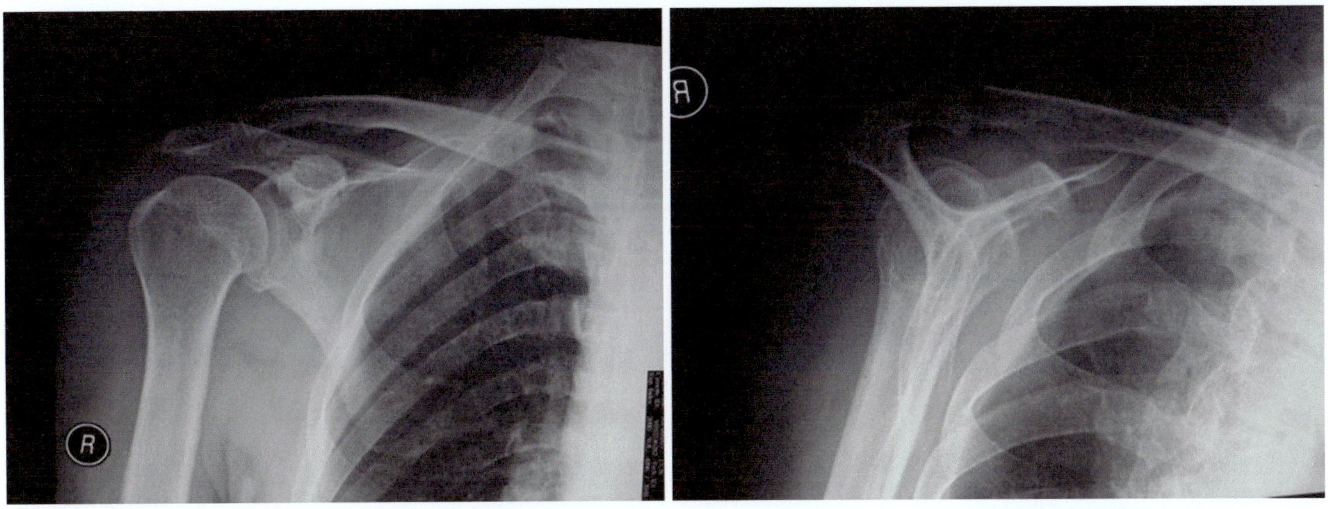

Fig. 6.7 X-ray shows a Type II acromion (Bigliani classification)

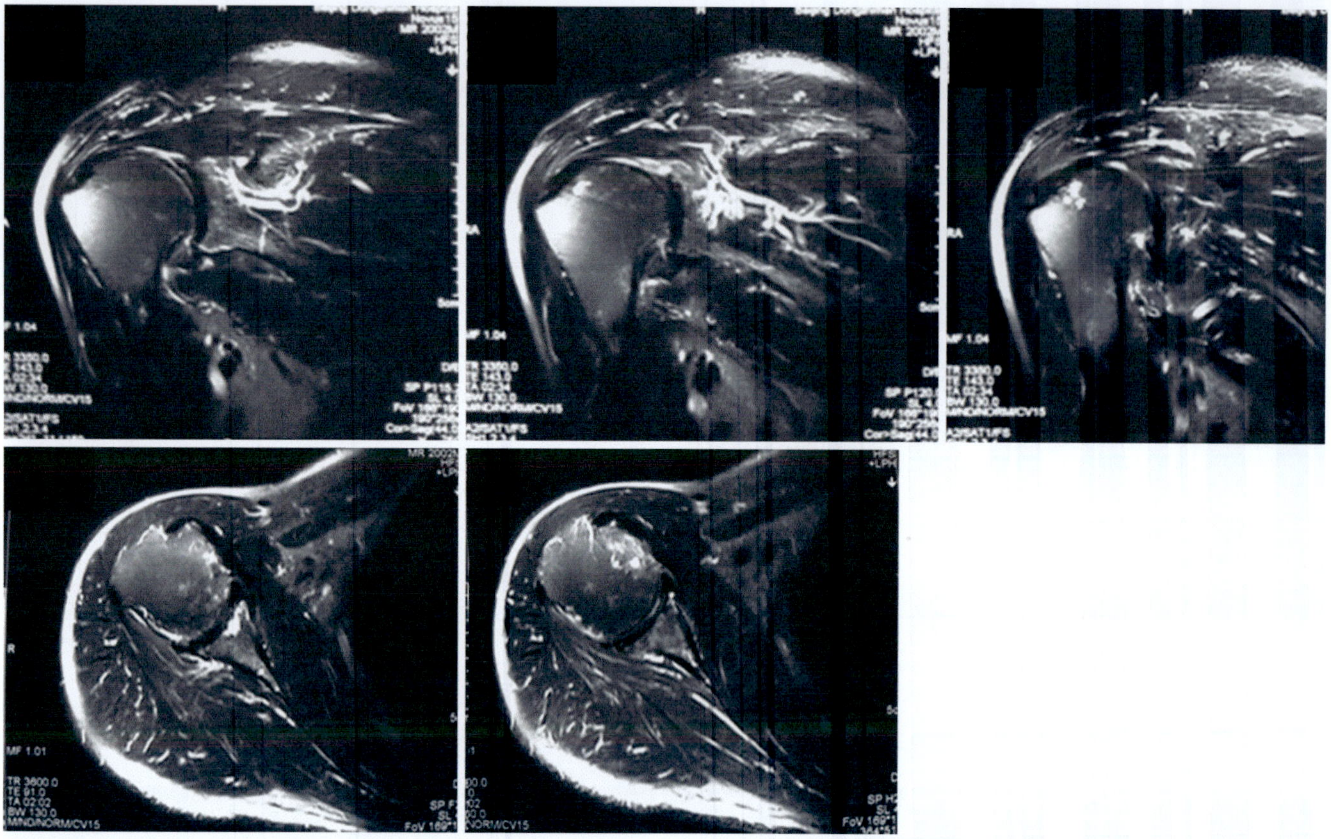

Fig. 6.8 High-signal areas in the subchondral bone of the greater tubercle of the humerus and anteroinferior part of the glenoid

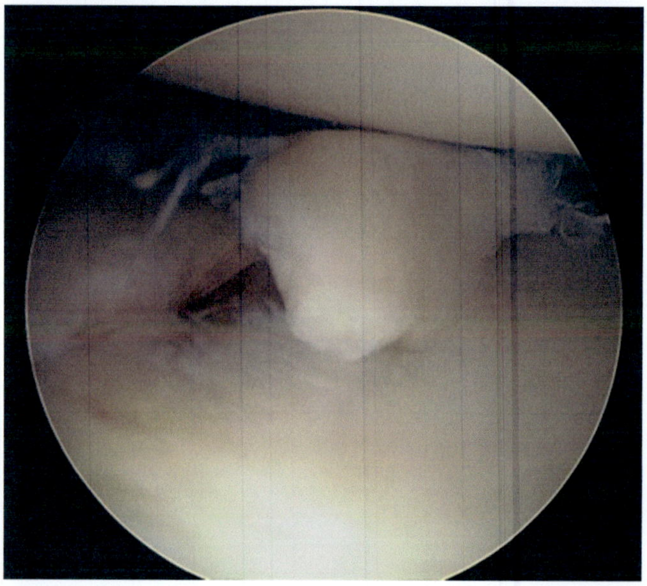

Fig. 6.9 GLAD injury

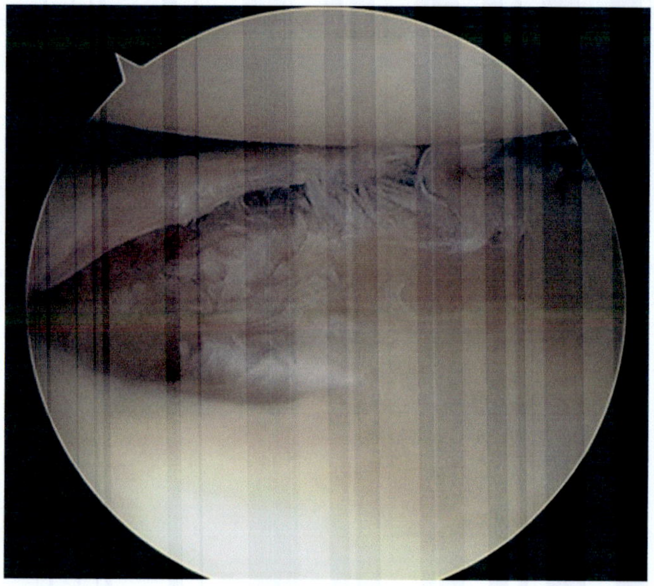

Fig. 6.10 A tear of the glenoid

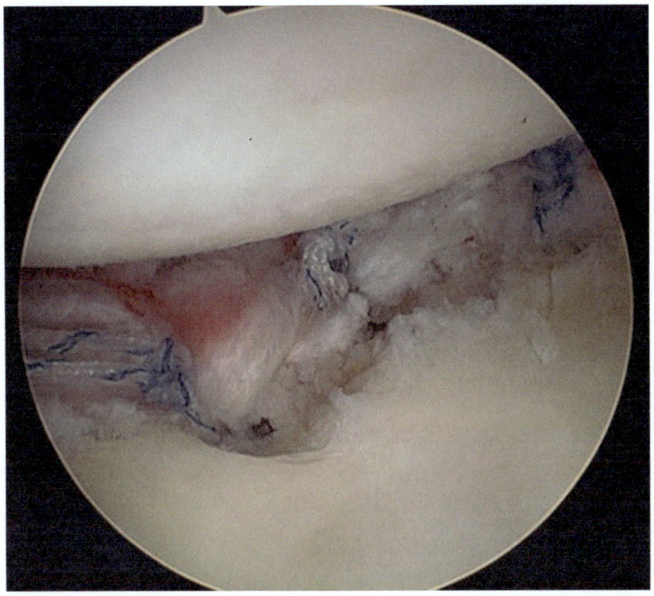

Fig. 6.11 Bankart repair

6.2 GLAD Lesion and Shoulder Instability

Reports of Glenolabral Articular Disruption (GLAD) injuries are rare, with an incidence of 1.5–2.9% in anteroinferior labrum injuries [1–3]. The majority of these injuries are caused by trauma [2, 4]. The shoulder joint is typically in an extreme position of abduction and external rotation at the time of injury. Patients experience significant pain, and most do not present with symptoms of shoulder dislocation or instability [2]. Physical examinations and imaging studies have certain limitations [2, 4], but MRI is more sensitive [5–7], showing high signals in the anteroinferior labrum and less obvious cartilage injury signals. This unique and concealed injury should be closely monitored to avoid misdiagnosis. The causal relationship between scapular cartilage damage and GLAD injuries is still unclear. Cartilage changes can also occur in patients without trauma.

Arthroscopic inspection plays a vital role in both diagnosis and treatment. Surgical treatment primarily involves suturing the labrum injury and performing a microfracture procedure after debriding cartilage fragments. This process creates a Fibrin clot covering the cartilage surface, which is beneficial for repairing the cartilage surface. There are also case reports where the torn cartilage flap is sutured simultaneously with the labrum repair [1]. For larger areas of cartilage damage, cartilage fixation techniques can also be used [3].

References

1. Agarwalla A, Puzzitiello RN, Leong NL, et al. Concurrent primary repair of a glenoid labrum articular disruption and a bankart lesion in an adolescent: a case report of a novel technique. Case Rep Orthop. 2019;1–6.
2. Neviaser TJ. The GLAD lesion: another cause of anterior shoulder pain. J Arthros Relat Surg. 1993;9(1):22–23.
3. Galano GJ, Weisenthal BM, Altchek DW. Articular shear of the anterior-inferior quadrant of the glenoid: a glenolabral articular disruption lesion variant. Am J Orthop. 2013;42(1):41–43.
4. Florian E, Sepp B, Christopher BD, et al. Glenohumeral joint preservation: current options for managing articular cartilage lesions in young, active patients. J Arthros Relat Surg. 2010;26(5):685–696.
5. Waldt S, Burkart A, Imhoff AB, et al. Anterior shoulder instability: accuracy of MR arthrography in the classification of anteroinferior labroligamentous injuries. Radiology. 2005;237(2):578–583.
6. Antonio GE, Griffith JF, Yu AB, et al. First-time shoulder dislocation: high prevalence of labral injury and age-related differences revealed by MR arthrography. J Magn Reson Imaging. 2007;26(4):983–991.
7. Boileau P, Villalba M, Héry JY, et al. Risk factors for recurrence of shoulder instability after arthroscopic bankart repair. J Bone Joint Surg. 2006;88(8):1755.

7 Complications Associated with Suture Anchor Repair for Shoulder Bankart Injury

Yu-jie Liu and Jun-liang Wang

7.1 Overview of the Diagnosis and Treatment Process

A basketball player, a 30-year-old male, suffered the right shoulder joint dislocation in the basketball game accident. Emergency X-ray examination revealed anterior dislocation of right shoulder joint (Fig. 7.1). 3D-CT showed fractures of anterior and inferior glenoid (Fig. 7.2) and depressed fracture of the greater tubercle of humerus (Fig. 7.3). An MRI of the shoulder joint showed bony Bankart injury, Hill-Sachs injury of the humerus, and bone edema of intertubercular sulcus (Fig. 7.4). Diagnosis revealed dislocation of right shoulder joint, bony Bankart injury, and Hill-Sachs lesion.

After completing the preoperative examination, shoulder arthroscopic exploration under general anesthesia revealed Bankart injury of the right shoulder joint (Fig. 7.5), with tear ranging from 1 o'clock to 6 o'clock and fracture pieces in the anterior and inferior shoulder glenoid. Bankart injury and Hill-Sachs lesion were repaired with multiple anchors (Fig. 7.6). Postoperative radiographs showed normal shoulder joint reduction, and some anchor ends were found to be higher than the margin of glenoid (Fig. 7.7). CT examination of shoulder joints showed that some anchors were closer to the humerus head (Fig. 7.8). After the operation, the right forearm was suspended, and the shoulder joint function was rehabilitated according to the rehabilitation procedure. The shoulder joint function returned to normal after operation.

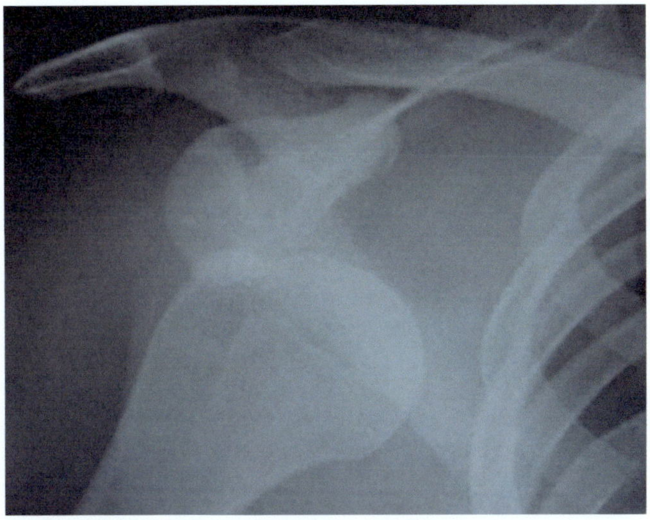

Fig. 7.1 The X-ray examination revealed anterior and inferior dislocation of shoulder joint

Six months after surgery, the patient fell down in a basketball game, and the right shoulder joint was dislocated again. An arthroscopic investigation revealed tears of labrum and sutures and exposed anchors in the first surgically repaired Bankart injury (Fig. 7.9). According to the examination, revision surgery was performed on the right shoulder joint. As the anchor occupied the glenoid space, it was not possible to implant the anchor again, so it was decided to remove the broken anchor and perform Bankart repair surgery.

Metal anchor screw (Fig. 7.10) could not be removed with screwdriver. Bone chisel was used to remove part of the bone (Fig. 7.11), and nucleus pulposus forceps was used to hold the tail end of the anchor screw (Fig. 7.12), then the anchor was removed through a channel (Fig. 7.13). Severe glenoid bone defect was shown (Fig. 7.14).

Y.-j. Liu
Orthopaedics, Chinese PLA General Hospital, Beijing, China

J.-l. Wang (✉)
Department of Orthopedics, Hainan Hospital of Chinese PLA General Hospital, Sanya, China

Y.-j. Liu et al. (eds.), *Pitfalls in Diagnosis and Treatment of Shoulder Joint Diseases*, https://doi.org/10.1007/978-981-96-2472-0_7

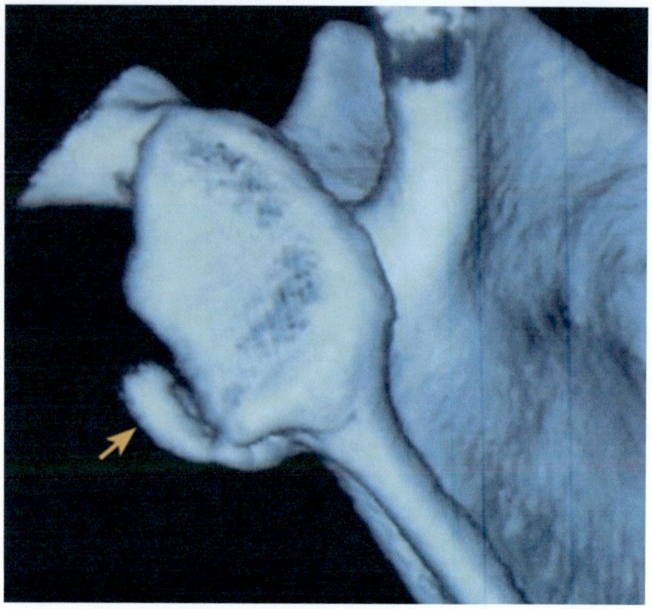

Fig. 7.2 3D CT showed the bone Bankart injury

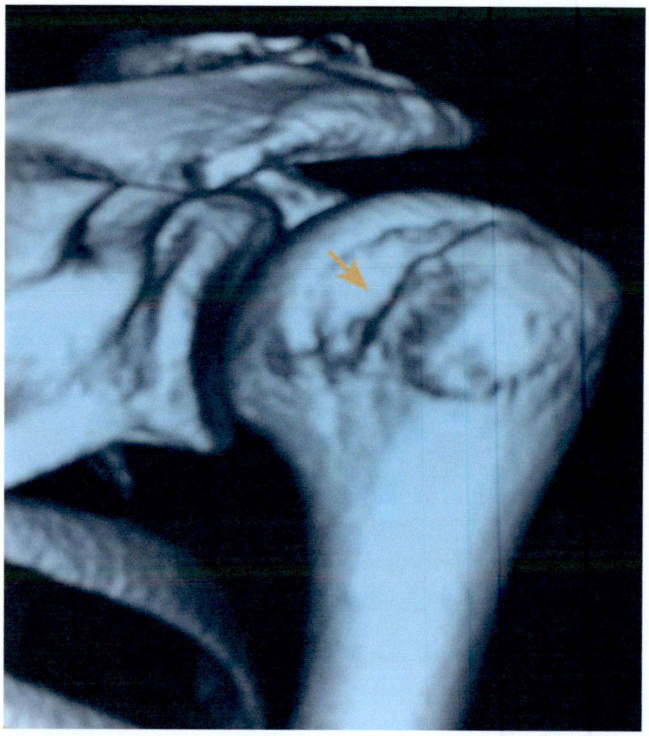

Fig. 7.3 3D CT of the right shoulder joint showed depressed fracture of the greater tubercle of humerus (Hill-Sachs injury)

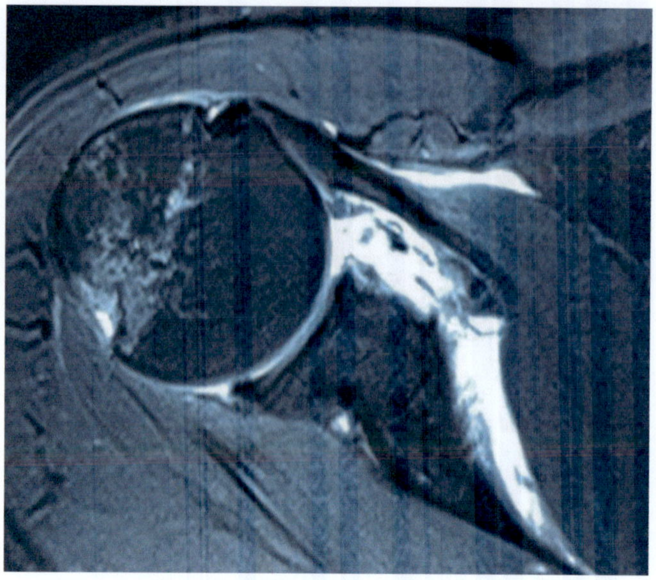

Fig. 7.4 An MRI of the shoulder joint showed Hill-Sachs injury and edema of the humerus head

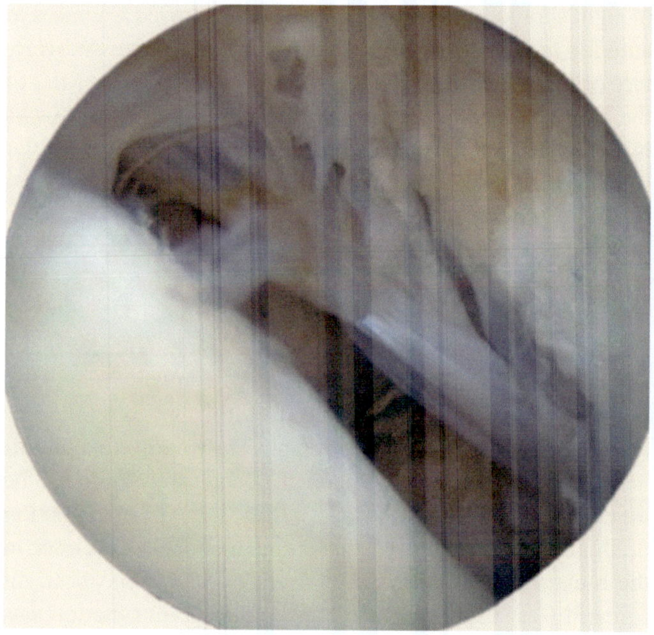

Fig. 7.5 Bankart injury was found arthroscopically

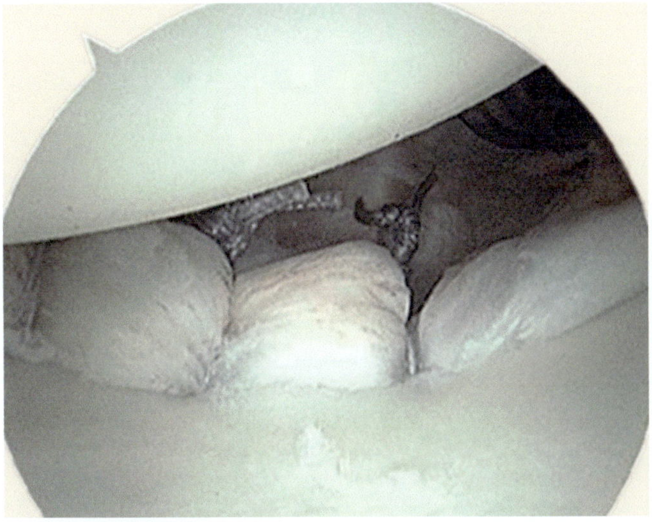

Fig. 7.6 Bankart injury was repaired with suture anchor

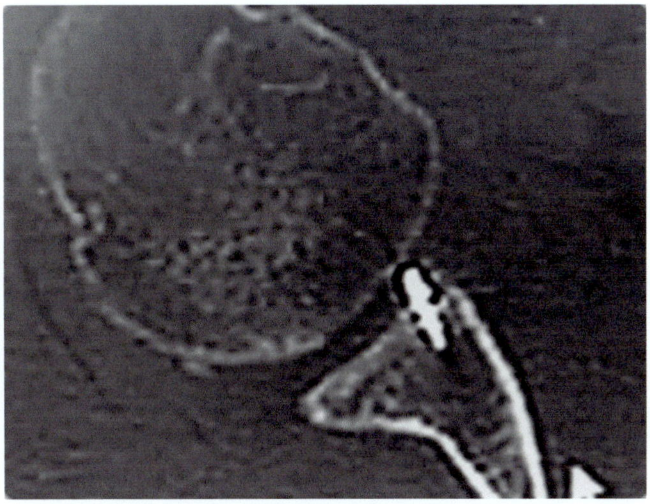

Fig. 7.8 CT examination of the shoulder joint showed that the end of the anchor was exposed outside the glenoid cortical bone, and the anchor was impinged on the head of the humerus

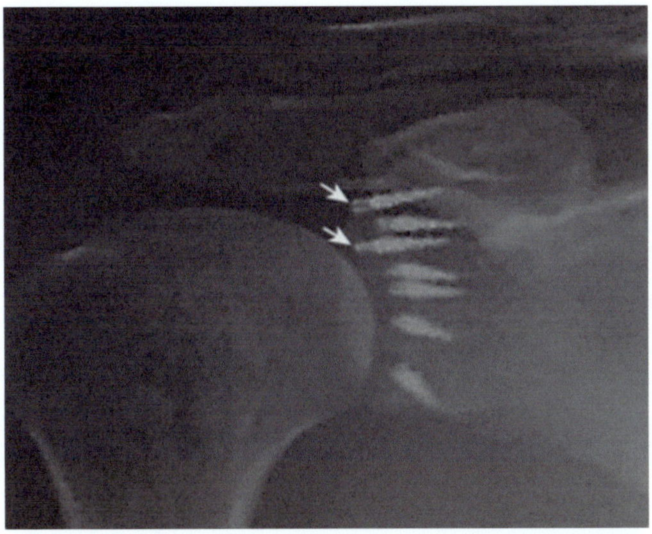

Fig. 7.7 The radiographs show that the ends of multiple metal anchors were exposed

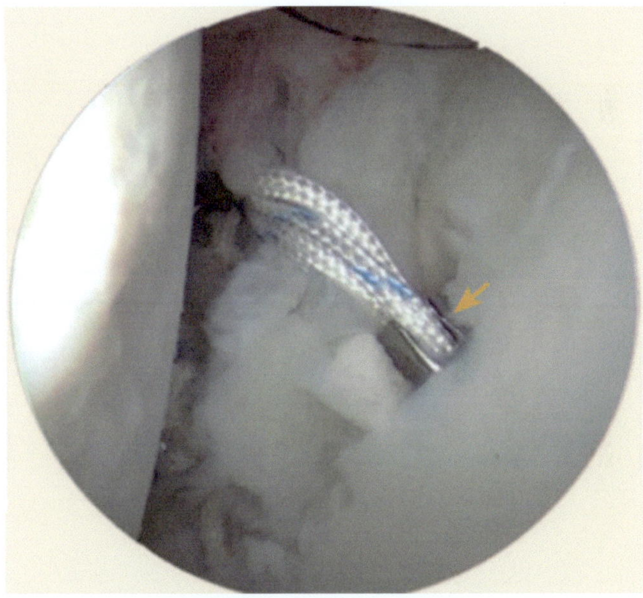

Fig. 7.9 Arthroscopic examination revealed that the end of the anchor was exposed and the suture was broken

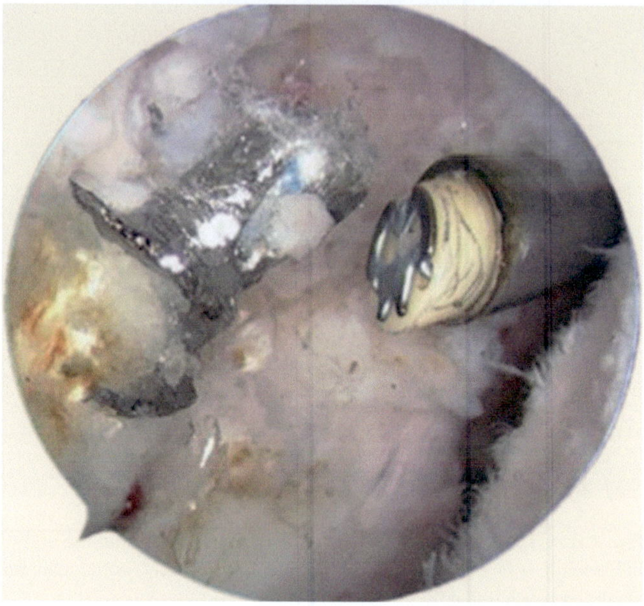

Fig. 7.10 Suture anchor slip was revealed

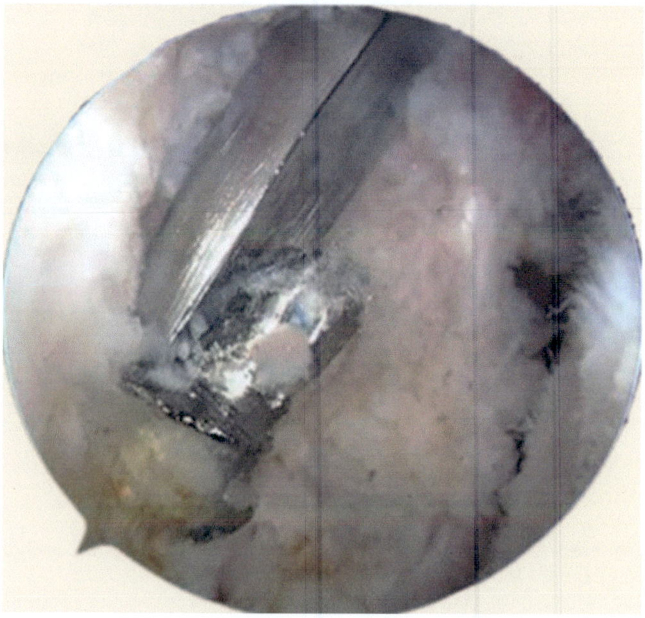

Fig. 7.11 Part of bone was removed with bone chisel

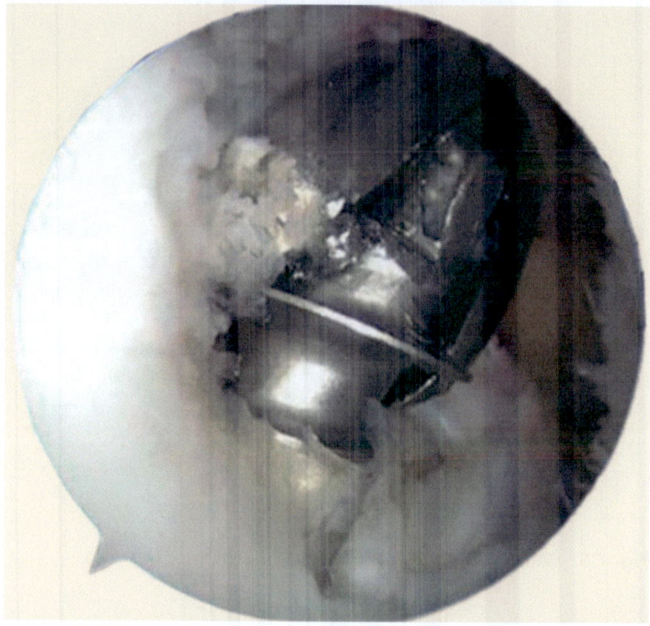

Fig. 7.12 The end of the anchor was hold with nucleus pulposus forceps

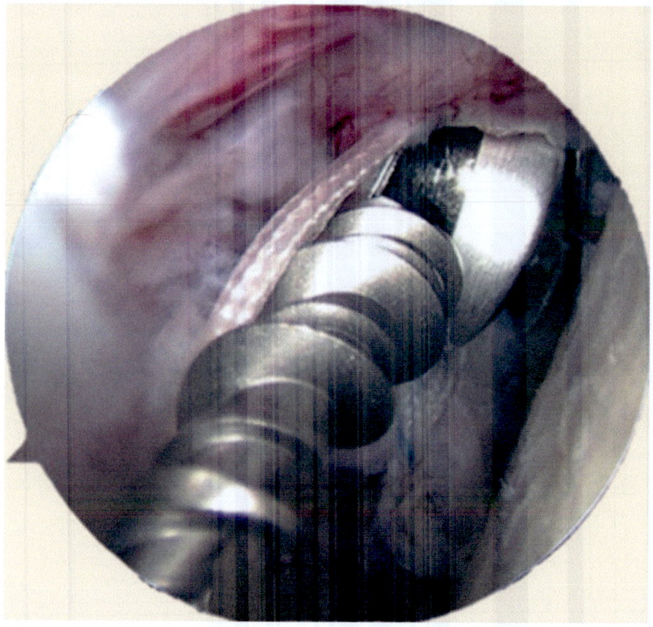

Fig. 7.13 The anchor was removed through a channel

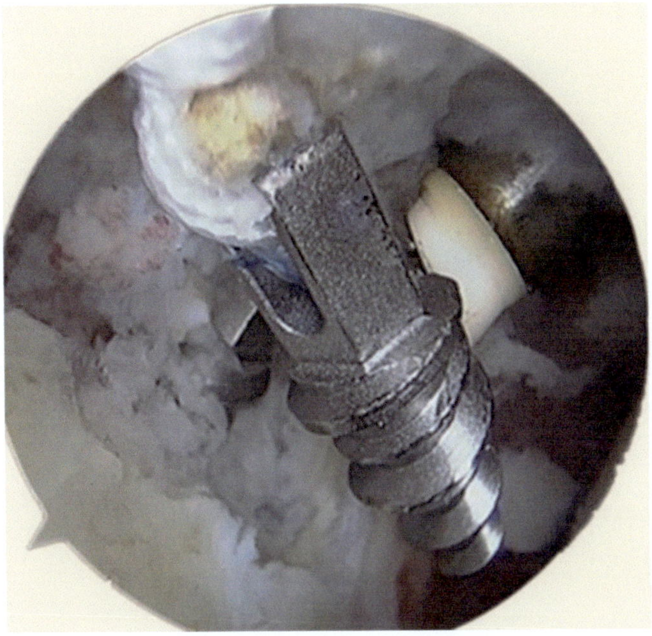

Fig. 7.14 Severe glenoid bone defect was shown

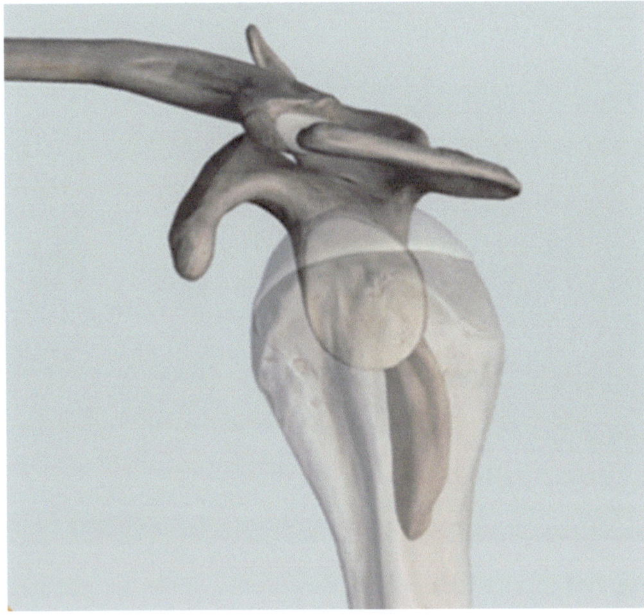

Fig. 7.15 Shoulder joint diagram

7.2 Discussion on Complications

The shoulder joint is characterized by large humerus head, shallow glenoid (Fig. 7.15), wide range of motion, and poor stability, so the shoulder joint is prone to dislocation. According to literature reports, shoulder dislocation accounts for 45% of total joint dislocation, and anterior dislocation accounts for 96~98% of all cases [1]. Shoulder dislocation will lead to shoulder glenoid labrum and joint capsule tear. These injuries need to be repaired in time, otherwise it will cause habitual shoulder dislocation. In the past, Latarjet surgery was used to treat scapular defects (Fig. 7.16). Due to factors such as technology and equipment, complications are very common [2]. With advances in arthroscopic technology, it has become routine to repair Bankart injuries with absorbable anchors, metal anchors, or PEEK anchors under arthroscopy [3] (Fig. 7.17).

During the operation, for example, due to technical irregularities, the nail path was drilled too shallow and the anchor was thick, the diameter of the nail and the anchor did not match, and the anchor was strongly screwed into the shoulder, causing the end of the metal anchor to slip, and the anchor was exposed to be too long (Fig. 7.18). The exposed part of the anchor collided with the humerus head of the shoulder joint and caused cartilage damage [4] (Fig. 7.19). In addition, if the anchor implantation angle is low, it may be implanted under the glenoid cartilage (Fig. 7.20). The nail path is thick and the anchor is thin, which is easy to pull out the anchor (Fig. 7.21).

The absorbable anchor was broken [5, 6] (Fig. 7.22) and exploded (Fig. 7.23), and the PEEK anchor was broken (Fig. 7.24) if not done properly.

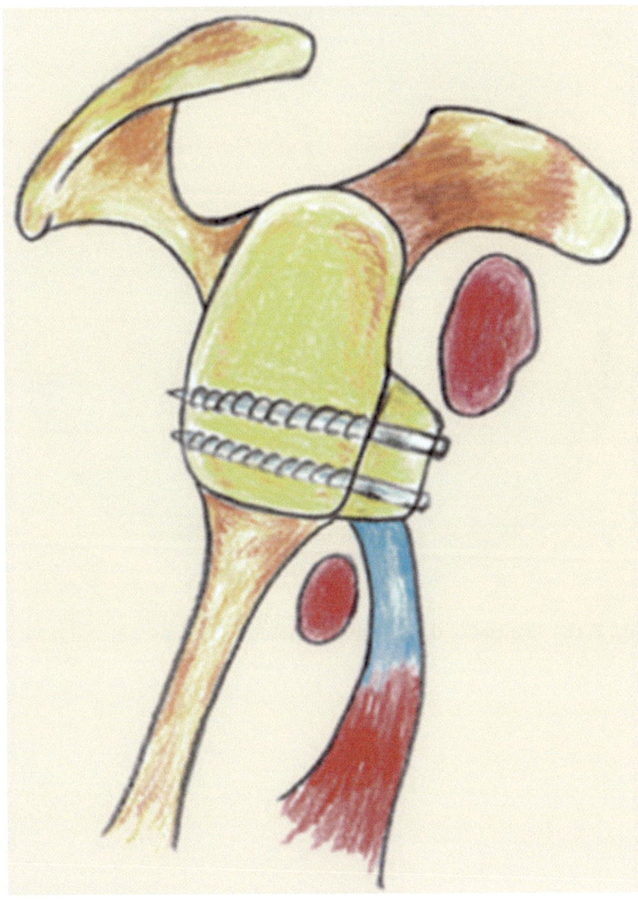

Fig. 7.16 Diagram of the Latarjet operation

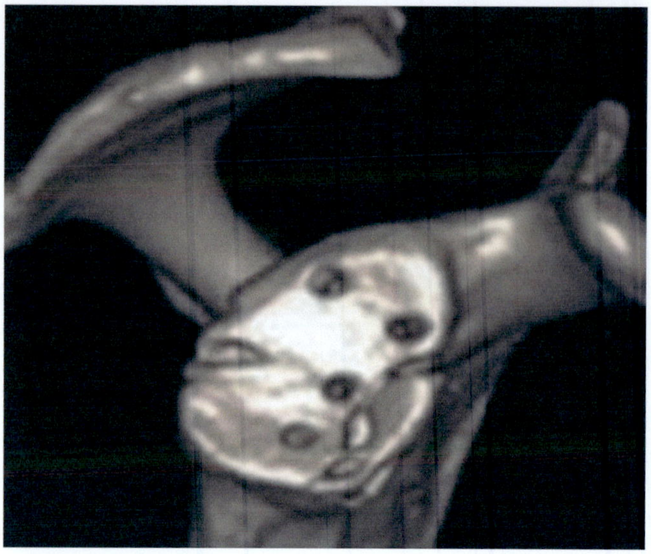

Fig. 7.17 3D-CT reconstruction showed clear anchor path and good reduction of glenoid fracture

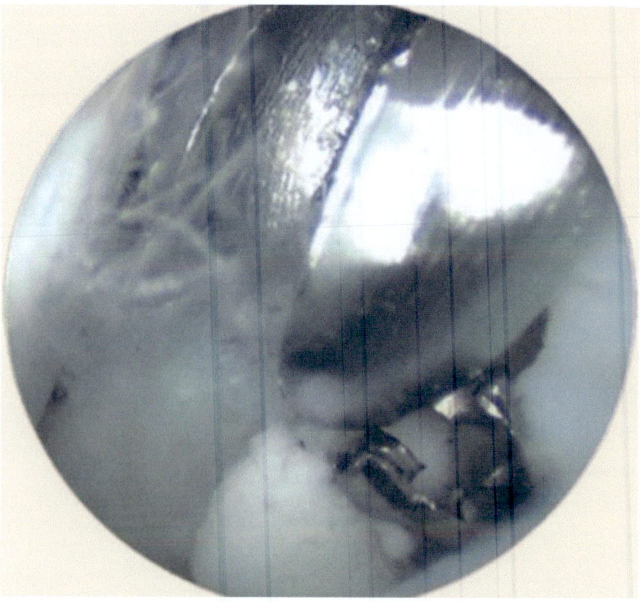

Fig. 7.18 The end of the anchor is exposed outside the glenoid bone

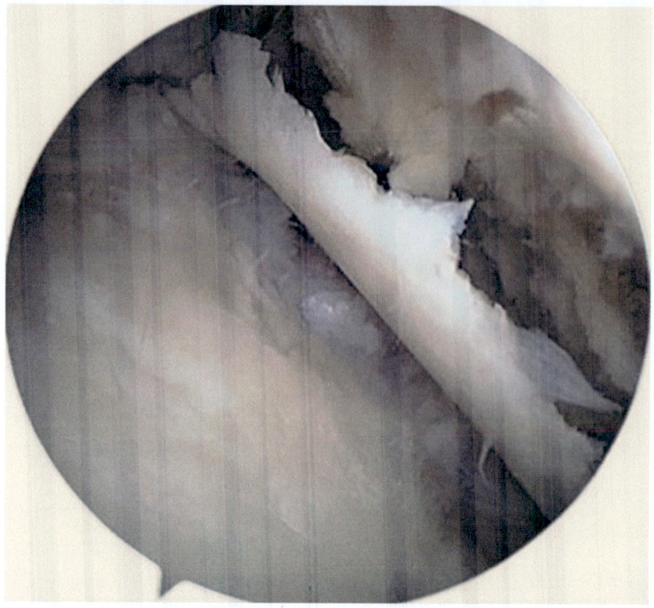

Fig. 7.19 The anchor caused extensive damage to the shoulder cartilage

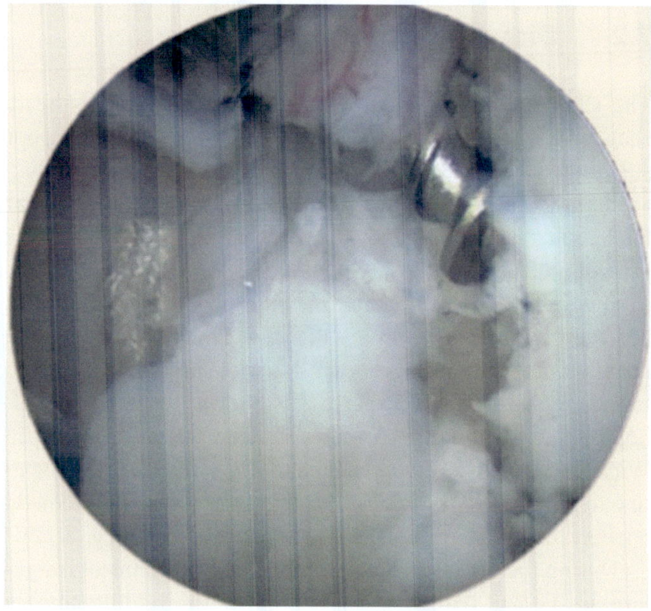

Fig. 7.20 The metal anchor was angled into the cartilage during the operation

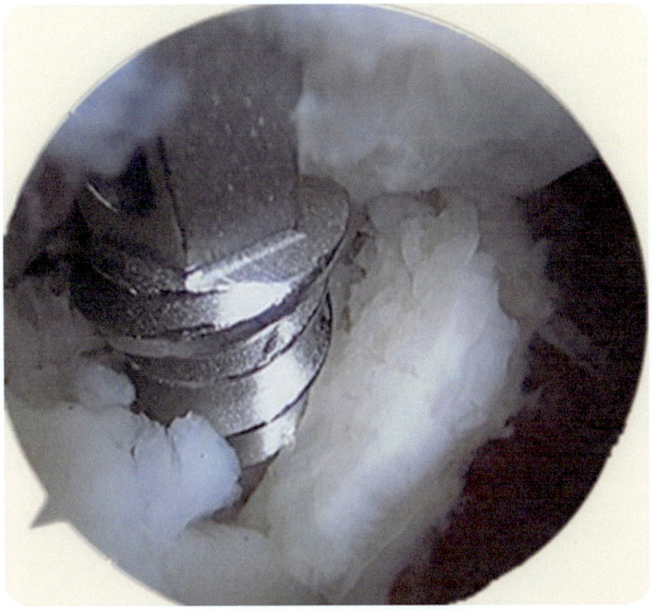

Fig. 7.21 A thick tack and a thin anchor cause the anchor to pull out

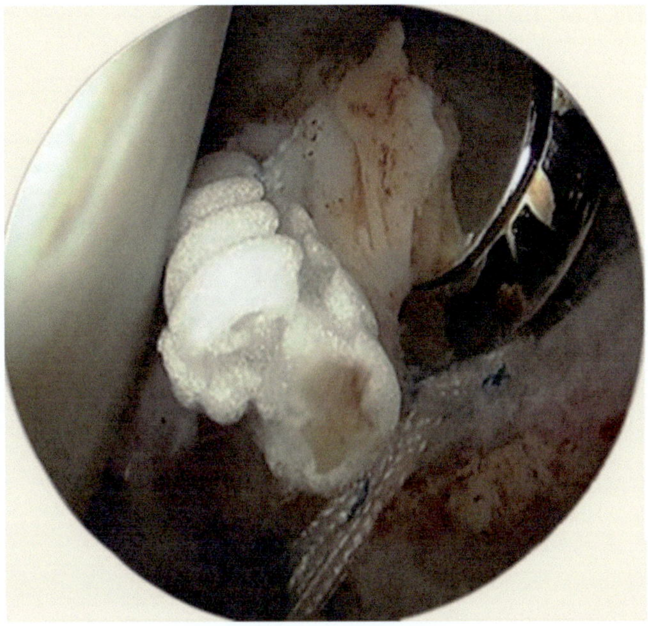

Fig. 7.23 Absorbable anchor fracture

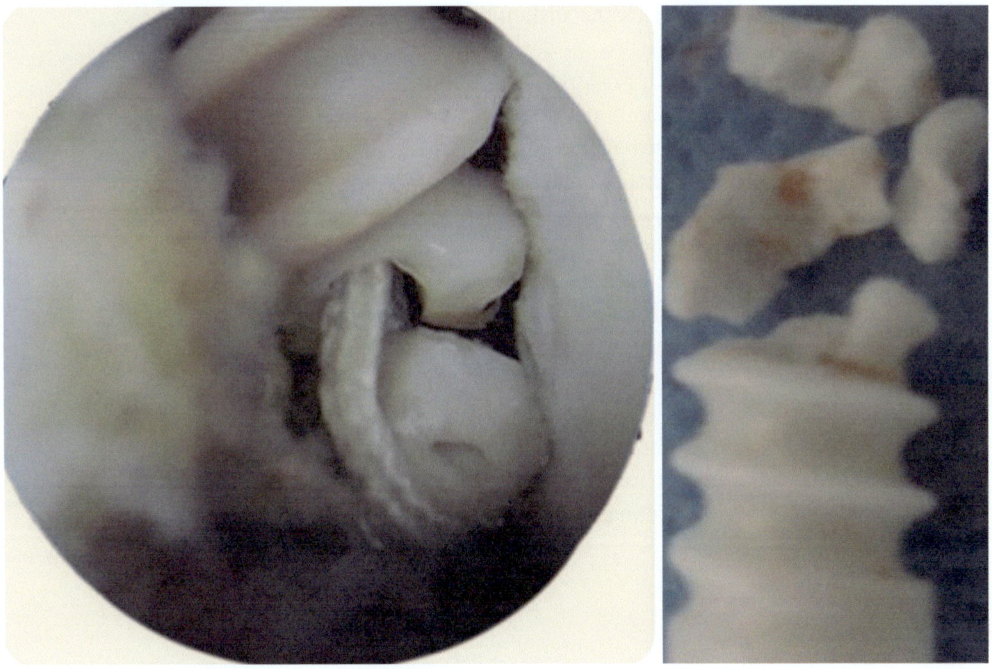

Fig. 7.22 Absorbable anchor was broken

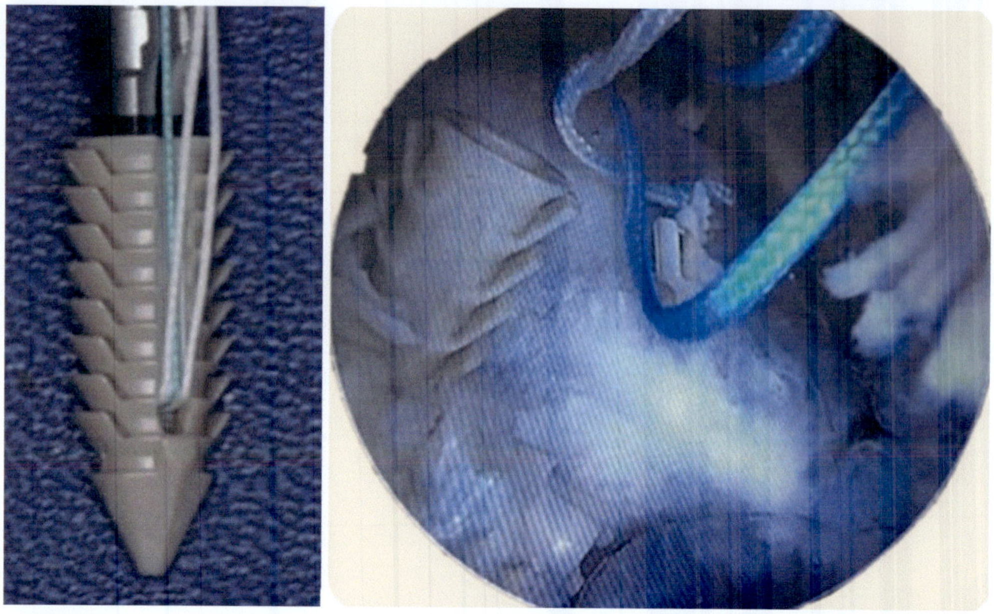

Fig. 7.24 The PEEK anchor was broken

After Bankart injury anchor fixation, the above common complications may affect the surgical effect. When the anchor is removed during revision surgery, the glenoid bone is easily destroyed, which increases the difficulty of revision surgery.

Especially for sports people, postoperative training may lead to reinjury [7–9]. How to facilitate the revision of shoulder joint instability, how to avoid anchor complications, and how to prevent glenoid damage and bone loss are important topics worthy of discussion.

The allograft bony anchor designed by the author (Fig. 7.25) has achieved good curative effect in the reconstruction of shoulder joint Bankart injury (Fig. 7.26). Allograft bony anchors were implanted into the shoulder glenoid (Fig. 7.27) to complete crawling replacement and osseous healing of the bone canal. This method is beneficial to the revision surgery of recurrent dislocation, does not affect the drilling of the anchor path in or around the anchor for surgical revision, and does not damage the anatomical structure of the glenoid.

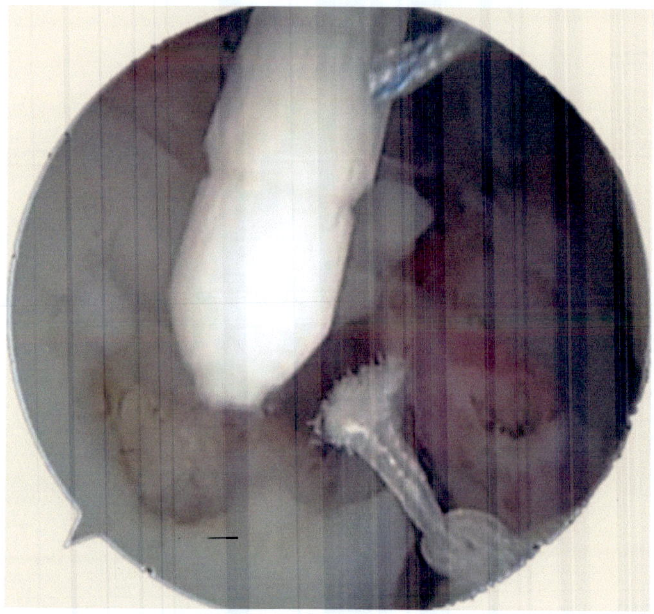

Fig. 7.25 The allograft bony anchor

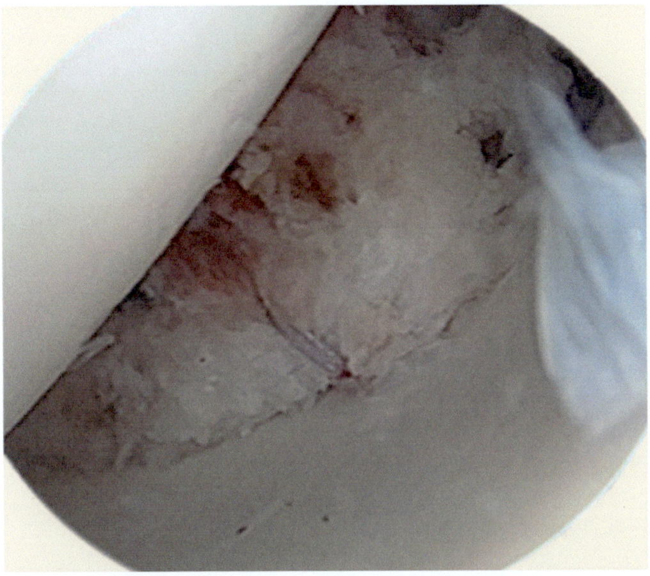

Fig. 7.26 Bankart injury was repaired with allograft bony anchor

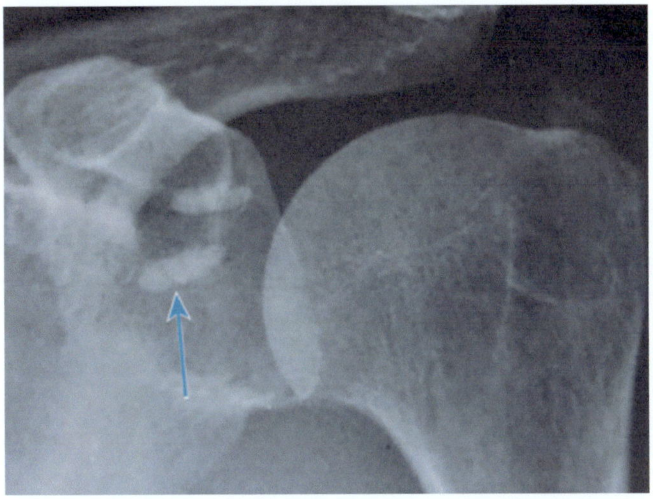

Fig. 7.27 Radiographs showing the results of implantation of the allograft bony anchors to repair Bankart injury in the shoulder glenoid

References

1. Khiami F, Gérometta A, Loriaut P. Management of recent first-time anterior shoulder dislocations. Orthop Traumatol Surg Res. 2015;101(1 Suppl):S51–7.
2. Domos P, Lunini E, Walch G. Contraindications and complications of the Latarjet procedure. Shoulder Elb. 2018;10(1):15–24.
3. Shea KP. Arthroscopic Bankart repair. Clin Sports Med. 1996;15(4):737–51.
4. Lorbach O, Wilmes P, Brogard P, et al. Complications related to implants in arthroscopic shoulder surgery. Orthopade. 2008;37(11):1073–9.
5. Dhawan A, Ghodadra N, Karas V, et al. Complications of bio-absorbable suture anchors in the shoulder. Am J Sports Med. 2012;40(6):1424–30.
6. Cobaleda Aristizabal AF, Sanders EJ, Barber FA. Adverse events associated with biodegradable lactide-containing suture anchors. Arthroscopy. 2014;30(5):555–60.
7. Alkaduhimi H, Van Der Linde JA, Willigenburg NW, et al. Redislocation risk after an arthroscopic Bankart procedure in collision athletes: a systematic review [J]. J Shoulder Elb Surg. 2016;25(9):1549–58.
8. Cho NS, Hwang JC, Rhee YG. Arthroscopic stabilization in anterior shoulder instability: collision athletes versus noncollision athletes. Arthroscopy. 2006;22(9):947–53.
9. Petrera M, Dwyer T, Tsuji MR, et al. Outcomes of arthroscopic Bankart repair in collision versus noncollision athletes. Orthopedics. 2013;36(5):e621–6.

Complications of Latarjet Surgery for Shoulder Instability Reflection and Countermeasures

8

Chang-ming Huang, Yu-jie Liu, and Yang-pan Fu

8.1 Overview of Disease Diagnosis and Treatment

The patient, a 32-year-old male worker, accidentally slipped his left hand while pulling a horizontal bar and was suspended in the air by gripping the horizontal bar with his right hand, resulting in dislocation of the right shoulder joint (Fig. 8.1). He was successfully repositioned using foot pedal traction technique in the emergency department of the local hospital. Two months later, the right shoulder joint experienced dislocation again, and CT examination showed bony Bankart injury and right glenoid bone defect (Fig. 8.2). Latarjet surgery was performed on the right shoulder joint. Two screws were used to fix the coracoid process bone block (Fig. 8.3), and postoperative functional rehabilitation was performed. Three months later, shoulder joint function returned to normal, and 1 year later, except for mild discomfort, there were no special symptoms in the shoulder joint. Before admission, suddenly felt pain and swelling in the right shoulder joint while moving a weight of 20 kg. and went to the hospital for emergency treatment. The X-ray examination revealed that two screws fixing the transplanted bone block were broken and displaced (Fig. 8.4). After admission, he underwent shoulder joint revision surgery.

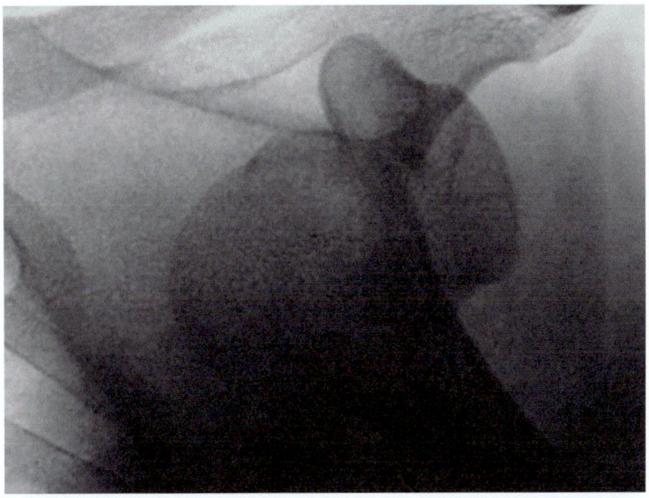

Fig. 8.1 X-ray fluoroscopy showing dislocation of the right shoulder joint

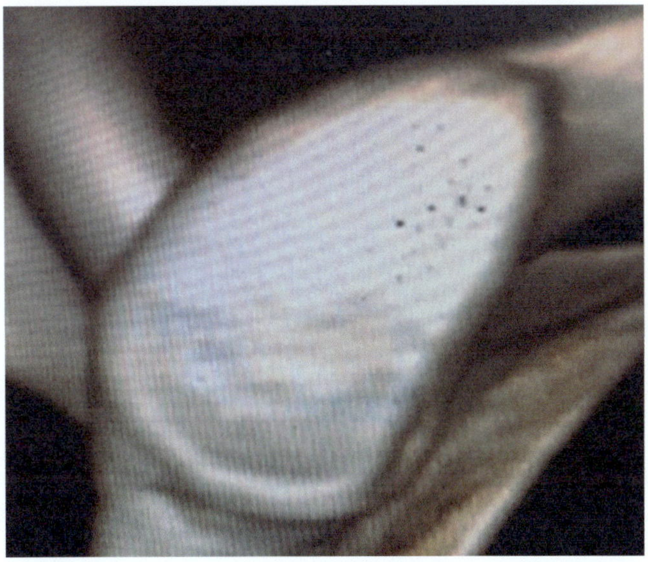

Fig. 8.2 CT 3D reconstruction showing right glenoid bone defect

C.-m. Huang (✉) · Y.-p. Fu
Department of Orthopedics, The 73rd Group Army Hospital, Chenggong Hospital Affiliated to Xiamen University, Xiamen, China

Y.-j. Liu
Orthopaedics, Chinese PLA General Hospital, Beijing, China

Y.-j. Liu et al. (eds.), *Pitfalls in Diagnosis and Treatment of Shoulder Joint Diseases*, https://doi.org/10.1007/978-981-96-2472-0_8

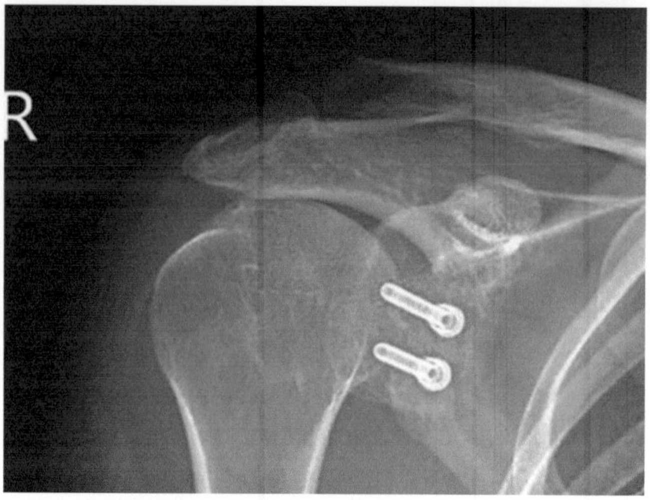

Fig. 8.3 Postoperative X-ray showing fixation of the coracoid process bone block with screws after Latarjet surgery

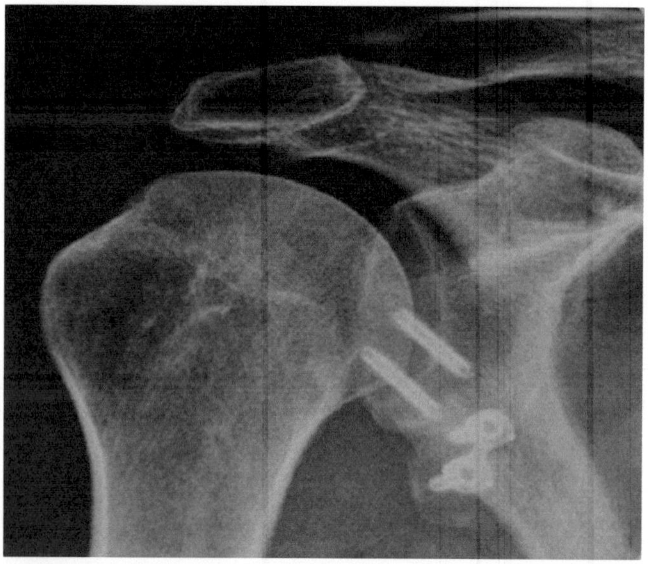

Fig. 8.4 X-ray images 1 year after surgery show fracture of the hollow screw and displacement of the bone block

8.2 Reflection on the Relationship Between Nail Breakage and Bone Nonunion After Latarjet Surgery

The shoulder joint is the most active and unstable joint in the human body. Shoulder joint dislocation accounts for 50% of total joint dislocation in the body. The recurrence rate of anterior dislocation of the shoulder joint after surgery is related to age. Andziora et al. [1] found a significant correlation between the recurrence rate of postoperative dislocation and the age at surgery (<20 years: 25%; 21–30 years: 20%; 31–40 years: 7.1%;>41 years: 0%). Porcellini et al. [2] found that 13.3% of 98 patients aged ≤22 years experienced redislocation, and 6.3% of 287 patients aged >22 years experienced redislocation. The younger the age, the higher the recurrence rate.

Bony Bankart injury is a avulsion fracture of the anterior lower part of the shoulder glenoid. In 2014, Kim classified bony Bankart injuries into three types: Type I, with bone defects <12.5%; Type II, with bone defects from 12.5% to 25%; Type III, with bone defect >25%. Shoulder glenoid bone defect >25% requires bone grafting in front of the shoulder glenoid to restore its anatomical structure. The conventional procedure for repairing shoulder and glenoid bone defects is the Latarjet surgery (Fig. 7.16), which involves transplanting the biceps brachii tendon with the coracoid process bone block. This procedure has the effects of suspension (sliding effect), strengthening the anterior shoulder joint capsule and repairing the shoulder and glenoid bone defects. Complications such as nerve injury, coracoid process fracture, and shoulder osteoarthritis after Latarjet surgery can reach up to 25–30%, the absorption rate of bone graft was 15–34%, and the recurrence rate was 15–17%. Therefore, the problems of coracoid bone graft and neurovascular injury, bone nonunion and broken nails have aroused great concern.

Why is it easy to experience bone graft nonhealing after Latarjet surgery? Why did the screw break? The author believes that without functional rehabilitation training after shoulder joint surgery, shoulder joint adhesion, disuse muscular atrophy, and osteoporosis will occur. In the early postoperative stage of Latarjet surgery, the biceps brachii muscle is used to contract and pull the bone block. Stress acts on the screw, causing slight movement of the bone graft and affecting the healing of the interface between the graft and the shoulder glenoid. Both metal hollow screws (Fig. 8.5) and solid screws (Fig. 8.6) have experienced fractures. Postoperative infection of the shoulder joint can lead to bone resorption, causing screw loosening, extraction, and even detachment into surrounding soft tissues (Fig. 8.7).

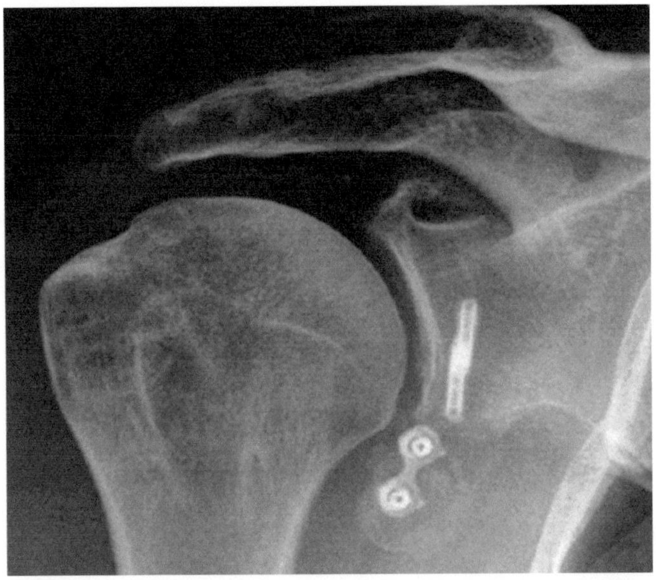

Fig. 8.5 Postoperative X-ray of right shoulder shows fracture of metal hollow screw and displacement of bone block after Latarjet surgery

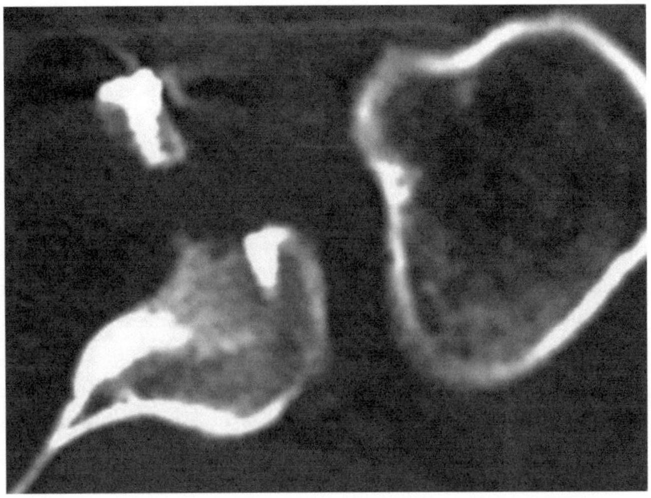

Fig. 8.6 Cross axial CT section of left shoulder after surgery shows solid screw fracture and bone displacement after Latarjet surgery

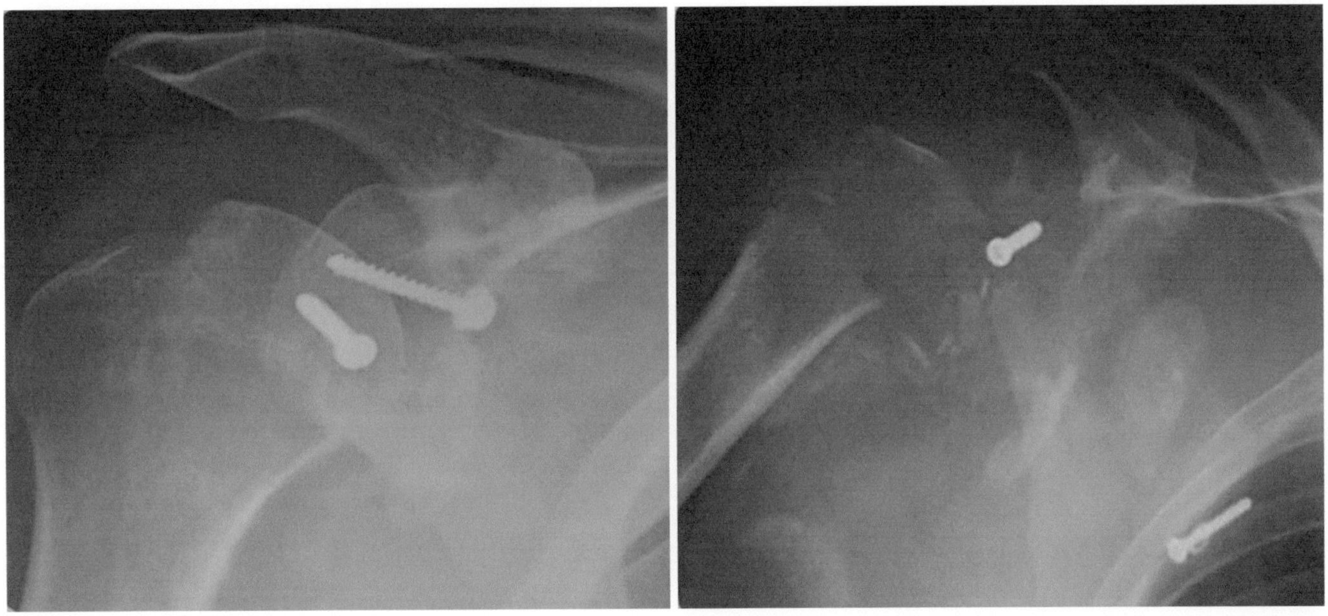

Fig. 8.7 Postoperative infection of the right shoulder joint X-ray shows postoperative bone resorption, with screws removed and released to the chest

8.3 Repair of Osteogenic Bankart Injury with Scapular Spine Bone Block Transplantation

Coracoid transplantation is routinely used to repair bony Bankart injuries. However, the removal of coracoid process affects the anatomic structure attached to it, such as tendons and ligaments, and affects the stability of the upper front shoulder joint. The author studied the anatomy of scapula and discussed the use of scapular spine bone as the graft material for repairing Bankart injury. The thickness, height, and usable length of bone mass at 4–8 cm of coracoid process and medial spine were measured by three-dimensional CT reconstruction of bilateral scapula in 60 adults (Fig. 8.8). Finite element and biomechanical studies have proved that the use of scapular spine bone as graft material can satisfy the repair of bone defects injured by bone Bankart.

Clinical surgical procedure: CT three-dimensional reconstruction of the affected shoulder joint was performed before surgery, and the area of the glenoid bone defect was measured (Fig. 8.9). Take autologous scapular spine bone block from the same side. After drilling holes for bone block repair, insert the threaded bone transverse nail into the bone block hole for later use (Fig. 8.10).

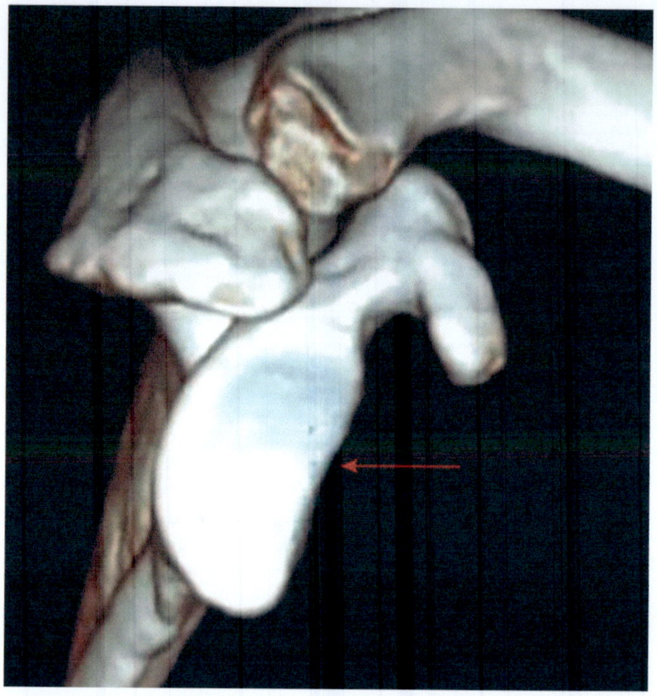

Fig. 8.9 CT three-dimensional reconstruction of the right shoulder joint showing the range of glenoid bone defect

Arthroscopic exploration (Fig. 8.11), debridement of the bony bed associated with the Bankart lesion, and preparation of the bony surface for optimal tissue repair. Cut the skin 2 cm along the anterior approach of the shoulder joint, separate the soft tissue, and reach the Bankart injury wound. Implant the bone block into the anterior bone defect of the shoulder glenoid, and pre-drill the nail hole along the bone block's passage in the shoulder glenoid. After resetting the bone block, the allogeneic cortical bone nail is inserted into the glenoid foramen (Fig. 8.12) to support and fix the bone block. The soft tissue in front of the glenoid bone is sutured and embedded (Fig. 8.13). Postoperative CT three-dimensional reconstruction examination showed good healing between the bone block and the recipient area (Fig. 8.14).

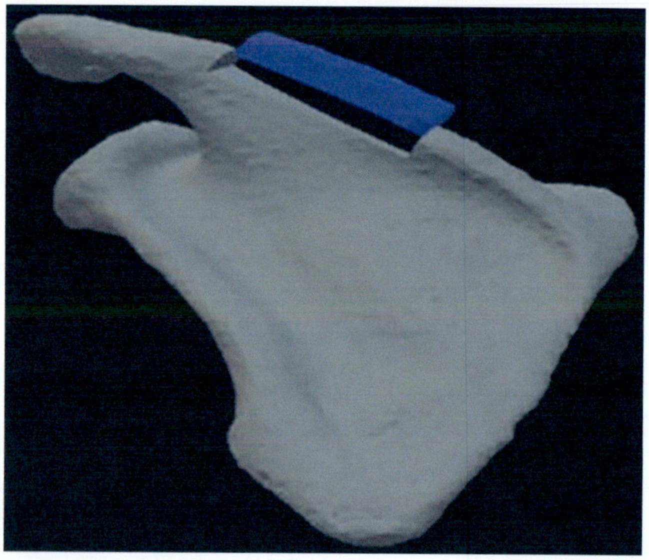

Fig. 8.8 Location and size of scapular spine bone graft

The position of the scapular spine bone block is superficial, adjacent to the surgical site of the shoulder joint, and does not affect the anatomical structure of the coronoid process and the stability of the shoulder joint. Through clinical application, the use of allogeneic cortical bone transverse nail fixation for repairing bone Bankart injuries is convenient and feasible. The bone graft and recipient area heal well, avoiding the use of high-value consumables and reducing the cost of consumables. The postoperative effect is satisfactory, and there are no metal or other chemical materials left after fracture healing, which is beneficial for recurrent patients undergoing revision surgery.

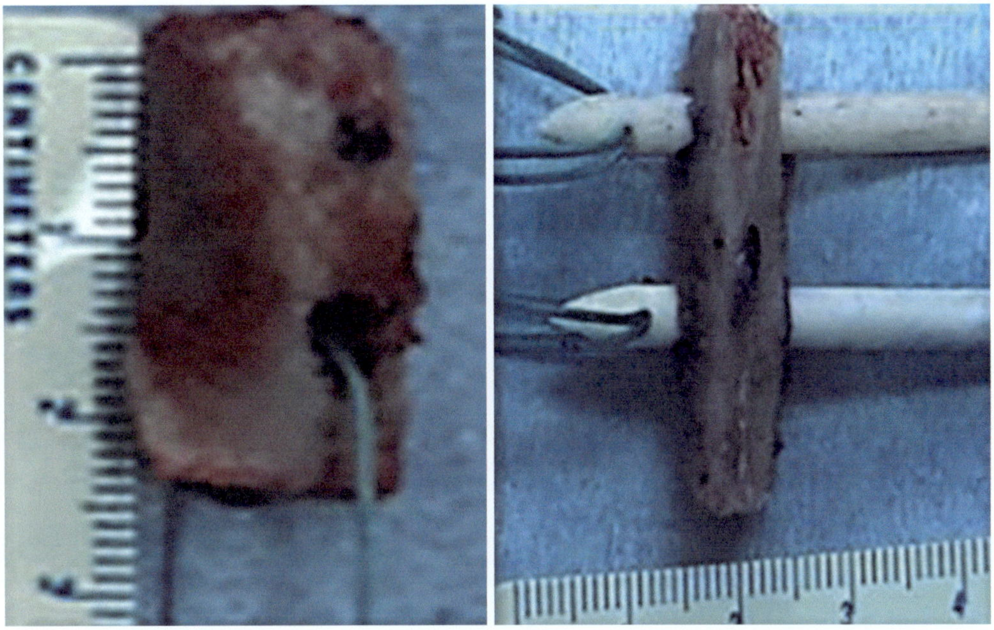

Fig. 8.10 Inserting a threaded bone nail into the foramen of the scapular spine bone block

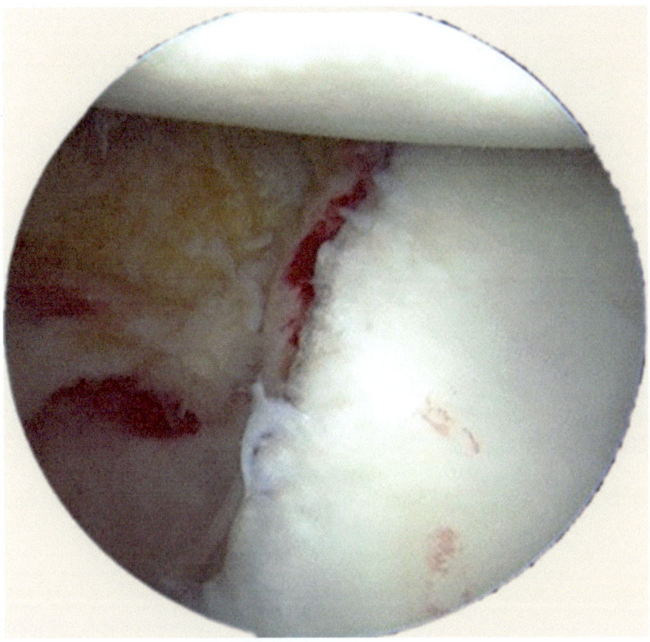

Fig. 8.11 Arthroscopic display of Bankart injury bone defect

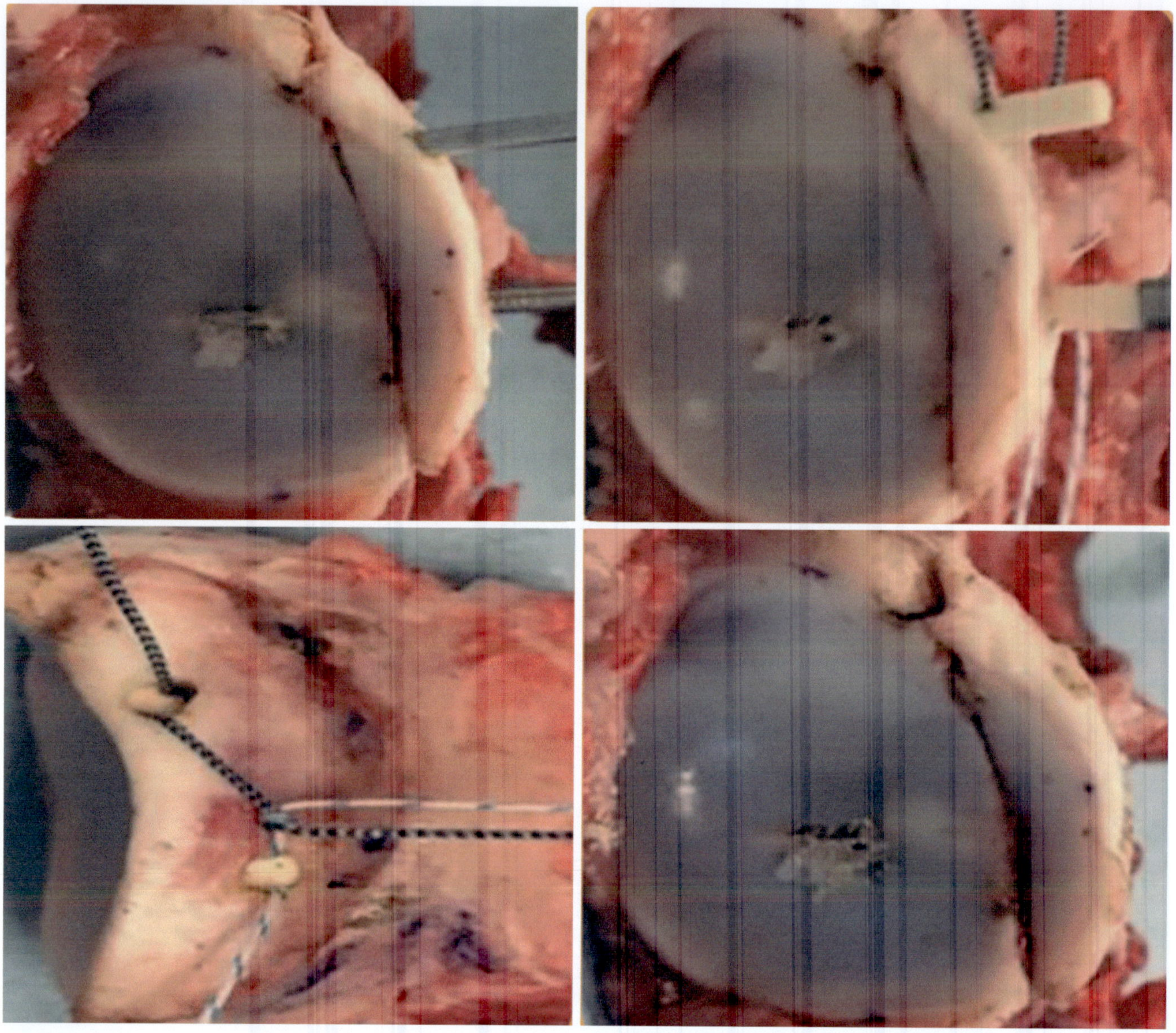

Fig. 8.12 Experimental schematic diagram of animal specimens: Repair of bone Bankart injury with bone block supported and fixed by bone transverse nails

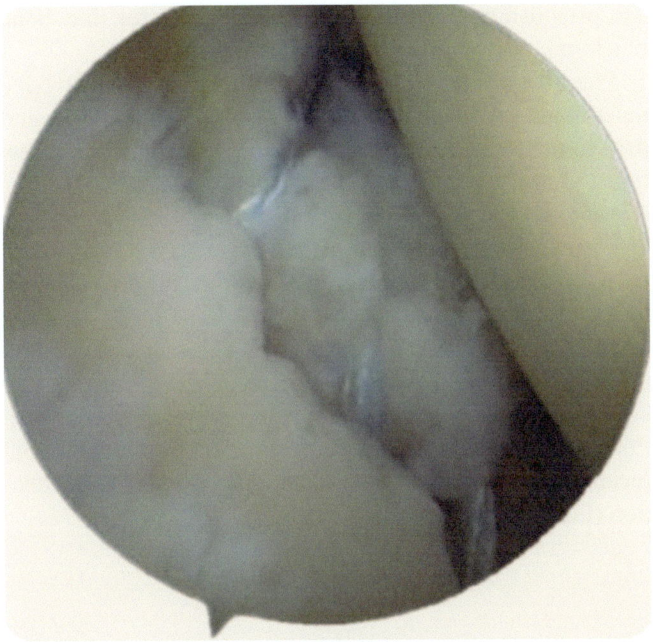

Fig. 8.13 After transplantation and fixation under the microscope, the scapular spine bone block is transplanted to the defect of the glenoid bone, soft tissue is sutured, and the bone block is embedded

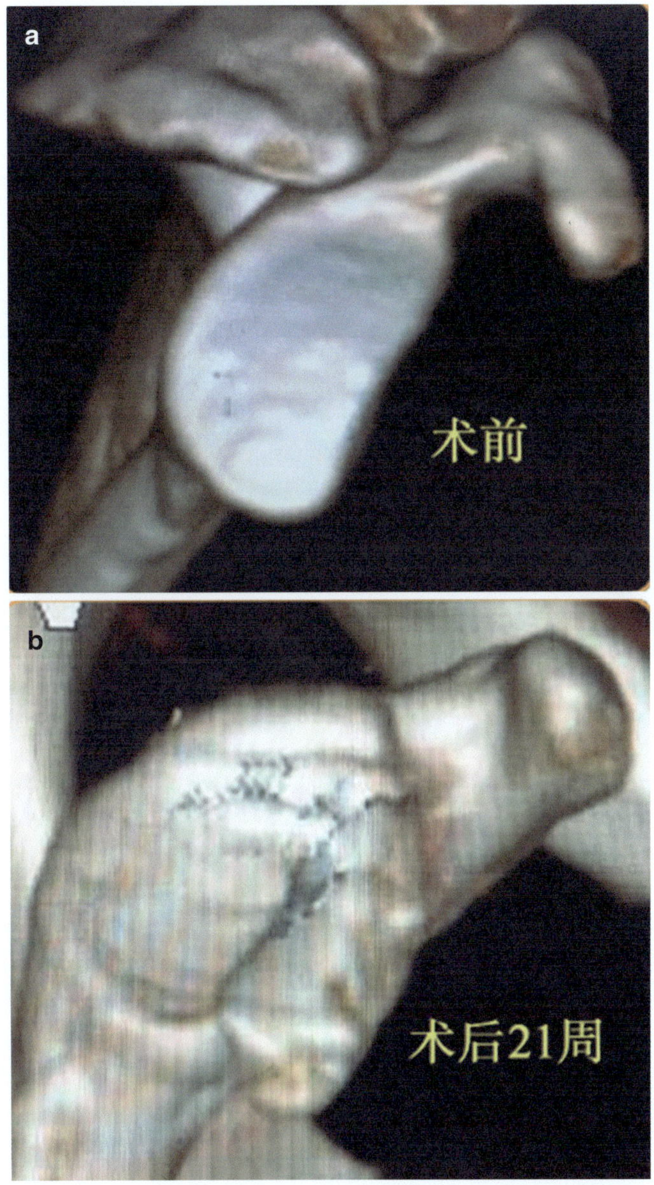

Fig. 8.14 Comparison of CT three-dimensional reconstruction of the right shoulder gleniod. (**a**) Preoperative bone Bankart injury with bone defects greater than 25%; (**b**) After transplantation and repair of scapular spine bone block

8.4 Iliac Bone Block Transplantation for Repairing Shoulder and Glenoid Bone Defects

The use of iliac bone blocks to reconstruct shoulder and glenoid bone defects is also one of the commonly used, simple, safe, and effective surgical methods with fewer complications in clinical practice [5]. General anesthesia was used, and the patient was placed in a lateral decubitus position with the affected limb pulled and disinfected and laid out. Design a surgical approach for the shoulder joint according to the surgical needs. The conventional approach is to use a posterior, anterosuperior, and anteroinferior portal. Soft tissue filling of the posterior joint capsule requires an additional posterior upper lateral approach. Insert arthroscopy through the posterior approach of the shoulder joint to explore the condition of shoulder joint injury. According to arthroscopic exploration and preoperative measurement of Bankart's injury to the glenoid bone defect, iliac bone blocks were cut and repaired for later use. Two Kirschner wires with a diameter of 1.2 mm were used to drill vertically into the iliac bone block. Two bone passages were drilled along the Kirschner wires, and hollow nuts were screwed in. Two fixing rods were screwed into the bone block along the double cannula, and the bone block was connected to the double cannula for later use (Fig. 8.15).

Locked anterior dislocation of the shoulder joint (Fig. 8.16) requires first reduction of the subscapular tendon and anterior glenoid lip in parallel with reduction of the shoulder joint (Fig. 8.17), followed by freshening of the bone defect site. For posterior bone defect, the soft tissue of the joint capsule is cleaned first, the wound is freshened, anchor holes are predrilled, and preparation work for soft tissue filling is performed (Fig. 8.18).

The exchange rod enters from the rear and passes through the shoulder joint surface, above the subscapular tendon, and outside the combined tendon of the coracoid process, releasing the rotator cuff space and subscapular tendon (Fig. 8.19), taking care not to damage the vascular and nerve bundles, and establishing a Halifax portal (Fig. 8.20) for iliac bone block implantation (Fig. 8.21).

Place the prepared bone block in front of the glenoid bone defect through the Halifax portal, insert a guide needle, and pass through the skin behind the shoulder joint. Drill screw holes along the guide needle (Fig. 8.22), implant hollow screws, and firmly fix the bone block (Fig. 8.23).

Check whether the position of the iliac bone block is flush with the surface of the glenoid joint from different angles. Grind and level the outer edge of the bone block with the surface of the glenoid joint. Anchor nail repair of joint capsule and glenoid humeral ligament complex (Fig. 8.24), and simultaneous repair if there is rotator cuff injury (Fig. 8.25). Postoperative follow-up X-ray and CT three-dimensional reconstruction observation of bone graft reduction and fixation (Fig. 8.26).

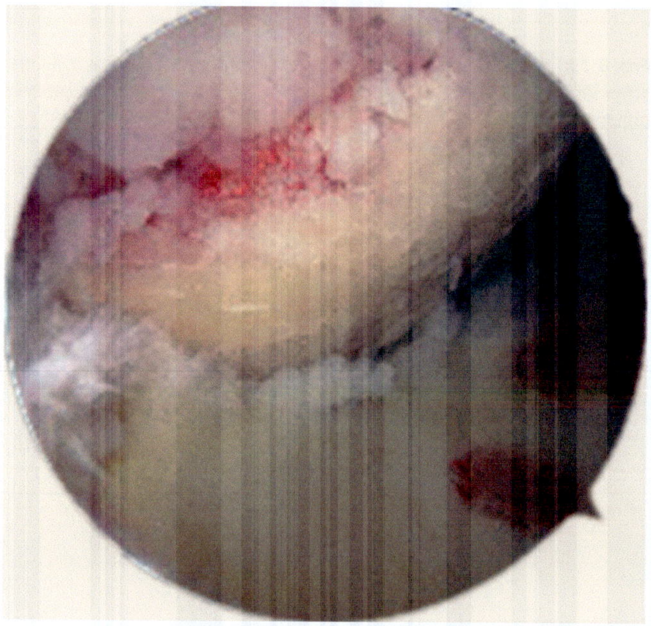

Fig. 8.16 Locked anterior dislocation of the shoulder joint

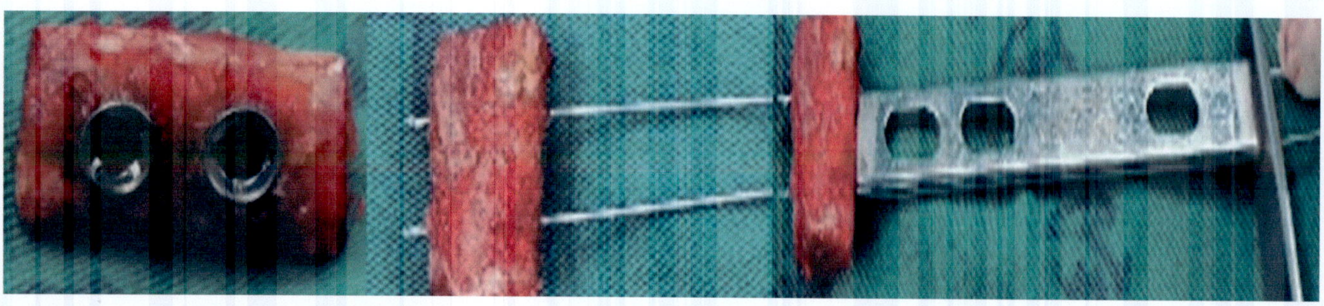

Fig. 8.15 Preparation of iliac bone blocks

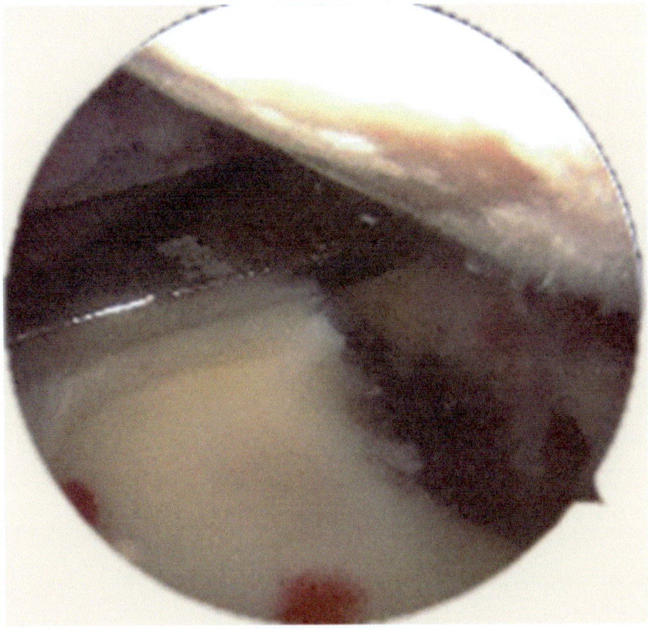

Fig. 8.17 Locked anterior dislocation of the shoulder joint release and reduction

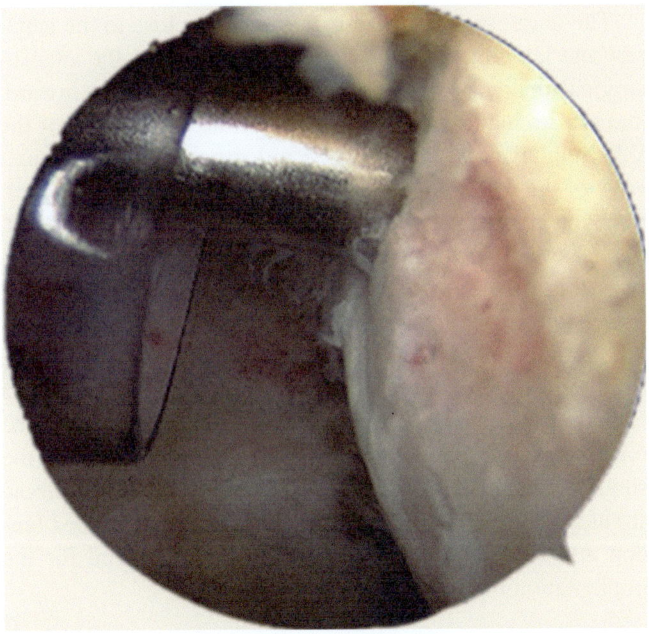

Fig. 8.18 Cleaning of the posterior joint capsule, predrilling anchor nail holes, and preparing for soft tissue filling

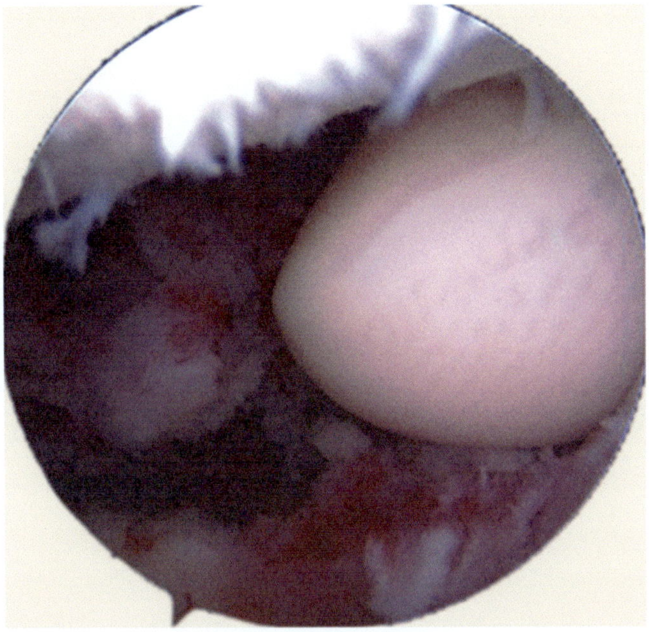

Fig. 8.19 Release of rotator cuff gap and subscapular tendon

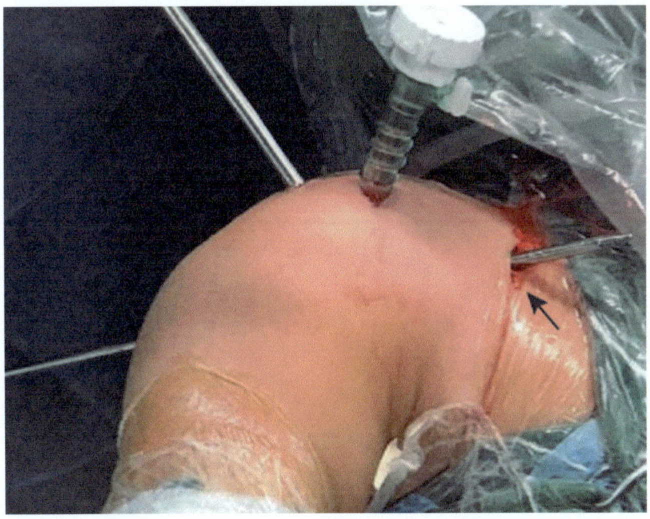

Fig. 8.20 Establishing Halifax portal (arrows)

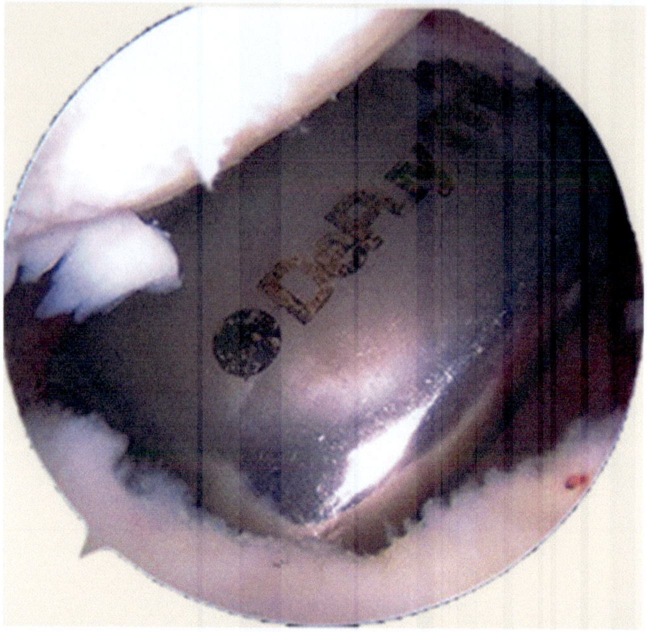

Fig. 8.21 Establishment of Halifax portal for iliac bone block and implant entry

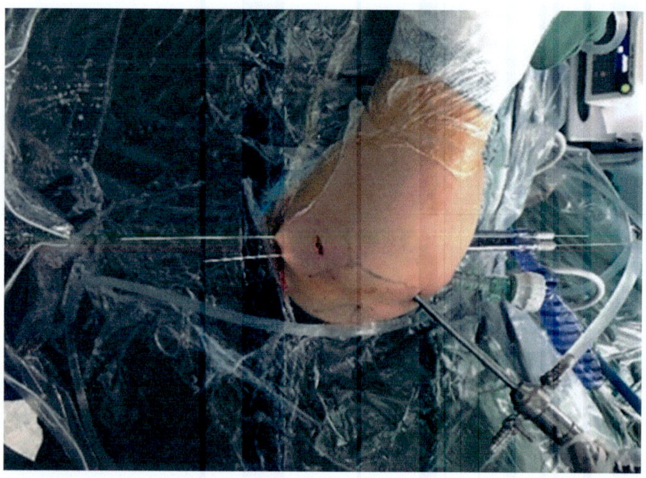

Fig. 8.22 Guide Pin Fixation of Iliac Bone Blocks

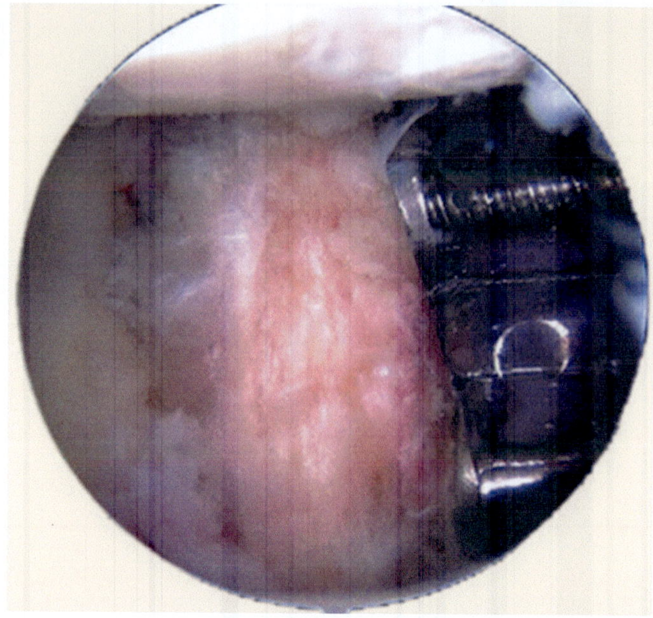

Fig. 8.23 Screw fixation of transplanted bone blocks

The anterosuperior portal should be as close to the superior and lateral as possible, making it easier for the anterior surgical operation. The Halifax portal needs to be inward, and the exchange rod passes through the upper edge of the subscapularis muscle, the coracoid process, and the outer edge of the combined tendon. Release to the 6 o'clock position and the surface of the subscapularis muscle in front, paying attention to the blood vessels below the front. The position of the iliac bone block should be accurate, without tilting upward or forward. Use an exchange rod parallel to the shoulder glenoid to press the iliac bone block through the back, and minimize the angle between the screw direction and the joint surface as much as possible. When the iliac bone block is implanted in the middle and lower parts of the shoulder glenoid, traction should be relieved and the elbow should be flexed to reduce the tension of the combined tendon and subscapularis muscle, which is beneficial for the implantation of the iliac bone block.

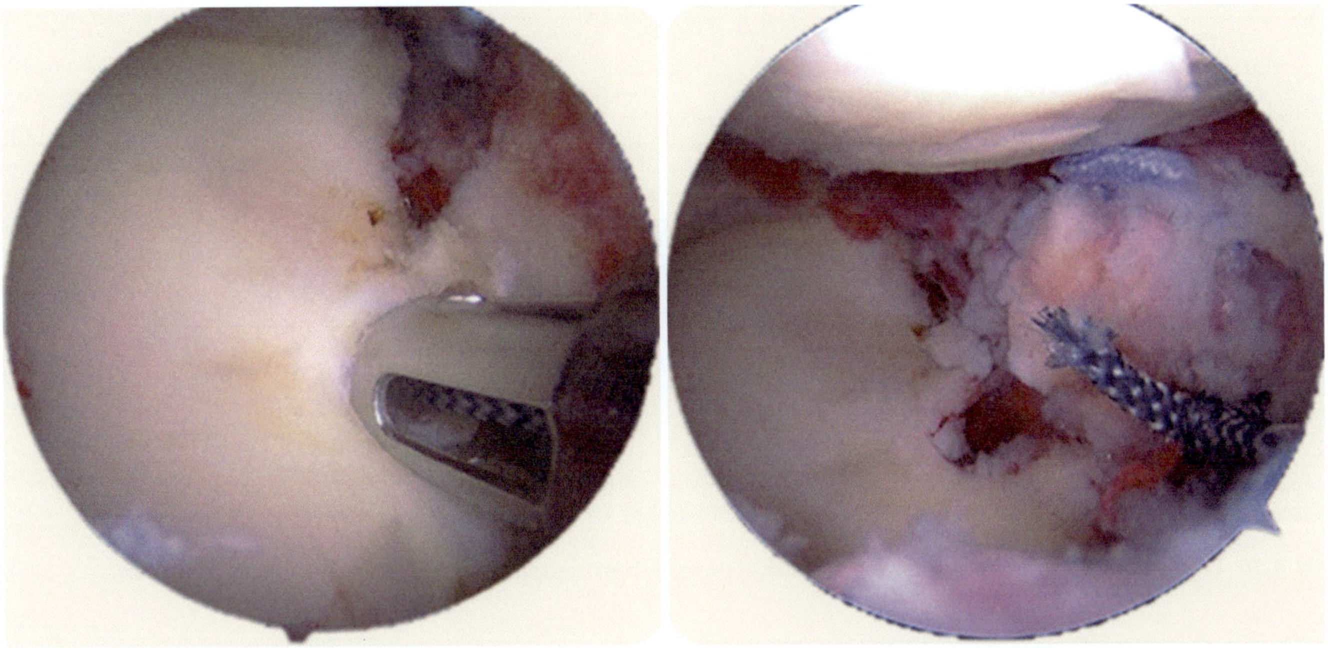

Fig. 8.24 Anchor nail repair of glenoid humeral ligament complex

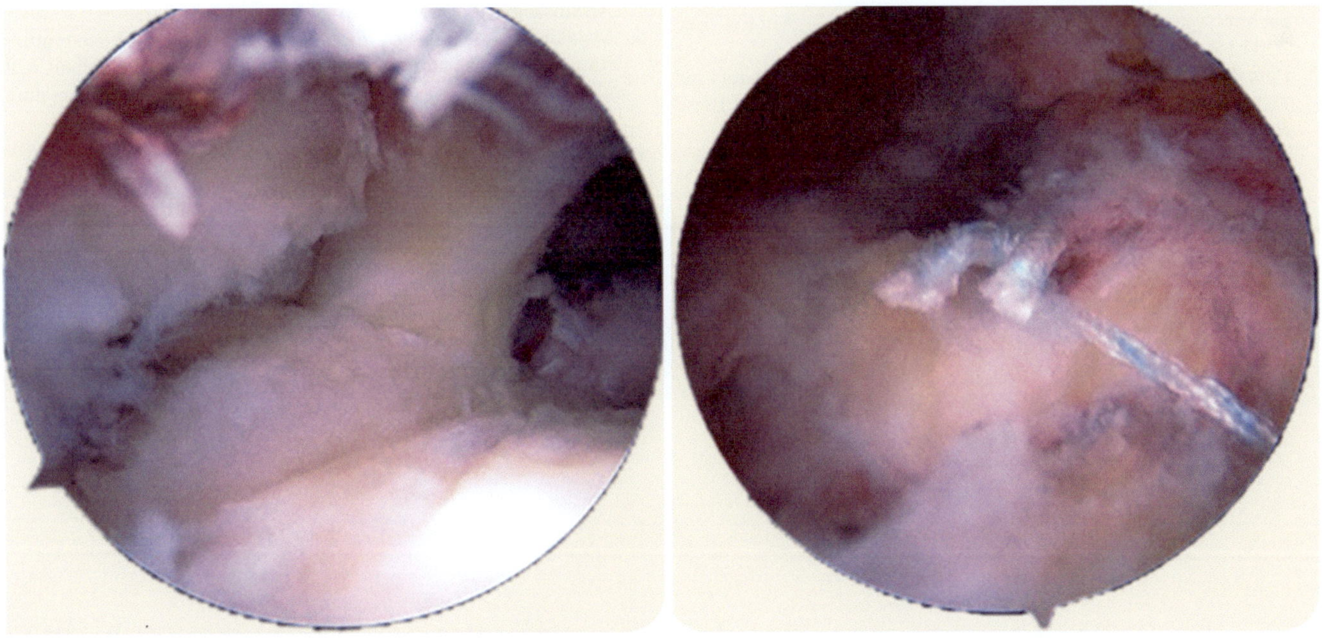

Fig. 8.25 Preoperative and postoperative for repairing rotator cuff injuries

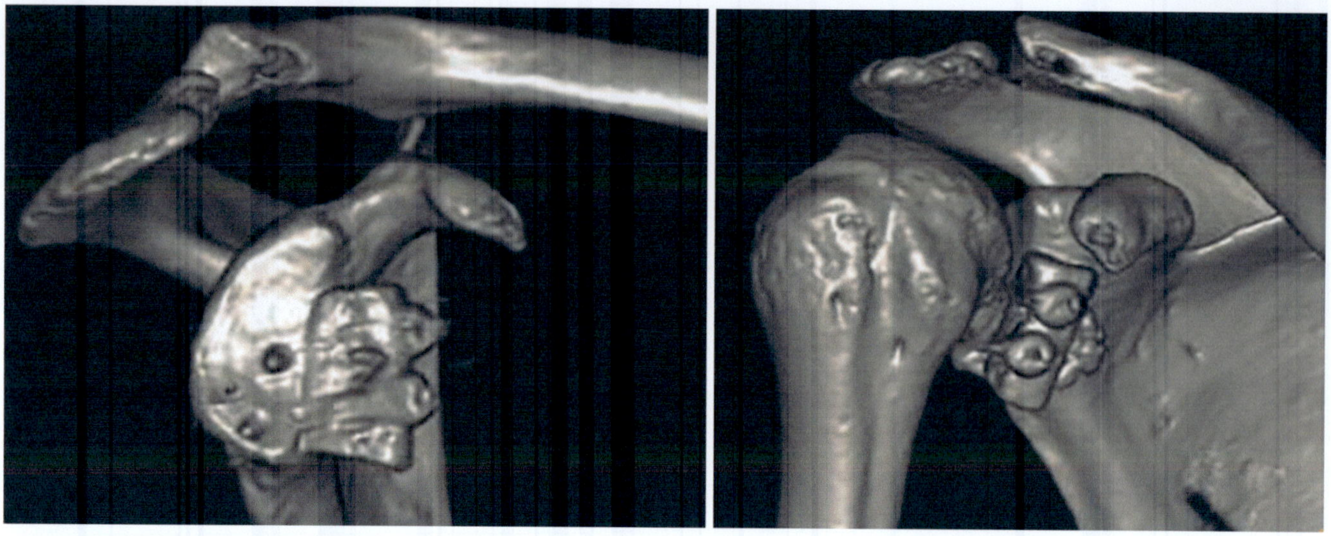

Fig. 8.26 Postoperative CT three-dimensional reconstruction of the right shoulder joint shows good position of the iliac bone block

References

1. Kandziora F, Jager A, Bischof F, et al. Arthroscopic labrum refixation for post-traumatic anterior shoulder instability: suture anchor versus transglenoid fixation technique. Arthroscopy. 2000;16(4):359–66.
2. Porcellini G, Campi F, Peg Reffifi F, et al. Predisposing factors for recurrent shoulder dislocation after arthroscopic treatment. J Bone Joint Surg Am. 2009;91(11):2537–42.
3. YK K, SH C, WS S, et al. Arthroscopic repair of small and medium-sized bony Bankart lesions. Am J Sports Med. 2014;42(1):86–94.
4. Lafosse L, Lejeune E, Bouchard A, et al. The arthroscopic Latarjet procedure for the treatment of anterior shoulder instability. Arthroscopy. 2007;23:1242.e1–5.
5. Malahias MA, Chytas D, Raoulis V, et al. Iliac crest bone grafting for the management of anterior shoulder instability in patients with glenoid bone loss: a systematic review of contemporary literature. Sports Med. 2020;6(1):12.

Part IV

Anterior Shoulder Dislocation: A Guide and Summary

Chang-ming Huang

Guides

This part analyzes cases of anterior dislocation of the shoulder joint, with a focus on the misconceptions of anterior dislocation of the shoulder joint, as well as the misconceptions of shoulder dislocation fractures combined with brachial plexus paralysis. Strategies for early diagnosis, treatment, and prevention of complications are formulated.

Summary

Shoulder dislocation is commonly seen in trauma, sports traction injury, electric shock injury, epilepsy, psychiatric seizures, etc. Carefully inquire about medical history and injury process, analyze injury mechanism, conduct comprehensive physical examination, carefully read examination materials, and if necessary, perform shoulder joint CT or MRI examination to clarify the diagnosis. When diagnosing and treating multiple injuries, it is crucial to avoid misdiagnosis or missed diagnoses, and not to focus on minor issues at the expense of overlooking more critical ones— "pick sesame seeds, while lose watermelons."

Patients with shoulder dislocation must have a shoulder X-ray film after diagnosis and before treatment, in order to determine whether shoulder dislocation is accompanied by humeral tuberosity avulsion fracture. Do not hastily reduce it to avoid medical disputes.

Manual reduction should be carried out under anesthesia to avoid muscle tension affecting the reduction or the occurrence of avulsion fractures, which can increase the patient's pain. After reduction, timely X-ray examination of the shoulder joint should be performed to observe whether it has been reduced and whether there are fractures.

After the reduction of shoulder dislocation and anesthesia recovery, the active and passive movement of the shoulder joint, limb sensation, and motor nerve function should be checked in a timely manner. If necessary, MRI and electromyography should be performed at an appropriate time to prevent brachial plexus injury and missed treatment of rotator cuff tear.

Shoulder dislocation and humeral head fracture can compress blood vessels, affecting blood circulation in the upper limbs. During physical examination, attention should be paid to pulse and peripheral circulation, and if necessary, ultrasound examination of blood vessels in the upper limbs and armpits should be performed to prevent thrombosis.

Whether patients should use anticoagulant drugs for treatment should be adjusted in a timely manner according to their condition to avoid bleeding that is difficult to control, affecting surgical treatment and venous reflux caused by hematoma compression.

C.-m. Huang (✉)
Department of Orthopedics, The 73rd Group Army Hospital,
Chenggong Hospital Affiliated to Xiamen University, Xiamen, China

Do not ignore the treatment of humeral tuberosity avulsion fracture. If the fracture is displaced and malunion occurs, the fracture block may collide with the acromion, leading to rotator cuff injury.

When dealing with emergencies, attention should not only focus on open wounds, organ injuries, or bleeding from fractures but also neglect shoulder joint examinations to avoid missed treatment.

9 Experience and Lessons Learned from Missed Diagnosis of Anterior Dislocation of the Shoulder Joint

Chang-ming Huang and Yang-pan Fu

9.1 Introduction

The main reasons for missed diagnosis of shoulder dislocation are: (1) multiple injuries, other injuries covering up the shoulder trauma, such as Case 1, an open trauma to the left elbow, where the doctor only paid attention to the condition of the elbow and did not conduct a detailed physical examination, resulting in missed diagnosis. (2) Suffering from certain diseases and unwilling to report to the doctor, the patient has a history of epilepsy, had functional impairment in the right shoulder after the seizure, and was unwilling to undergo follow-up X-rays after reduction, resulting in missed diagnosis. Patients with mental illness and elderly people may miss diagnosis due to unclear perception and sensation, mistaking them for soft tissue damage [1]. At the same time, patients with financial difficulties are reluctant to go to the hospital for examination and treatment, which is also one of the reasons for missed diagnosis.

9.2 Overview of Disease Diagnosis and Treatment Process

9.2.1 Case 1

The patient is a 24-year-old male who suffered from a fall and experienced pain in the left shoulder and elbow joints, with limited lifting activity for 2 months. When injured, there is an open injury to the elbow joint, which requires emergency debridement and suturing. After surgical treatment, routine physical and imaging examinations were not performed on the shoulder joint. The postoperative elbow joint wound healed well, and the function was normal. After injury, shoulder joint lifting, internal rotation, and external rotation activities are significantly restricted.

Physical examination revealed atrophy of the left shoulder joint supraspinatus, infraspinatus, and deltoid muscles, presenting with a square shoulder deformity and Dugas sign (+). Active and passive obstacles in lifting, internal rotation, external rotation, and outward movement.

The X-ray (Fig. 9.1) and CT three-dimensional reconstruction (Fig. 9.2) show anterior dislocation of the left shoulder joint with fracture of the greater tuberosity of the humerus.

9.2.2 Case 2

The patient is a 48-year-old male who had a right shoulder dislocation caused by an epileptic seizure 1 year ago. He underwent manual reduction and recovered on his own. No shoulder joint imaging examination was performed after reduction. After the injury, the right shoulder joint has been

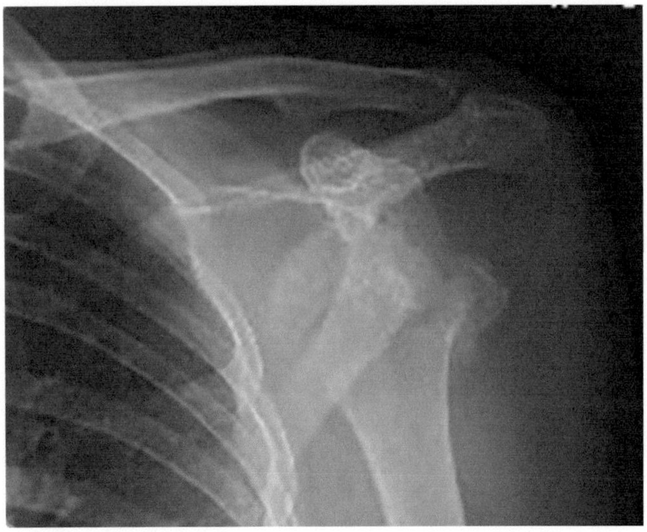

Fig. 9.1 Left shoulder joint anterior X-ray image

C.-m. Huang (✉) · Y.-p. Fu
Department of Orthopedics, The 73rd Group Army Hospital, Chenggong Hospital Affiliated to Xiamen University, Xiamen, China

Y.-j. Liu et al. (eds.), *Pitfalls in Diagnosis and Treatment of Shoulder Joint Diseases*, https://doi.org/10.1007/978-981-96-2472-0_9

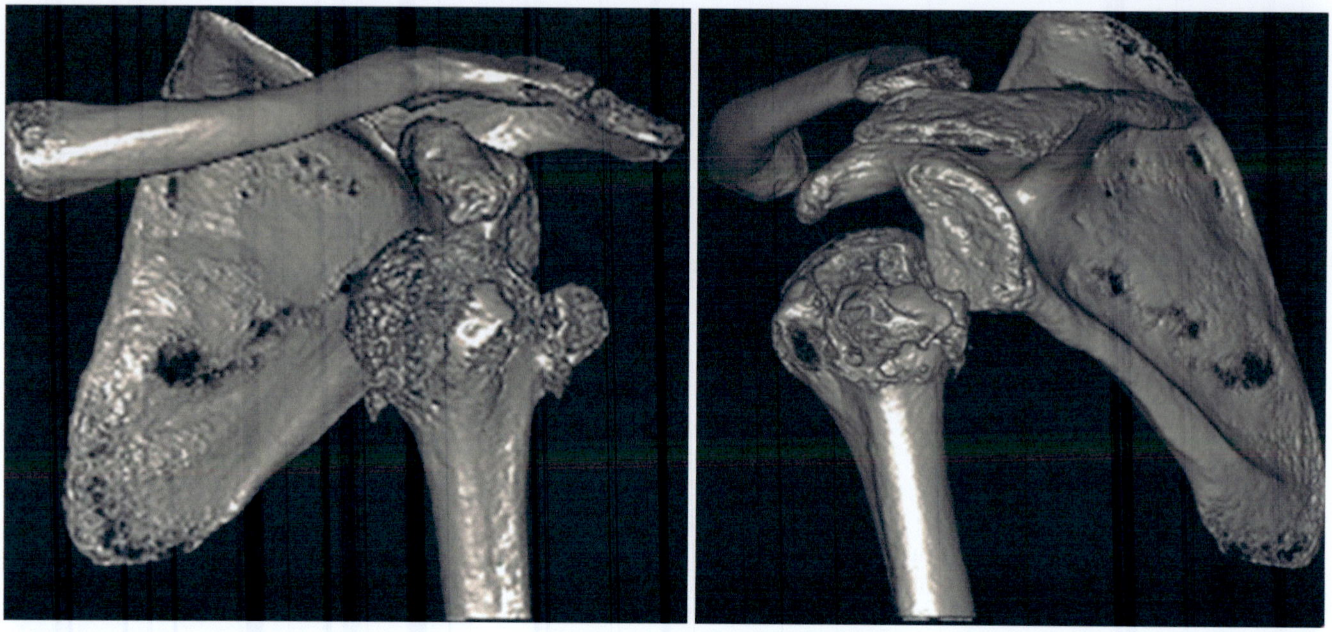

Fig. 9.2 CT three-dimensional reconstruction image of the left shoulder joint

experiencing continuous pain and limited mobility. Follow-up medical history revealed that the patient has a history of epilepsy for many years, attacks 2–3 times a year, and shoulder dislocation occurs after each attack, which can be manually reduced.

Physical examination revealed mild deformity of the right shoulder joint, atrophy of both the supraspinatus and deltoid muscles, square shoulder joint, empty shoulder joint, Dugas sign (+), and limited active and passive movement of the shoulder joint in multiple directions. The X-ray film of the shoulder joint (Fig. 9.3) and CT three-dimensional reconstruction (Fig. 9.4) showed anterior dislocation of the right shoulder joint. CTA (Fig. 9.5) shows displacement and compression of the right axillary artery.

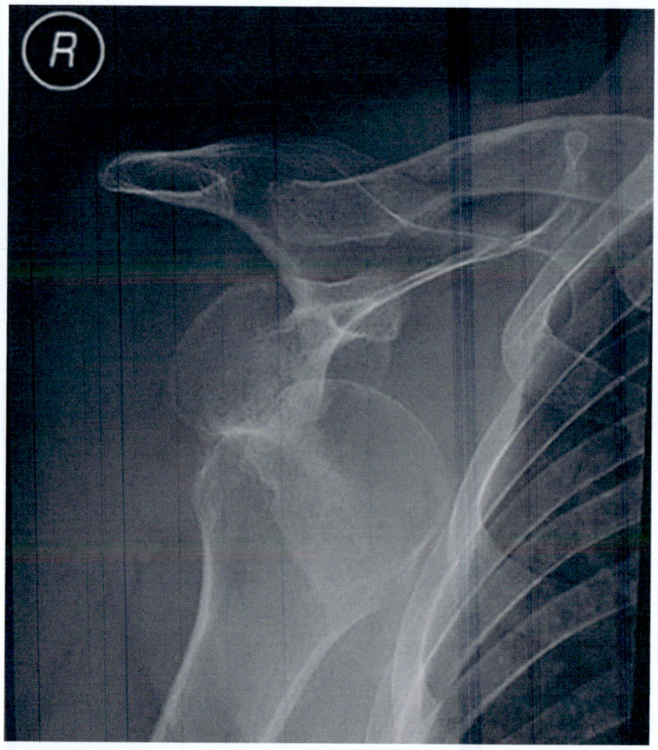

Fig. 9.3 Right shoulder joint anteroposterior X-ray showing anterior inferior dislocation of the right shoulder joint

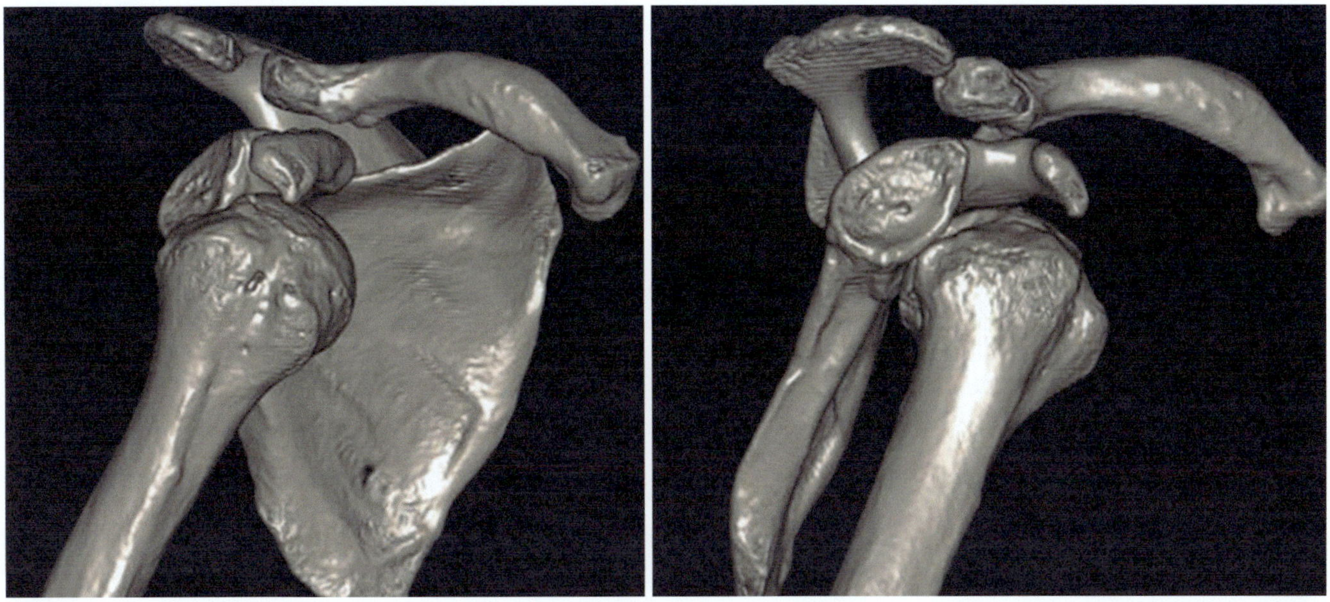

Fig. 9.4 CT 3D reconstruction showing anterior dislocation of the right shoulder joint

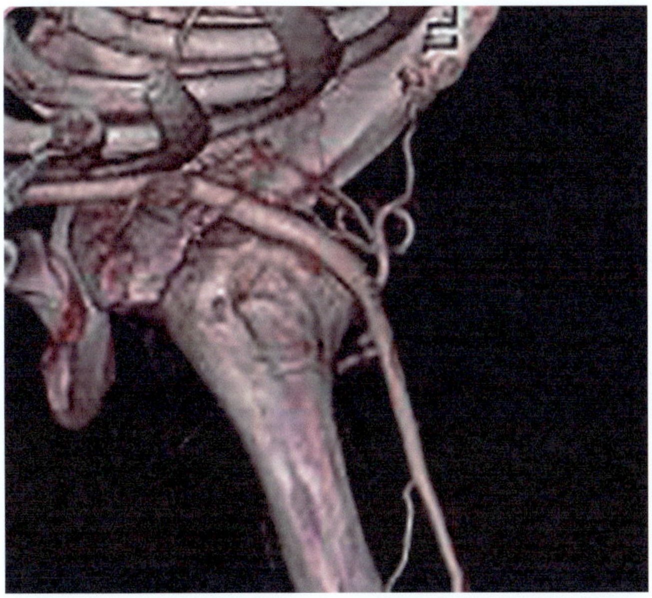

Fig. 9.5 CTA of the right shoulder joint shows the right axillary artery being displaced by the humeral head

9.3 Reasons and Countermeasures for Missed Diagnosis

To avoid missed diagnosis of shoulder dislocation, it is crucial to carefully inquire about medical history, especially whether there is a history of epilepsy, electric shock, mental illness, or hypoglycemia [2, 3]. At the same time, when accompanied by multiple injuries, it is necessary to inquire in detail about the process of the injury, analyze the mechanism of the injury, and conduct a serious physical examination. It is important not to be overshadowed by other easily observable injuries and to settle for only a single diagnosis..

Shoulder dislocation is commonly seen in trauma, sports traction injury, electric shock injury, epilepsy, psychiatric seizures, etc. Carefully inquire about medical history and injury process, analyze injury mechanism, conduct comprehensive physical examination, carefully read examination materials, and if necessary, perform shoulder joint CT or MRI examination to clarify the diagnosis. When diagnosing and treating multiple injuries, reduce misdiagnosis or missed diagnosis; do not neglect one aspect and lose the other—"pick sesame seeds, lose watermelons."

After receiving and before treatment, patients with shoulder dislocation must have a shoulder X-ray film to determine whether shoulder dislocation is accompanied by humeral tuberosity avulsion fracture. Do not hastily reduce it to avoid medical disputes.

Shoulder dislocation and humeral head fracture can compress blood vessels, affecting blood circulation in the upper limbs. During physical examination, attention should be paid to pulse and peripheral circulation, and if necessary, ultrasound examination of blood vessels in the upper limbs and armpits should be performed to prevent thrombosis.

References

1. Novi M, Tarallo L. Locked anterior glenohumeral dislocation: is it always recommendable a conservative treatment. Musculoskel Surg. 2022;106(3):239–45.
2. John R, Coady CM, Wong I. Arthroscopic revision with autologous iliac crest bone graft for failed anatomic glenoid reconstruction using distal tibia allograft. Arthroscopy Tech. 2019;8(11):e1333–8.
3. Jeong JY, Yoo YS, Kim T, et al. Arthroscopic iliac bone block augmentation for glenoid reconstruction: transglenoid fixation technique using an all-suture anchor. Arthroscopy Tech. 2020;9(3):e351–6.

10 Misdiagnosis of Anterior Shoulder Dislocation Accompanied by Vascular and Nerve Injury

Yu-jie Liu and Jun-liang Wang

10.1 Overview of the Diagnosis and Treatment Process

A 79-year-old female patient accidentally fell down with left upper limb outstretching. After the injury, the left shoulder joint was painful, swollen, and limited in movement. The doctor of local hospital gave external application of drugs for the injury, but the symptoms did not improve. So, the patient went to the hospital again. The dislocation was reduced with Hippocrates manipulation and immobilized with triangular scarf suspension. X-rays showed avulsion fracture of the greater tubercle of humerus after reducing anterior dislocation of the left shoulder joint (Fig. 10.1). However, the patient felt severe pain and swelling of the shoulder joint. 3D CT revealed a displaced fracture of the greater tubercle of the humerus (Fig. 10.2). The physical examination revealed swelling and dropping of the left wrist, dysfunction of the thumb, finger, and wrist extension (Fig. 10.3), Soft tissue swelling of the left shoulder joint, tenderness in the greater tubercle of the humerus (++), decreased sensation of the back and palm of hand, and positive paper pinch test. Active and passive movements of the shoulder joint were significantly limited. Electromyography suggested left brachial plexus injury. Diagnosis: dislocation of left shoulder joint and avulsion fracture displacement of greater tubercle of humerus combined with left brachial plexus injury.

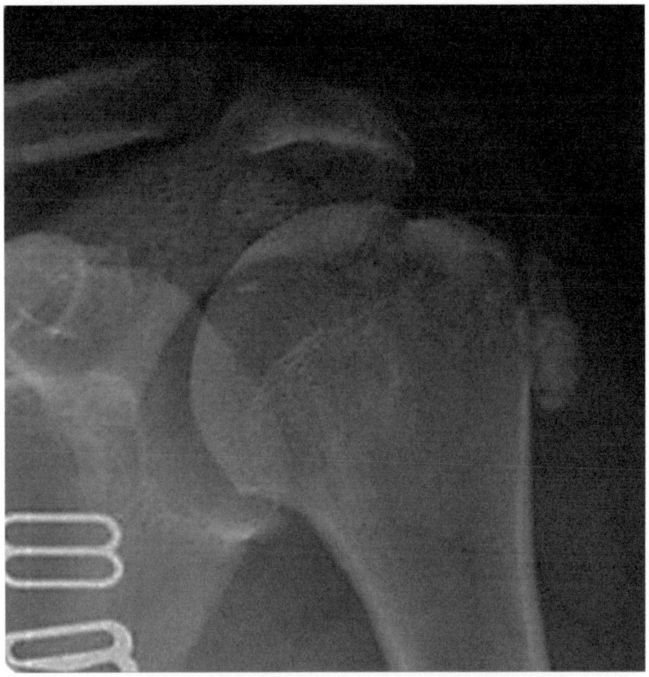

Fig. 10.1 X-rays showed avulsion fracture of the greater tubercle of humerus after reducing anterior dislocation of the left shoulder joint

Y.-j Liu
Orthopaedics, Chinese PLA General Hospital, Beijing, China

J.-l. Wang (✉)
Department of Orthopedics, Hainan Hospital of Chinese PLA General Hospital, Sanya, China

Y.-j. Liu et al. (eds.), *Pitfalls in Diagnosis and Treatment of Shoulder Joint Diseases*, https://doi.org/10.1007/978-981-96-2472-0_10

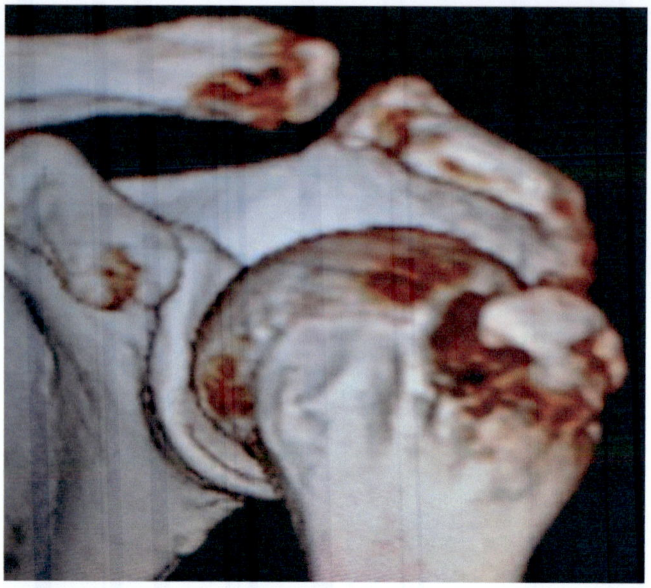

Fig. 10.2 CT 3D reconstruction shows displacement of the greater tubercle fracture

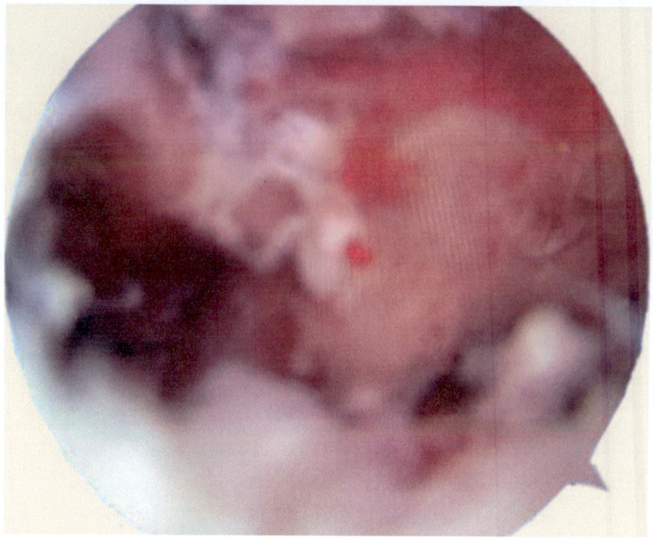

Fig. 10.4 Comminuted fracture of greater tubercle of humerus

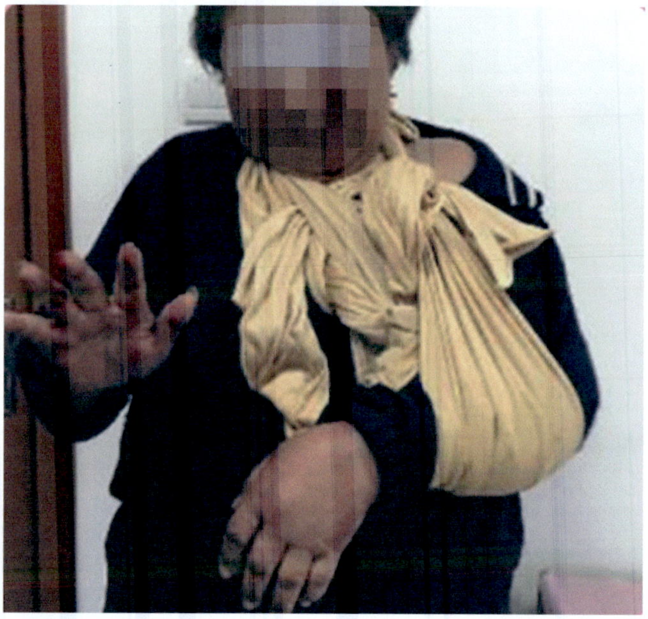

Fig. 10.3 Swelling and dropping of the left wrist, dysfunction of the thumb, finger, and wrist extension

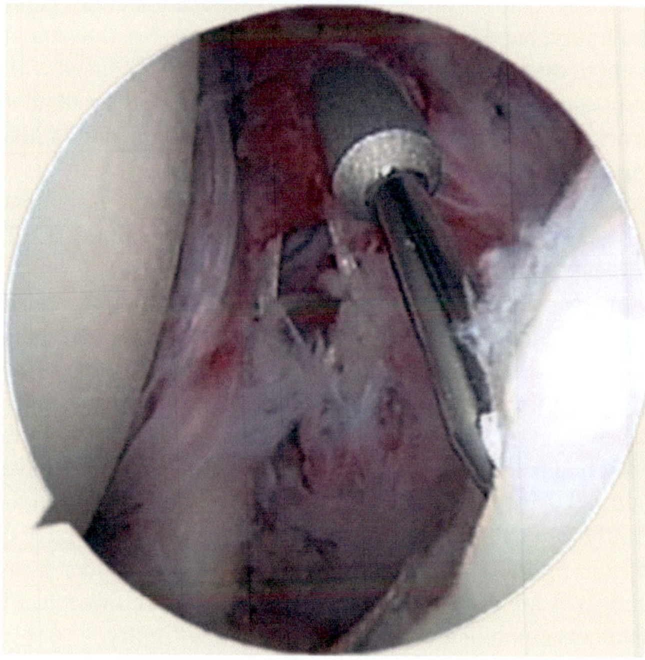

Fig. 10.5 Bankart injury of shoulder joint

10.2 Surgical Treatment

Arthroscopic exploration of the left shoulder revealed comminuted fracture of the greater tubercle of the humerus (Fig. 10.4), anterior and inferior dislocation of the humerus head, and injury of the anterior inferior glenoid labrum (Fig. 10.5). Hematoma, bone debris, and synovitis were debrided arthroscopically. Glenohumeral joint were reduced to relief the compression of brachial plexus. Injury of anterior and inferior glenoid labrum was repaired with suture anchor (Fig. 10.6). Osteochondral debris was removed from the greater tuberosity area (Fig. 10.7). Two suture anchors were implanted, and the sutures were knotted through the supraspinatus tendon to fix and repair the rotator cuff tissue. The sutures of anchors were netted over the surface of the supraspinatus tendon (Fig. 10.8), and two external rows of

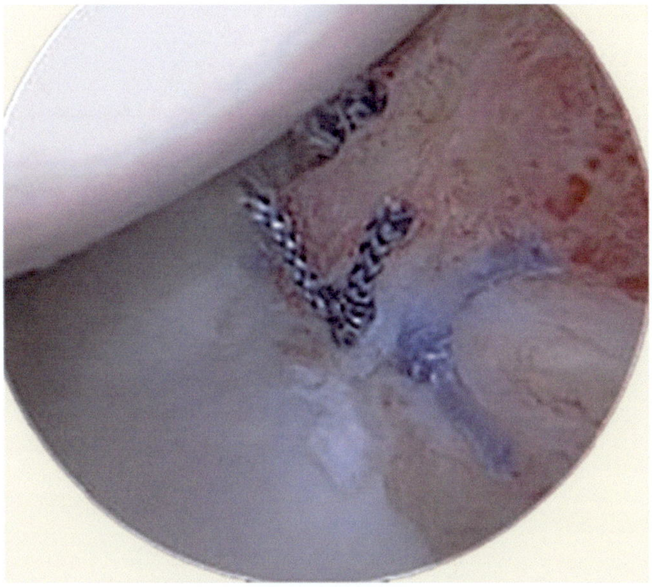

Fig. 10.6 Repair Bankart injury with suture anchors

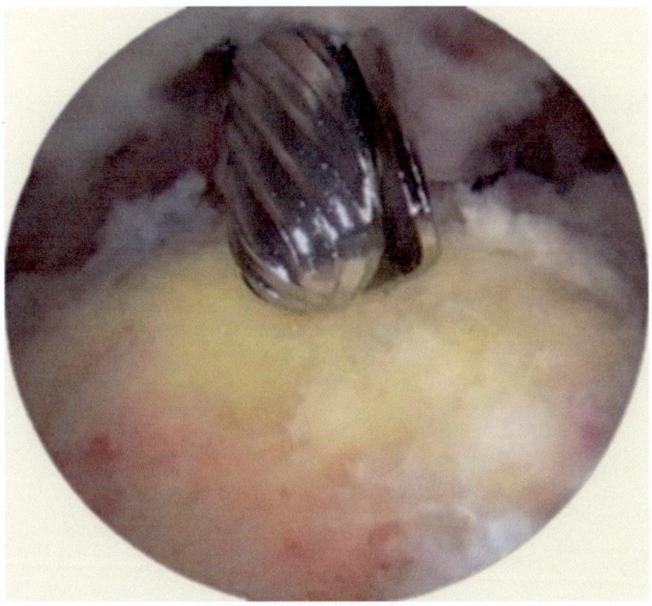

Fig. 10.7 The cartilage of intertubercular sulcus was removed

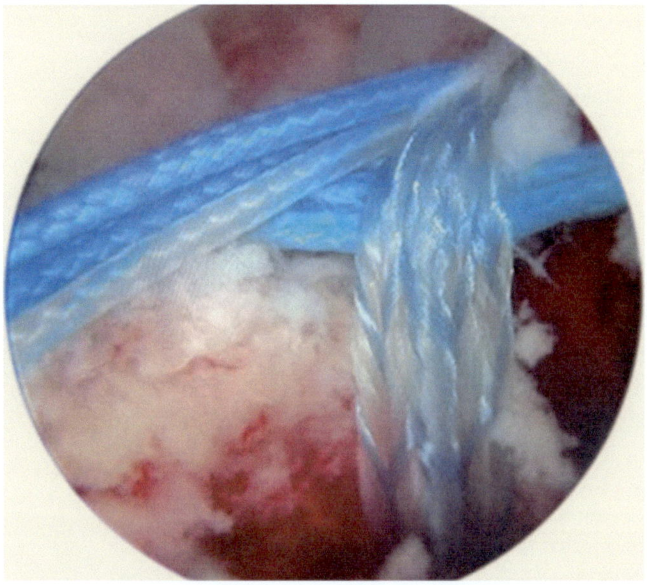

Fig. 10.8 The supraspinatus tendon was secured with the sutures

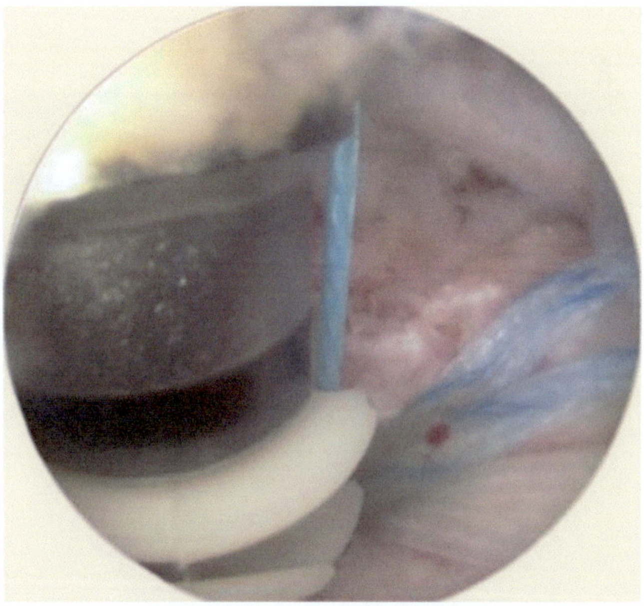

Fig. 10.9 A lateral row of anchors holds the sutures in place, securing the rotator cuff and bone mass in a network

anchors were implanted 1 cm away from the fracture of the greater tubercle of the humerus (Fig. 10.9) to fix the sutures (Fig. 10.10), and the affected limb was immobilized at 45° with a brace after surgery (Fig. 10.10). Preoperative MRI showed that the supraspinatus tendon pulled and displaced the greater tubercle of the humerus (Fig. 10.11a), and post-operative MRI showed that the reconstructed rotator cuff and the fragments were well fixed (Fig. 10.11b). After operation, neurotrophic drugs were given, and functional rehabilitation training was carried out according to rehabilitation procedures. Swelling of affected limb gradually subsided and brachial plexus function returned to normal 1 month after operation.

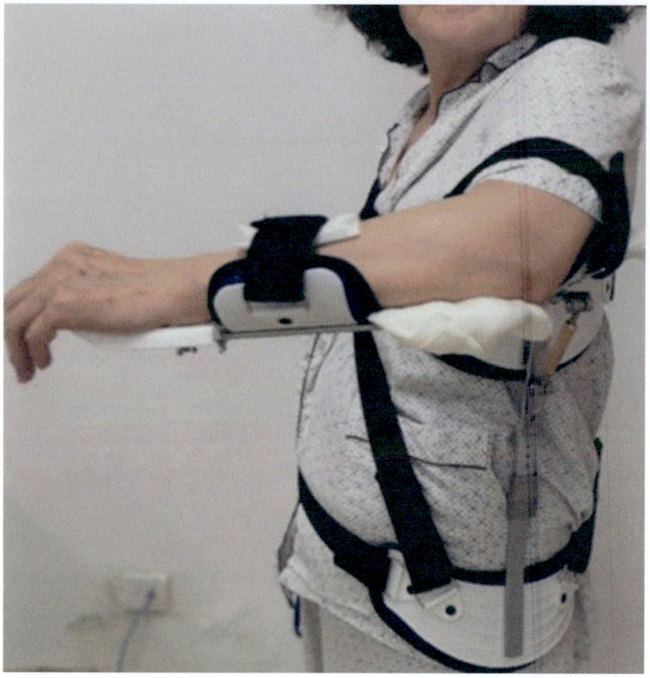

Fig. 10.10 After surgery, the affected limb was fixed with a brace

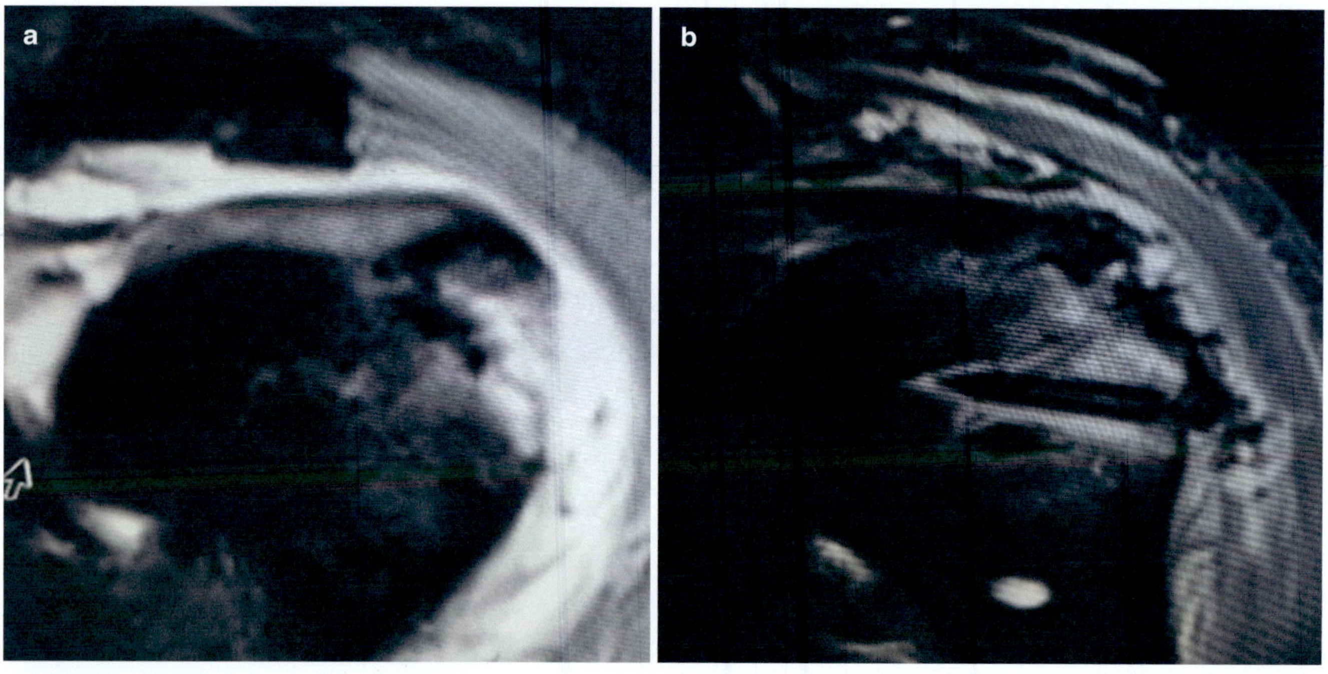

Fig. 10.11 MRI image. (**a**) Preoperative MRI revealed a displaced fracture of the greater tubercle of humerus. (**b**) Postoperative MRI showed that the rotator cuff was reconstructed with suture anchors fixed in a mesh

10.3 Lessons from Missed Diagnosis

Humeral greater tubercle fractures are caused by shoulder dislocation in 5–57%, while humeral greater tubercle fractures can occur in 15–30% of anterior shoulder dislocation [1]. Most elderly people have osteoporosis. When they fall, the palm support the ground, and the violence is transmitted from the wrist joint to the shoulder joint. The shoulder dislocation with avulsion fracture of the greater tubercle of humerus is more common, so we should pay attention to the health education of the elderly to prevent falls and injuries. The patient failed to make accurate diagnosis and effective treatment at an early stage in all three visits. Some doctors do not grasp the basic professional knowledge, and some doctors are sloppy in diagnosis and treatment, resulting in missed diagnosis. It is very necessary to strengthen the training of basic knowledge of young doctors. The training of basic clinical skills cannot be learned overnight. It is necessary to study intensively under the help, guidance of the older generation of experts. Doctors should strengthen the summary of experience and lessons and train the basic clinical skills. The doctor must be close to the clinic, must carefully ask the history, and carefully examine the patient. Combined with the analysis of imaging data, a definitive diagnosis and correct management can be obtained. Some doctors only look at imaging data and do not check the patient during the diagnosis and treatment process, which is very terrible.

For shoulder dislocation, whether manual reduction or surgical treatment, routine imaging must be performed before surgery to determine the location of shoulder dislocation, avulsion fracture of the greater tubercle of humerus, or glenoid fracture. Ogawa's [2] study of 163 humerus greater tubercle fractures of the shoulder joint showed that most of the fractures (57%) involved the supraspinatus and infraspinatus muscles, thereby shifting the fracture fragments upward and backward. When the infraspinatus tendon is intact, the fracture mass is displaced backward. The degree of backward displacement of the fracture is difficult to assess with standard radiographs alone, even with axillary radiographs. Therefore, CT 3D reconstruction is the best method to evaluate the degree of backward displacement of the fracture mass. If no imaging data were available prior to treatment and subsequent imaging findings of avulsion fracture or bony Bankart injury of the greater tubercula of the humerus were observed after treatment, it is difficult to distinguish whether the fracture occurred at the time of injury or as a result of operative treatment. Before diagnosis and treatment, patients and their families should be truthfully explained in detail about the condition, treatment plan, postoperative prognosis and functional rehabilitation training, and informed consent should be signed.

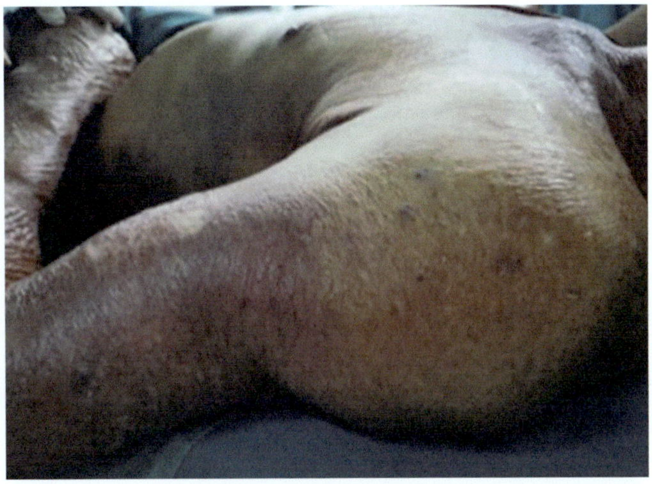

Fig. 10.12 A dislocation of the shoulder joint with a fracture of the greater tubercle of the humerus leads to venous thrombosis

Due to shoulder dislocation combined with greater tubercle fracture of the humerus, local bleeding and compression of the humerus head may cause compression of axillary vascular nerve bundles, resulting in nerve conduction and blood circulation disorders. If the limbs are swollen, watch out for venous thrombosis (Fig. 10.12). Anterior and inferior shoulder dislocation squeezing the brachial plexus nerve (Fig. 10.13) can lead to sensory and motor dysfunction of the forearm and hand. Therefore, special attention should be paid to the detection of brachial plexus paralysis, when imaging findings of shoulder dislocation accompanied by avulsion fracture displacement of the greater tubercle of humerus are found [3–5].

10.4 Diagnosis and Treatment Strategy

During the physical examination of shoulder dislocation, it is important to pay attention to swelling, skin color, and pulse of the affected limb. If abnormalities are found, vascular ultrasound and nervous system related examinations should be performed in time to identify vascular and nerve damage as soon as possible.

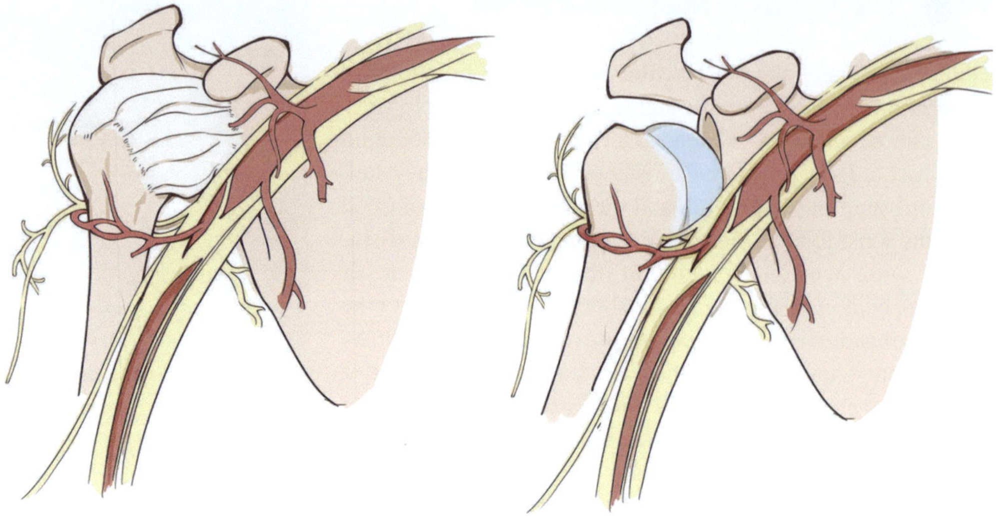

Fig. 10.13 Humerus head of shoulder dislocation compresses brachial plexus neurovascular bundle

References

1. Yanmiş İ, Kömürcü M, Oğuz E, et al. The role of arthroscopy in chronic anterior shoulder dislocation: technique and early results. J Arthros Relat Surg. 2003;19(10):1129–32.
2. Rowe CR, Zarins B. Chronic unreduced dislocation of the shoulder. J Bone Joint Surg Am. 1982;64(4):494–505.
3. Litchfield JC, Subhedar VY, Beevers DG, et al. Bilateral dislocation of the shoulders due to nocturnal hypoglycaemia. Postgrad Med J. 1988;64(752):450–2.
4. George MS. Fractures of the greater tuberosity of the humerus. J Am Acad Orthop Surg. 2007;15:607–13.
5. Ogawa K, Yoshida A, Ikegami H. Isolated fractures of the greater tuberosity of the humerus: solutions to recognizing a frequently overlooked fracture. J Trauma. 2003;54(4):713–7.

Part V

Posterior Dislocation of the Shoulder Joint and Diseases that Are Easily Confused with Posterior Dislocation: An Introduction and Summary

Jing Xue

Introduction

This part focuses on cases of posterior dislocation of the shoulder joint, analyzes the causes of missed diagnosis and misdiagnosis, particularly highlighting posterior shoulder dislocation secondary to brachial plexus birth palsy injury and injection-induced deltoid muscle contracture. It also proposes countermeasures to avoid missed diagnosis and mistreatment.

Summary

1. To prevent missed diagnosis of posterior shoulder dislocation, it is crucial to thoroughly inquire about medical history, especially regarding epilepsy or electrical injuries. Additionally, a meticulous physical examination should be conducted along with necessary auxiliary examinations while carefully reviewing X-ray films. When Light-Bulb sign is present, CT or MRI scans can provide a definitive diagnosis.
2. Posterior shoulder dislocations caused by birth palsy injuries are relatively uncommon but prone to being overlooked or improperly treated. In cases where unexplained chronic shoulder dislocations occur in children, obtaining information about the mother's delivery history is highly valuable for reference purposes. If shoulder dislocation is caused by dystocia, it is necessary to check the sensory and motor functions of the upper limb to rule out brachial plexus nerve injury.
3. Injection-induced deltoid muscle contracture occurs due to contraction of the posterior bundle of the deltoid muscle, which results in prolonged abduction and external rotation of the shoulder joint, affecting its adduction and internal rotation functions. This condition can be mistakenly diagnosed as posterior shoulder dislocation due to Light-Bulb sign observed on X-ray films. Three-dimensional CT reconstruction is helpful for differential diagnosis.

J. Xue (✉)
Orthopaedics, Air Force Medical Center of Chinese PLA, Beijing, China

Diagnosis and Treatment Misconceptions of Posterior Dislocation of the Shoulder Joint

11

Chang-ming Huang, Xun-wu Huang, and Yu-jie Liu

11.1 Introduction

Shoulder dislocation is commonly caused by trauma, traction injury, epilepsy, electrical injury, psychosis, and other reasons. Especially in multiple injuries, attention is focused on open wounds, bleeding, organ damage, or fractures when treating patients. Anterior shoulder dislocation is relatively common compared to posterior shoulder dislocation, with a prevalence of 1–4% [1, 2]. Posterior shoulder dislocation is prone to missed diagnosis, with a missed diagnosis rate of up to 50–79%, with 34% of shoulder dislocation fractures, 2–13% of rotator cuff injuries, and 29–86% of reverse Hill-Sachs injuries [3, 4].

The posterior dislocation of the shoulder joint is often misdiagnosed, primarily due to the neglect of shoulder joint examination, mistakenly assuming it to be mere soft tissue damage or other injuries in the shoulder, leading to delayed treatment and subsequent misdiagnosis [5, 6]. To prevent the misdiagnosis of posterior dislocation of the shoulder joint, it is crucial to diligently inquire about the medical history, including whether there is a history of epilepsy, electrical injury, mental illness, or hypoglycemia [7].

11.2 Overview of Medical Diagnosis and Treatment

The patient is a 48-year-old male who suffered a left shoulder joint injury while riding a motorcycle. The pain was accompanied by limited lifting and external rotation activities for more than 3 months. After the injury, X-ray examination of the shoulder joint was performed at the local hospital. At the initial diagnosis, no dislocation of the shoulder joint was noticed, and local treatment was carried out according to the soft tissue injury of the shoulder joint. The patient went home for recuperation. Since the injury, the patient has been experiencing pain and limited mobility in the left shoulder joint.

Physical examination revealed multiple skin scars on the left shoulder joint (Fig. 11.1), prominent protrusion of the coronoid process and anterior outer corner of the acromion, empty front of the shoulder joint, and full back (Fig. 11.2). The shoulder joint is in an internal rotation position, with significant limitations in lifting and external rotation. The double shoulder X-ray shows a light bulb sign in the left shoulder joint (Fig. 11.3). CT imaging shows a locked posterior dislocation of the left shoulder joint, and CT three-dimensional imaging reveals a locked posterior dislocation of the left shoulder joint, accompanied by an anterior counter-Hill-Sachs lesion (Figs. 11.4 and 11.5).

C.-m. Huang (✉)
Department of Orthopedics, The 73rd Group Army Hospital, Chenggong Hospital Affiliated to Xiamen University, Xiamen, China

X.-w. Huang
Department of Orthopedics, The Eighth Medical Center of the Chinese PLA General Hospital, Beijing, China

Y.-j. Liu
Orthopaedics, Chinese PLA General Hospital, Beijing, China

Y.-j. Liu et al. (eds.), *Pitfalls in Diagnosis and Treatment of Shoulder Joint Diseases*, https://doi.org/10.1007/978-981-96-2472-0_11

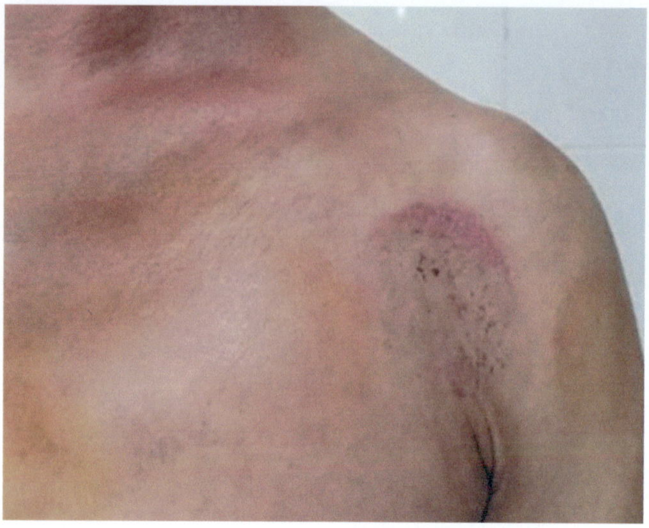

Fig. 11.1 Skin scar on left shoulder joint

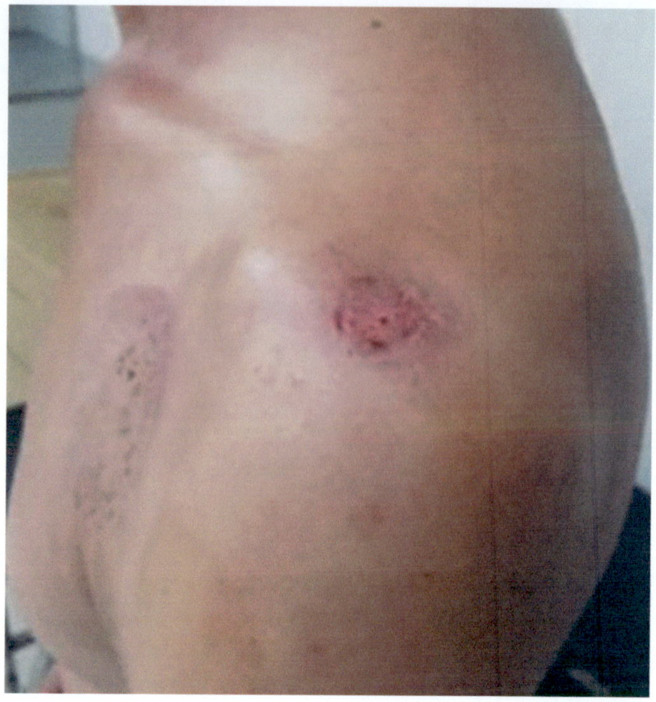

Fig. 11.2 Left shoulder front empty, rear full, protruding coracoid process, and acromion

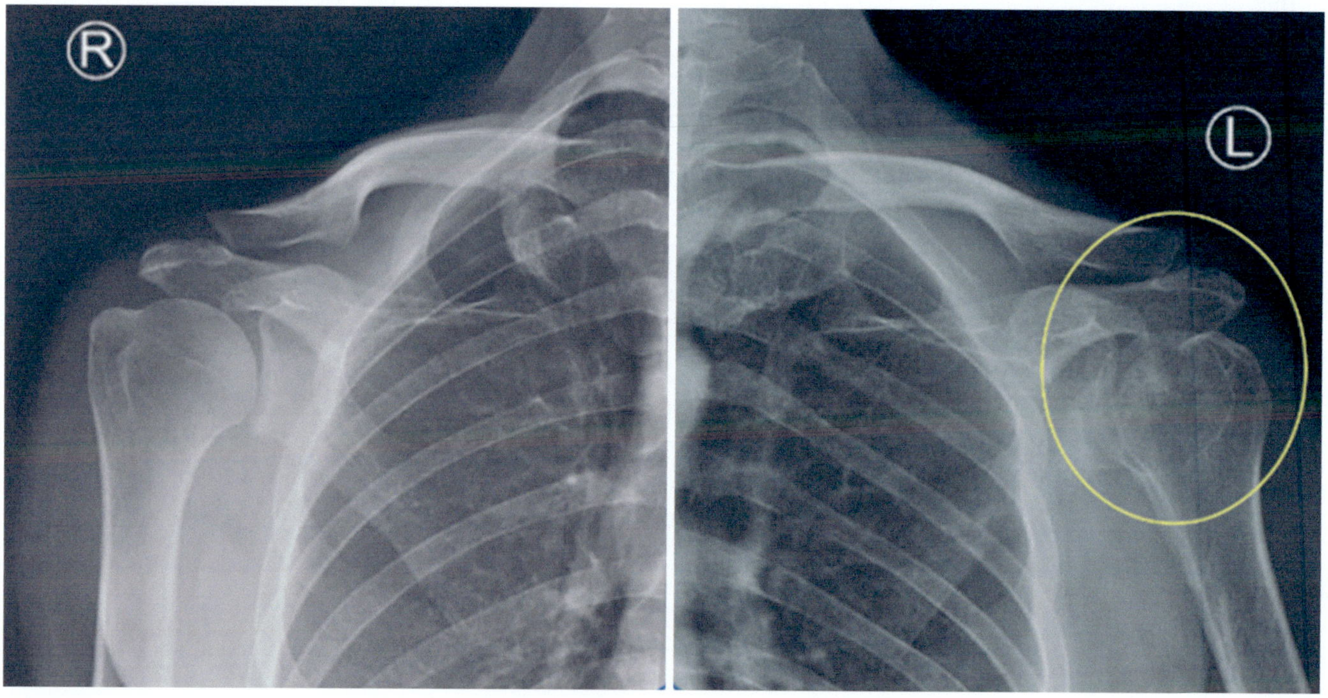

Fig. 11.3 X-ray shows light bulb sign in the left shoulder joint and normal in the right shoulder joint

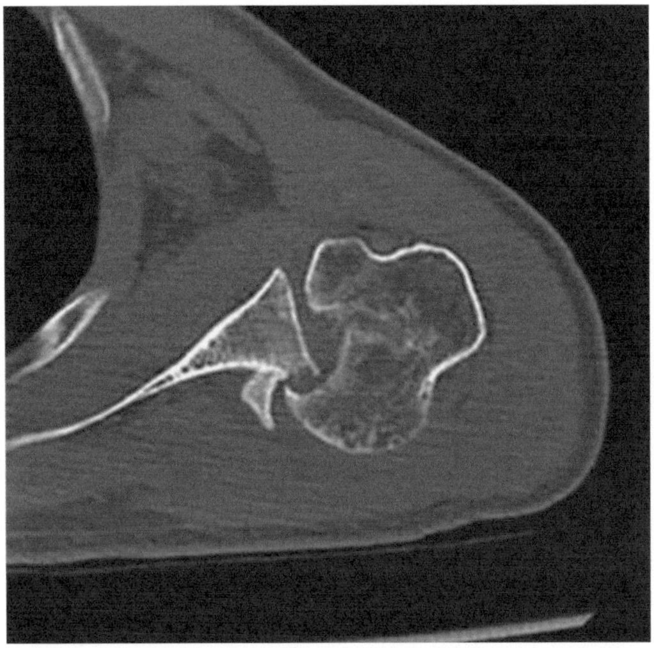

Fig. 11.4 CT scan of the left shoulder joint shows posterior dislocation of the left shoulder humeral head and occlusion of the posterior lip of the glenoid bone

11.3 Diagnosis and Treatment Strategies for Posterior Dislocation of the Shoulder Joint

The main signs of posterior dislocation of the shoulder joint are prominent anterior lateral angle and coracoid process on the affected side compared to the healthy side, full posterior soft spot, and significantly restricted external rotation activity.

The typical X-ray features are light bulb sign of the humeral head, internal rotation of the humerus, and empty joint (Fig. 11.6); edge sign, with a distance of ≥6 mm between the anterior edge of the joint and the humeral head; slot line sign, humeral head fracture forms a vertical line (Fig. 11.7).

When dealing with multiple injuries, doctors tend to focus on obvious injuries such as open wounds, heavy bleeding, organ injuries, or fractures, while neglecting physical examinations of the shoulder joint area. Doctors should inquire in detail about the process and mechanism of the injury, conduct a thorough physical examination, carefully read imaging examination reports, refer to auxiliary examination

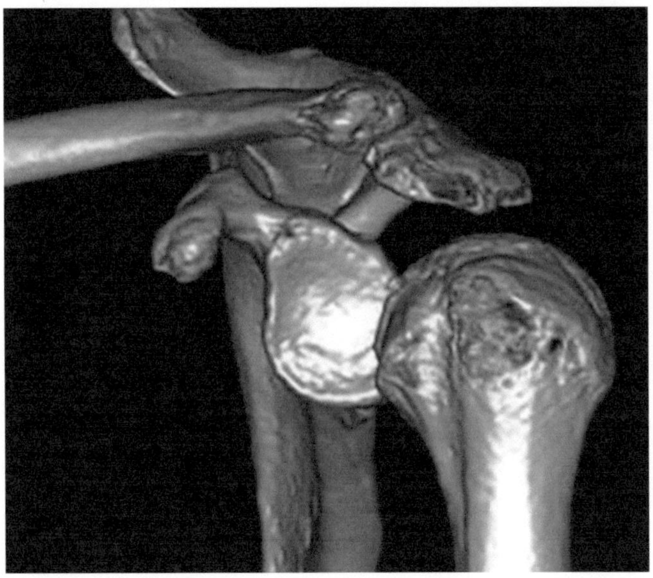

Fig. 11.5 CT three-dimensional reconstruction of the left shoulder joint showing posterior dislocation of the humeral head

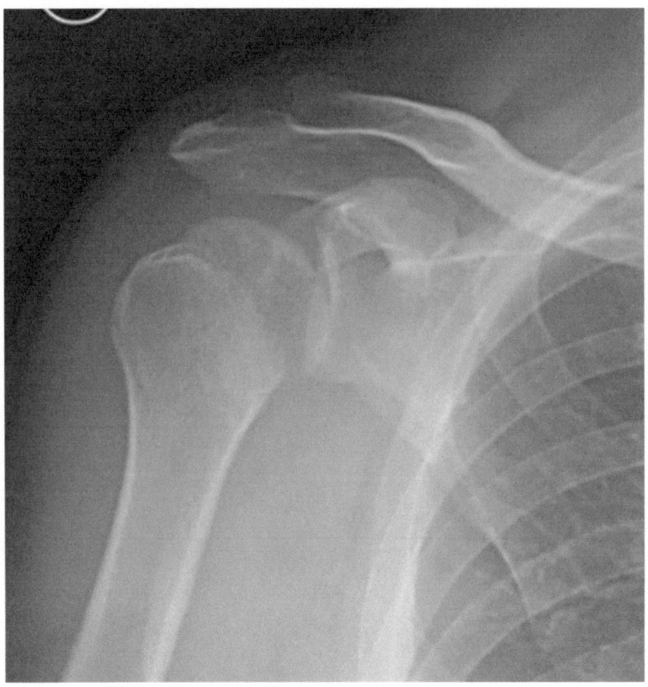

Fig. 11.6 Internal rotation of humerus and light bulb sign of humeral head

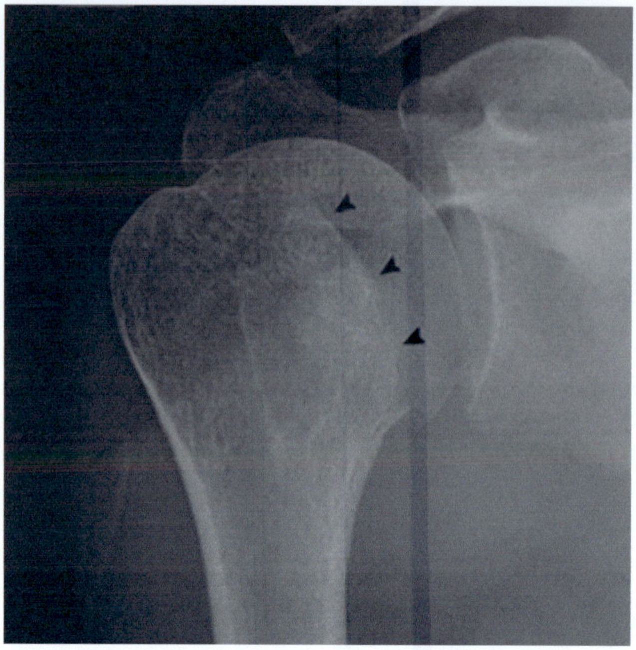

Fig. 11.7 Slot line sign: vertical line formed by humeral head fracture

results, and see the essence through phenomena. Do not be deceived by phenomena. X-ray shows light bulb sign, and CT three-dimensional reconstruction can provide a clear diagnosis.

In summary, to avoid missed diagnosis of posterior dislocation of the shoulder joint, the key is to carefully inquire about the history, especially if there is a history of epilepsy or electric shock. At the same time, carefully carry out a physical examination, do necessary auxiliary examinations, and carefully read the X-ray film. When light bulb sign appear, a CT or MRI examination can be performed to make a definitive diagnosis.

References

1. Benhamida MK, Ouertatani M, Hasayri I, et al. Locked posterior dislocation of the shoulder: a report of three cases. Chir Main. 2015;34(2):98–101.
2. Schoenfeld AJ, Lippitt SB. Rotator cuff tear associated with a posterior dislocation of the shoulder in a young adult: a case report and literature review. J Orthop Trauma. 2007;21(2):150–2.
3. Rowe CR, Zarins B. Chronic unreduced dislocations of the shoulder. J Bone Joint Surg Am. 1982;64(4):494–505.
4. Robinson CM, Aderinto J. Posterior shoulder dislocations and fracture-dislocations. J Bone Joint Surg Am. 2005;87(3):639–50.
5. Espag MP, Back DL, Baroni M, et al. Diagnosing shoulder dislocations: time for a change of view. Ann R Coll Surg Engl. 2002;84(5):334–7.
6. Rouleau DM, Hebert-Davies J. Incidence of associated injury in posterior shoulder dislocation: systematic review of the literature. J Orthop Trauma. 2012;26(4):246–51.
7. Cicak N. Posterior dislocation of the shoulder. J Bone Joint Surg. 2004;86(3):324–32.

12 Posterior Dislocation of Shoulder Joint in the Birth Injury

Yu Zhou and Yu-jie Liu

12.1 Overview of the Diagnosis and Treatment Process

The patient was male, aged 14. His parents found that the patient's bilateral upper limbs were unequal in length since childhood, and the left upper limb was shorter than the right upper limb. Because there are no obvious obstacles in the daily life of the patient and no significant influence on the motor function of the upper limbs, so parents did not pay attention to it. As the age increased, the parents found that the asymmetry of bilateral upper limb length became more obvious. Before the local hospital prepared to perform bone extension surgery on the left upper limb, the patient came to our department for further consultation. After investigation of medical history, we found that the patient was born with a dystocia, and the left upper limb was exposed first. The midwife pulled the left upper limb out of the birth canal.

Physical examination: Bilateral upper limbs were asymmetrical. The left side was shorter than the right side, the left shoulder joint abduction, external rotation, and lifting activities were slightly limited, while the right side was normal (Figs. 12.1 and 12.2). The left shoulder joint is with anterior void, rear full. Bilateral upper limbs' sensation and muscle strength were not significantly abnormal.

Medical image examination: Three-dimension (3D) computed tomography (CT) reconstruction of the left shoulder joint showed that the caput humeri had the light bulb sign (Fig. 12.3), with a posterior dislocation of the left caput humeri (Fig. 12.4).

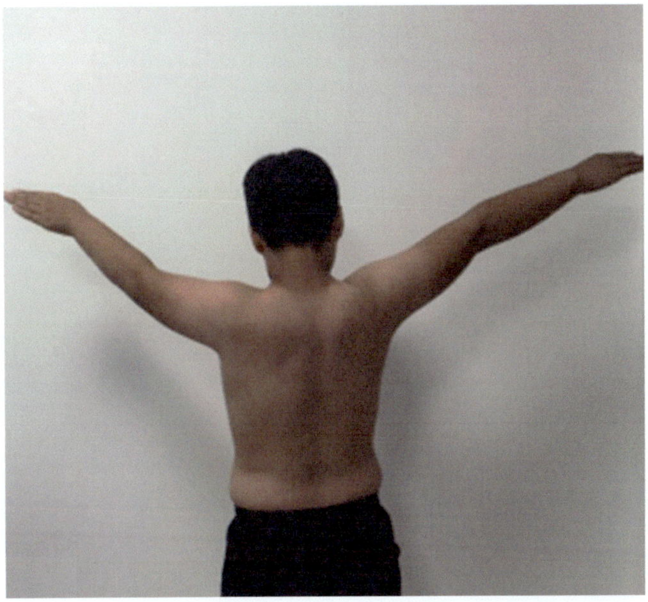

Fig. 12.1 Bilateral upper limbs abduction showed slight limitation on the left side compared to the right

Y. Zhou (✉)
Department of Orthopaedics, Beijing Chaoyang Hospital, Capital Medical University, Beijing, China

Y.-j. Liu
Orthopaedics, Chinese PLA General Hospital, Beijing, China

Y.-j. Liu et al. (eds.), *Pitfalls in Diagnosis and Treatment of Shoulder Joint Diseases*, https://doi.org/10.1007/978-981-96-2472-0_12

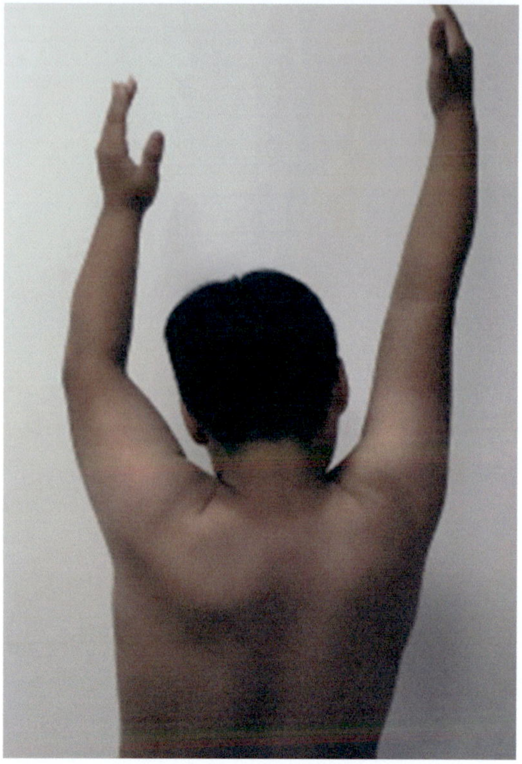

Fig. 12.2 The uplifting of both upper limbs showed that the left side was restricted more than the right side, and the left upper limb was shorter

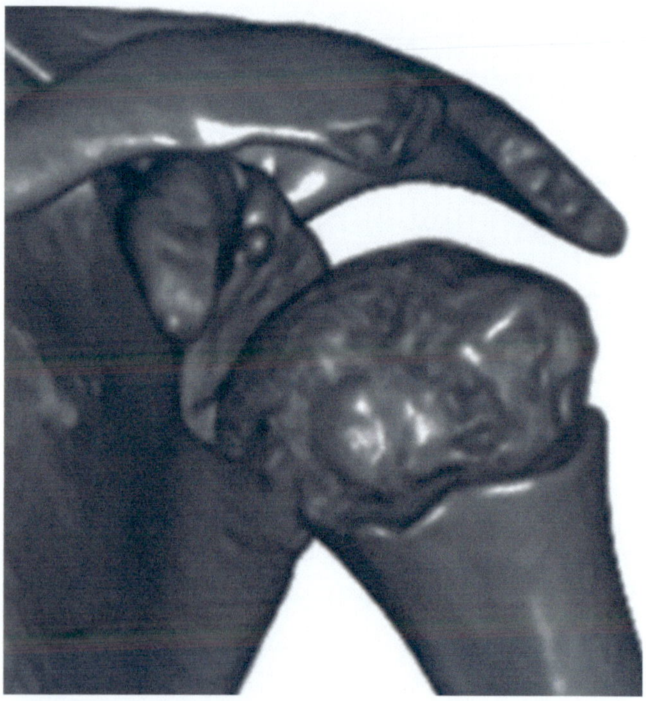

Fig. 12.3 Three-dimensional CT reconstruction of the left shoulder joint shows that the left caput humeri has a lightbulb sign

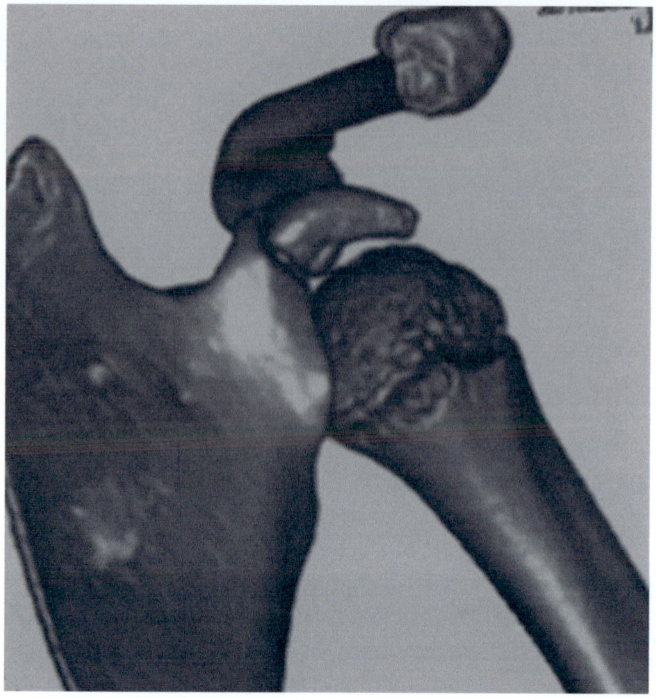

Fig. 12.4 Three-dimensional CT reconstruction of the left shoulder joint shows a posterior dislocation of the caput humeri

12.2 Exploration of Diagnosis and Treatment of Posterior Dislocation of Shoulder Joint

Posterior dislocation of shoulder joint caused by birth injury is rare, and it is easy to misdiagnose or mistreat. In this case, the patient was treated in local hospital. The doctor only found that the patient's limb length was asymmetrical, but did not find the posterior dislocation of shoulder joint. When children's unexplained old shoulder joint dislocation happens, mother's childbearing history has important reference value. If shoulder dislocation is caused by dystopia, we should pay attention to the sensory and motor function of the upper limbs and the injury of the external brachial plexus [1, 2].

The reduction of shoulder joint by orthopedic treatment? Or by conservative treatment? Which one is better? Although the length of the two upper limbs is asymmetrical, but the function of the left shoulder joint does not affect daily life. So operated osteotomy to lengthen the upper limbs is impractical. The patient has been experienced shoulder joint dislocation since childhood, and the caput humeri remained in this position for 14 years. Although it is not in a normal anatomical position, the anatomical structure and morphology of the caput humeri, glenoid, and the anteversion angle have been matured. The function of shoulder joint has adapted to such kind of anatomical structure. If osteotomy and orthopedic procedures were performed to correct the angle of the glenoid, caput humeri and anatomical neck, it would destroy the anatomical structure and function of the shoulder joint, and be opposite with no improvement of the shoulder joint. Through medical examination to find out the reasons for the unequal length of the upper limbs, based on the motor function of the patient, conservative treatment is the better choice. After years of clinical tracking, the patient's shoulder joint function does not affect his life and work.

The accurate treatment is based on the accurate diagnosis, while accurate diagnosis is originated from accurate medical history, examination, analysis, and judgment. Doctors cannot only take stopgap measures. The principle of orthopedic treatment has priority in the stability in the lower limbs and flexibility in the upper limbs, aiming to function first.

References

1. Moukoko D, Ezaki M, Wilkes D, et al. Posterior shoulder dislocation in infants with neonatal brachial plexus palsy. J Bone Joint Surg Am. 2004;86(4):787–93.
2. Torode I, Donnan L. Posterior dislocation of the humeral head in association with obstetric paralysis. J Pediatr Orthop. 1998;18(5):611–5.

13 Misdiagnosis of Posterior Dislocation of the Shoulder Joint Due to Injection-Induced Deltoid Muscle Contracture

Yu-jie Liu and Jing Xue

13.1 Overview of the Diagnosis and Treatment Process

The patient, a 28-year-old female who works as an elementary school teacher, presents with a history of bilateral shoulder joint limitations in internal rotation and adduction since childhood without any identifiable cause. Additionally, she reports experiencing popping sounds and scapular elevation when raising her shoulders. Further inquiry with the patient's parents revealed that she had a frequent history of colds, fevers, and pneumonia during childhood. Consequently, long-term benzylpenicillin injections were administered bilaterally into the gluteal muscles; however, poor absorption in this region resulted in the formation of local nodules and medication leakage from the injection site. Subsequently, injections were switched to both deltoid muscles. At the age of 5, it was noted that her upper limbs exhibited abduction by 20° along with limited internal rotation and adduction movements. This led to stiffness in shoulder joint mobility where both forearms could not be brought close to the trunk. The patient had received a diagnosis of bilateral posterior shoulder dislocation at multiple medical facilities.

The physical examination revealed the presence of multiple dimpled depressions in the posterior lateral region of both deltoid muscles (Fig. 13.1). When the upper limbs were adducted, scapular protrusion was observed (Fig. 13.2), accompanied by shoulder joint snapping during movement and limited abduction and lifting of the shoulder joint. The upper limbs cannot achieve full adduction (Fig. 13.3).

The patient exhibits an out-toe gait and experiences bilateral hip joint clicking during squatting. In addition, the patient demonstrates limited range of motion while attempting to cross their legs (Fig. 13.4) and when performing

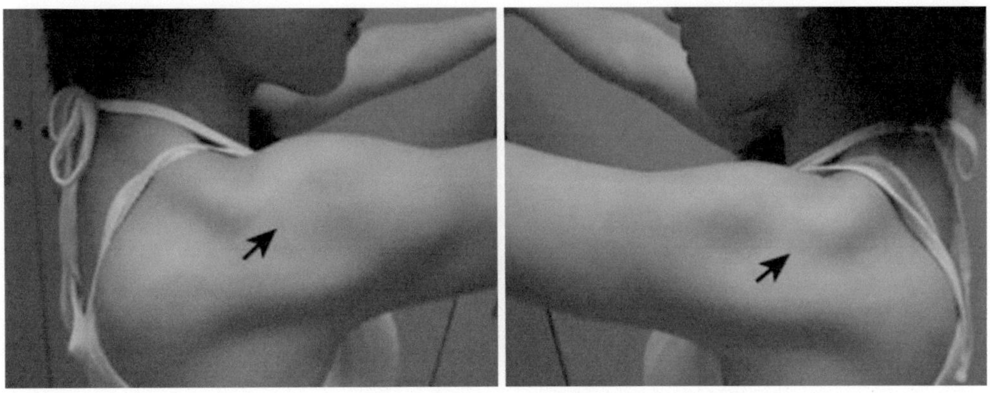

Fig. 13.1 The presence of depressed contracture bands in the posterior lateral region of both deltoid muscles

Y.-j. Liu
Orthopaedics, Chinese PLA General Hospital, Beijing, China

J. Xue (✉)
Orthopaedics, Air Force Medical Center of Chinese PLA, Beijing, China

Y.-j. Liu et al. (eds.), *Pitfalls in Diagnosis and Treatment of Shoulder Joint Diseases*,
https://doi.org/10.1007/978-981-96-2472-0_13

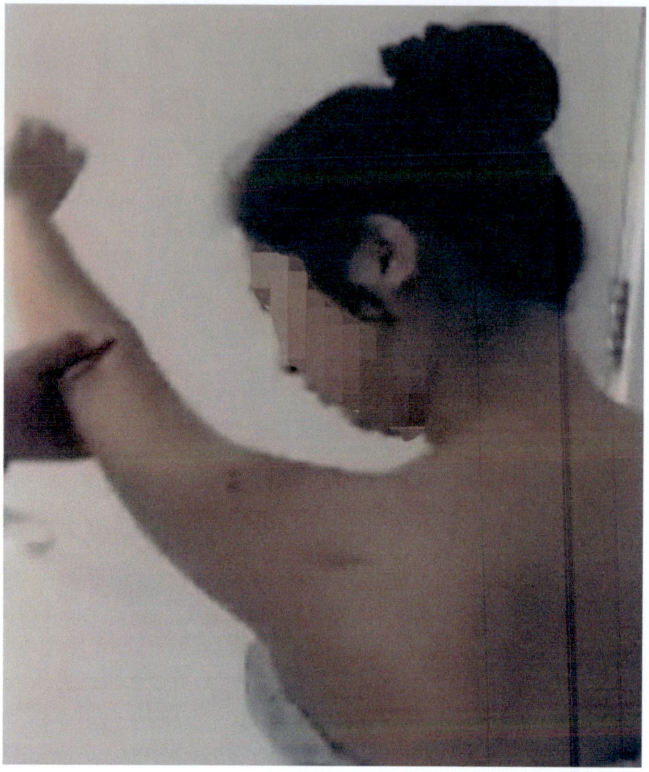

Fig. 13.2 Restricted internal rotation observed in the left shoulder joint

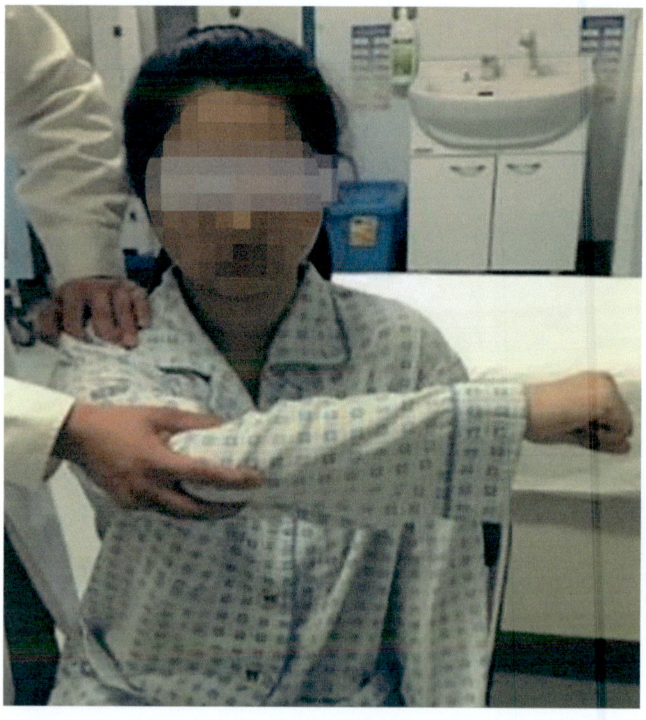

Fig. 13.3 The inability of the right upper limb to descend in the adducted position of the shoulder joint

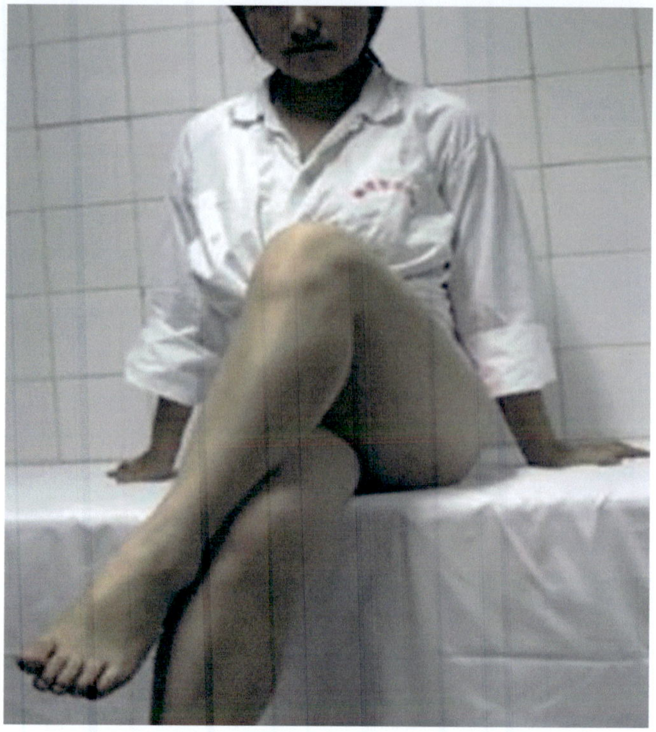

Fig. 13.4 Limited range of motion in crossing the legs bilaterally

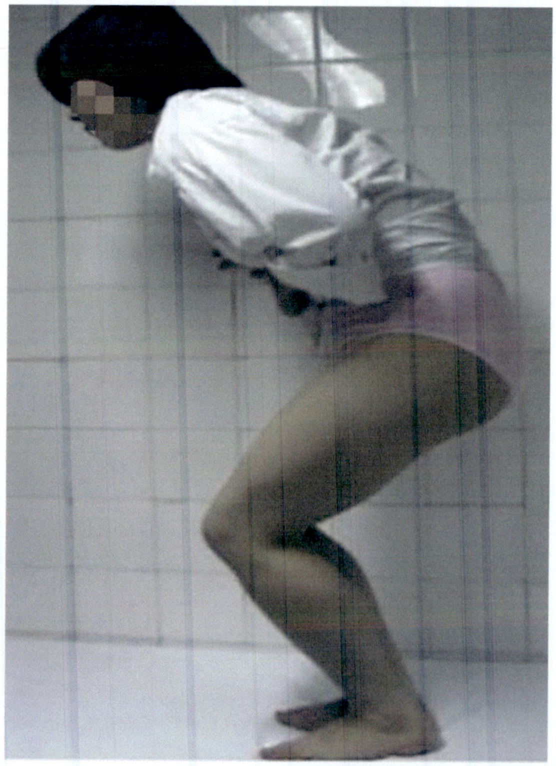

Fig. 13.5 Limited squatting capacity attributed to gluteal muscle contraction

squats (Fig. 13.5). Atrophy of the gluteal muscles is observed, presenting as a monkey-butt-like change (Fig. 13.6). X-ray examination reveals abnormal anatomical structures in both shoulder joints, resembling a light bulb sign (Fig. 13.7).

The patient was clinically diagnosed with deltoid and gluteal muscle contractures induced by injections. Under general anesthesia, arthroscopic procedures were carried out to release bilateral deltoid contracture and gluteal muscle contracture. During the examination under anesthesia, it was discovered that both shoulder joints exhibited stiffness, accompanied by snapping and a sensation of bouncing during passive movement. Additionally, there was limited range of motion in shoulder adduction and internal rotation.

A 2-cm arthroscopic approach was performed below the acromion, along the anterior and posterior borders of the deltoid muscle (Fig. 13.8). Utilizing arthroscopic guidance, shaving and debridement of contracted adipose tissue and fibrous tissue were conducted (Fig. 13.9), revealing a cord-like appearance of the contracted deltoid muscle beneath the acromion (Fig. 13.9). The radiofrequency blade is used to cut the contracted band along the inferior and posterior border of the acromion, while preserving muscle tissue (Fig. 13.10). The posterior bundle the posterior deltoid fasciculus contracture band is released along the posterior and inferior border of the acromion (Fig. 13.11). Postoperative functional

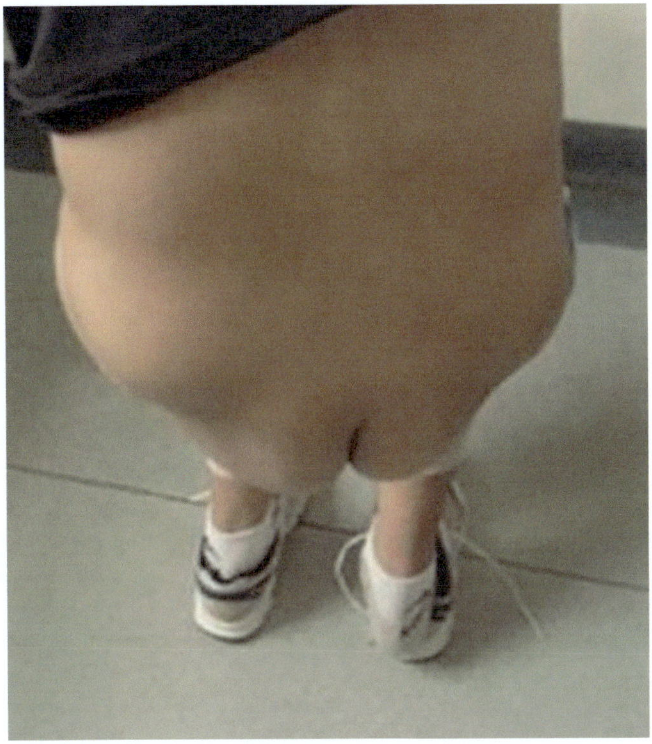

Fig. 13.6 The patient exhibited deformities in the buttock area, displaying changes resembling those seen in monkeys

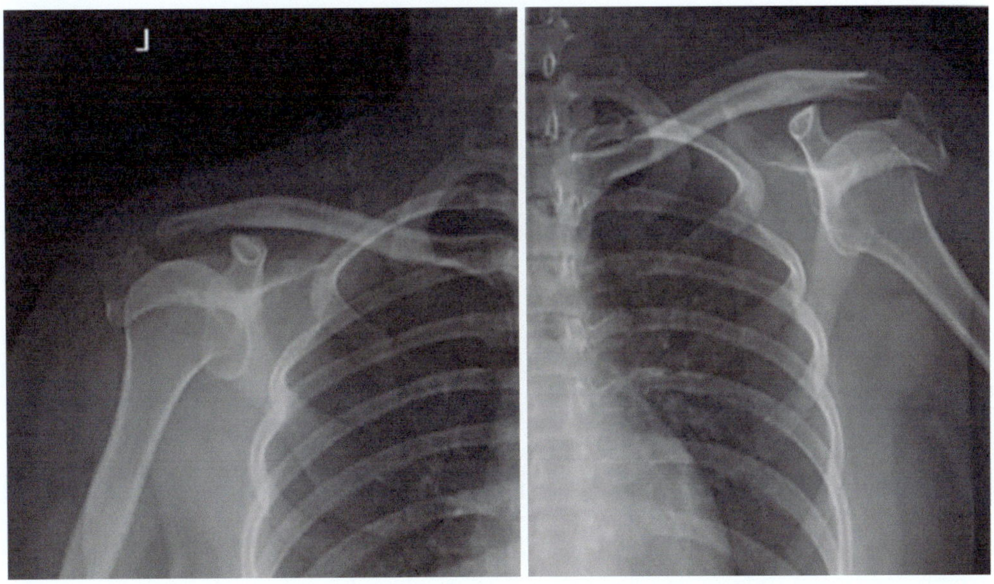

Fig. 13.7 Radiographs showed bulb-like signs in both shoulders

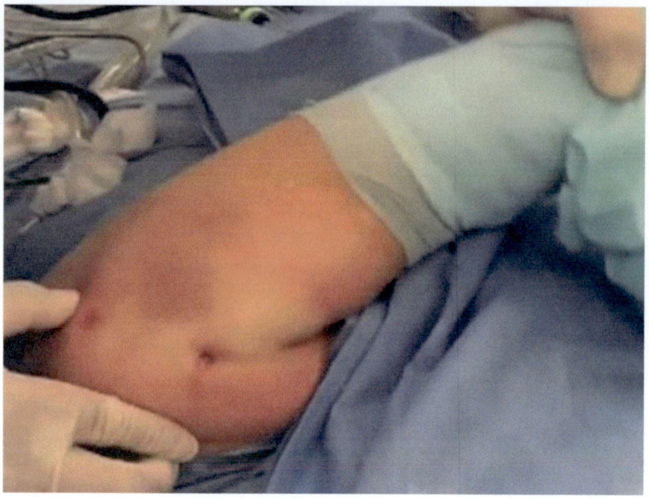

Fig. 13.8 Surgical approaches for arthroscopic release of deltoid contracture

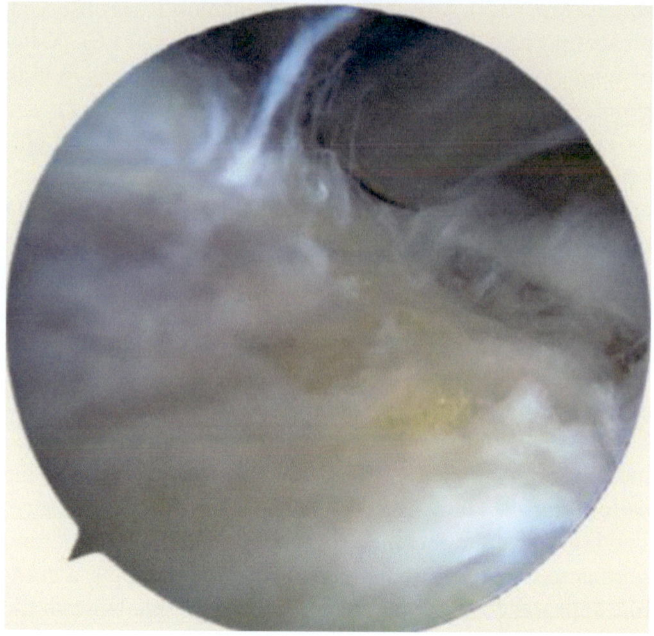

Fig. 13.9 The adipose fibrous tissue on the surface of the deltoid contracture band was debrided to make a working field for arthroscopic intervention

Fig. 13.10 Arthroscopic release of the subacromial deltoid contracture band using a radiofrequency blade

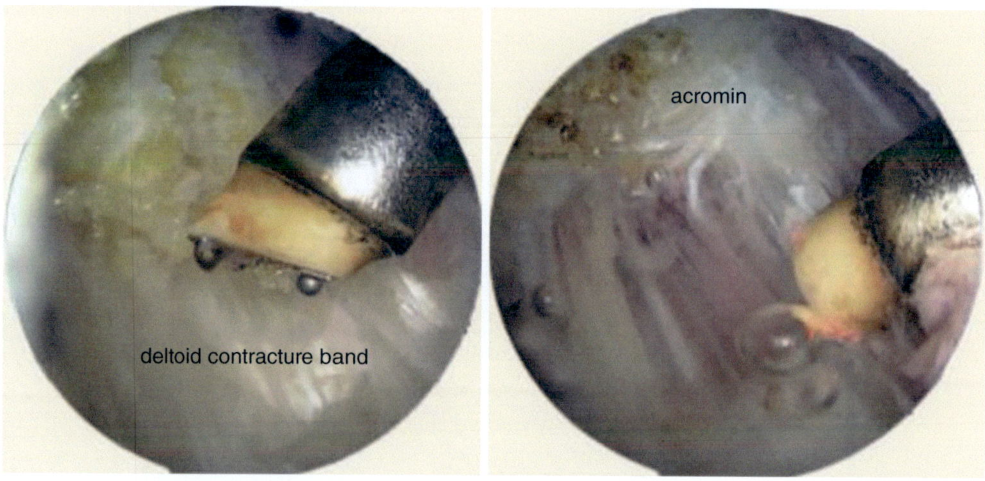

rehabilitation training is conducted. A comparison between preoperative (Fig. 13.12) and postoperative (Fig. 13.13) images demonstrates that after 6 months, the deltoid muscle exhibits enhanced fullness and has returned to its normal state. There are no limitations observed in shoulder joint abduction, external rotation, adduction, or internal rotation. Shoulder joint range of motion and function have been completely restored.

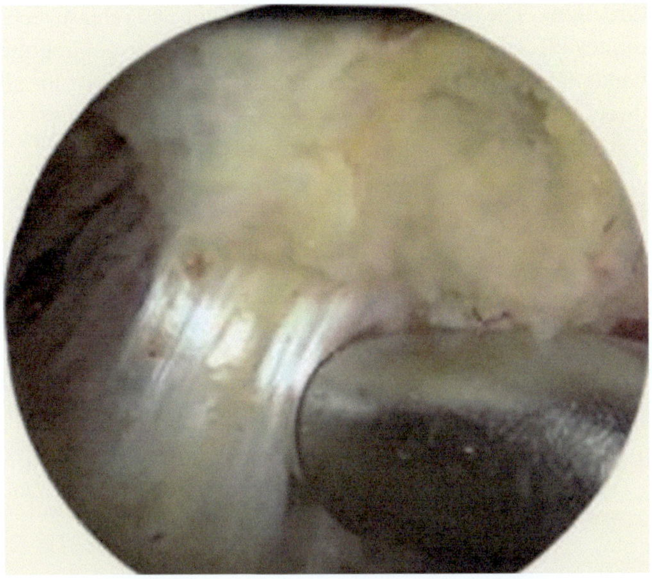

Fig. 13.11 Release of the contracture band of the posterior deltoid bundle along the posterior inferior border of the acromion

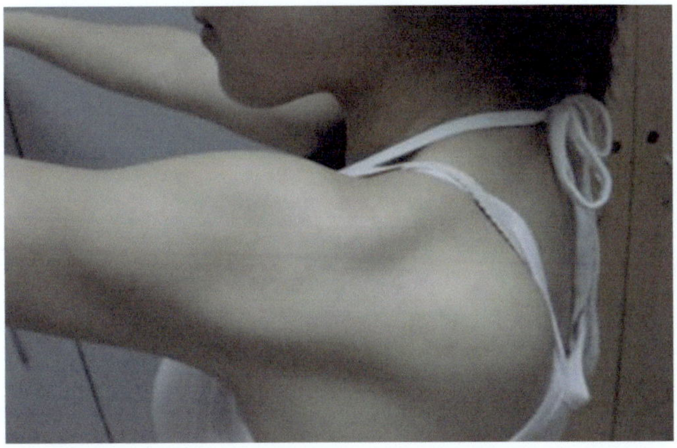

Fig. 13.12 Preoperatively, the patient presents depression in the posterior lateral region of the deltoid

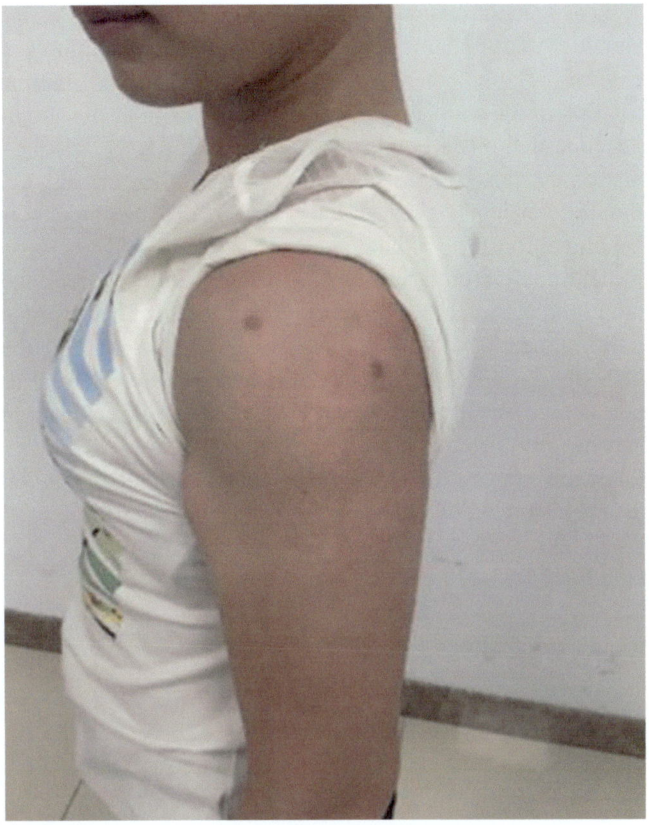

Fig. 13.13 Postoperatively, the deltoid muscle regained its full shape, and the function of the shoulder joint returned to normal

13.2 Misunderstandings in Diagnosis and Treatment, As Well as Their Countermeasures

Injection-induced gluteal muscle contracture is a common condition, whereas injection-induced deltoid muscle contracture is rare, and the majority lacks sufficient knowledge of this condition. Most patients were caused by the long-term and repeated intramuscular injection of benzyl penicillin due to frequent colds, fevers, pneumonia, or other chronic diseases in childhood. The presence of a history of deltoid injection should be inquired about and the possibility of deltoid muscle contracture should be assessed when dealing with patients presenting gluteal muscle contracture [1–3].

Due to contracture of the posterior deltoid bundle, the shoulder joint remains in a prolonged state of abduction and external rotation, thereby impeding adduction and internal rotation of the shoulder joint. The X-ray image of the shoulder joint exhibits a bulb sign, which can easily be misdiagnosed as posterior dislocation. The utilization of CT three-dimensional reconstruction and MRI techniques is beneficial for differential diagnosis [3].

The contracture band should be meticulously debrided along the acromial border at the deltoid attachment using a radiofrequency blade, with utmost care taken to preserve the integrity of the deltoid musculature during surgery. The axillary nerve, which extends 4 cm beyond the acromion, should be carefully considered and protected during surgical release. After the surgery, a comprehensive passive range of motion assessment should be conducted for the shoulder joint in all directions. The application of joint massage and release techniques effectively may alleviate any small fiber contracture bands until unrestricted movement was achieved in all directions.

References

1. Ko JY, An KN, Yamamoto R. Contracture of the deltoid muscle. Results of distal release. J Bone Joint Surg Am. 1998;80(2):229–38. https://doi.org/10.2106/00004623-199802000-00010.
2. Ogawa K, Inokuchi W, Naniwa T. Subacromial impingement associated with deltoid contracture. A report of two cases. J Bone Joint Surg Am. 1999;81(12):1744–6. https://doi.org/10.2106/00004623-199912000-00013.
3. Ogawa K, Takahashi M, Naniwa T. Deltoid contracture: MR imaging features. Clin Radiol. 2001;56(2):146–9. https://doi.org/10.1053/crad.2000.0589.

Part VI

Clavicular Fracture: A Guide and Summary

Chang-ming Huang

Guides

This part focuses on introducing cases of delayed brachial plexus paralysis caused by old clavicle fractures, misdiagnosis and missed diagnosis of distal clavicle fractures, and errors in loop plate suspension fixation for distal clavicle fractures. The causes of these errors are analyzed, and relevant complications of titanium cable strong internal fixation between the coracoid and clavicle for distal clavicle fractures, as well as postoperative precautions and revision methods for failed loop plate suspension fixation are proposed.

Summary

Middle clavicle fracture should pay attention to whether it is accompanied by brachial plexus or vascular injury. Due to the brachial plexus nerve passing through the scalene triangle and intercostal space before reaching the upper arm, it may be damaged due to displaced clavicle fracture or upper limb traction. Detailed examination is the key to avoiding missed diagnosis.

Distal clavicle fractures are prone to misdiagnosis and missed diagnosis. In addition to routine X-ray examination, CT three-dimensional reconstruction is crucial for diagnosis and fracture classification before surgery. Distal clavicle fractures are fixed with strong titanium cables between the coracoid and clavicle, which can lead to complications such as cutting the coracoid process and cable breakage. Early postoperative attention should be paid to the immobilization of the affected shoulder, and the affected limb should be immobilized with an abduction brace to avoid limb sagging, which can reduce the occurrence of postoperative complications of internal fixation.

The use of plate or coracoclavicular loop plate suspension fixation for distal clavicle fractures is a commonly used surgical method by scholars both domestically and internationally. Postoperative loop rupture is relatively rare, and the reason may be related to early excessive movement. The clavicle hook plate has unique complications, and it is recommended to use it as little as possible. It should only be used as a substitute when combined with coracoid process fractures or coracoid process loop plate fixation failure. Arthroscopic assisted double fixation of the coracoid process and clavicle can improve fracture healing rate and reduce complications.

C.-m. Huang (✉)
Department of Orthopedics, The 73rd Group Army Hospital,
Chenggong Hospital Affiliated to Xiamen University, Xiamen, China

Clavicle Fracture

14

Yu-jie Liu, Jun-liang Wang, and Chang-ming Huang

14.1 Introduction

This chapter mainly introduces the cases of old clavicular fracture complicated with brachial plexus delayed palsy, missed diagnosis and misdiagnosis of distal clavicular fracture, and the error of loop plate suspension fixation of distal clavicular fracture, analyzes the causes of occurrence, and puts forward the complications related to the rigid internal fixation of coracoclavicular titanium cable, the attention after loop plate suspension fixation, and the revision methods after failure.

14.1.1 Old Clavicular Fracture Complicated with Brachial Plexus Delayed Paralysis

14.1.1.1 Overview of the Diagnosis and Treatment Process

A 64-year-old man suffered a left clavicle fracture from a fall 5 months ago and was treated conservatively. Recently, the patient felt numbness and distension in the left upper limb, weakness in elbow flexion, upward lifting, and abduction. The sensation in the left hand is dull, with reduced palmar sensation in the thumb, index finger, and middle finger, as well as diminished dorsal skin sensation in the thumb and index finger.

Physical examination revealed: Bone eminence in the middle of the left clavicle, proximal tip of clavicle lift up, Tinel sign (+). Left upper limb muscle atrophy compared to the contralateral. Weak flexion, abduction and wrist extension of the left shoulder joint. No abnormalities were found in the abduction, adduction, and palmar function of the left thumb. Biceps reflex (−), triceps reflex (−), paper clamp test (−), left wrist flexion muscle strength 4−, wrist extension muscle strength 4, elbow flexion muscle strength 3+, elbow extension muscle strength 3+, shoulder shrug muscle strength 5, shoulder joint abduction and adduction muscle strength 3, internal rotation and external rotation muscle strength 3, forward flexion and extension muscle strength 3, and left hand grip strength 5.

Electromyography showed that the amplitude of sensory nerve conduction velocity (SCV) decreased in the left median nerve and ulnar nerve. The amplitude of motor nerve conduction velocity (MCV) on the left median nerve was lower than that on the right. F-wave detection: The F-wave latency of the left median nerve was longer than that of the right.

Imaging examination: CT three-dimensional reconstruction showed displacement of the fracture end of the clavicle, malunion, and callus formation at the fracture end of the fracture (Fig. 14.1); MRI showed clear structure of brachial plexus nerve roots, continuous nerves, abnormal signals below the fracture end of the clavicle, and compression of the brachial plexus nerve at the fracture end (Fig. 14.2).

After exploration under general anesthesia, it was found that the brachial plexus at the end of the fracture was compressed, the hyperplasia of the callus and scar tissue were removed, the brachial plexus was explored and released, and the clavicular fracture was fixed with anatomic reduction plate and screw. Postoperative X-rays showed good alignment and alignment of the fracture (Fig. 14.3). After 2 weeks, the numbness of the left hand gradually disappeared, and the sensory and motor function of the left upper limb gradually recovered.

Y.-j. Liu
Orthopaedics, Chinese PLA General Hospital, Beijing, China

J.-l. Wang (✉)
Department of Orthopedics, Hainan Hospital of Chinese PLA General Hospital, Sanya, China

C.-m. Huang
Department of Orthopedics, The 73rd Group Army Hospital, Chenggong Hospital Affiliated to Xiamen University, Xiamen, China

Y.-j. Liu et al. (eds.), *Pitfalls in Diagnosis and Treatment of Shoulder Joint Diseases*,
https://doi.org/10.1007/978-981-96-2472-0_14

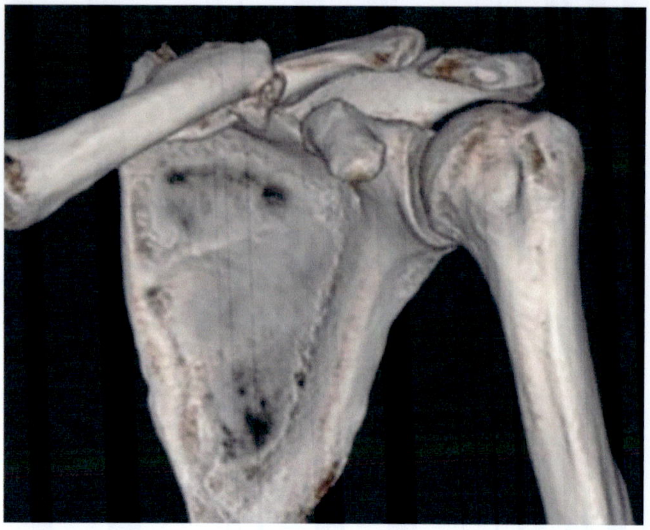

Fig. 14.1 3D-CT reconstruction shows displacements and malunion of the clavicle fracture

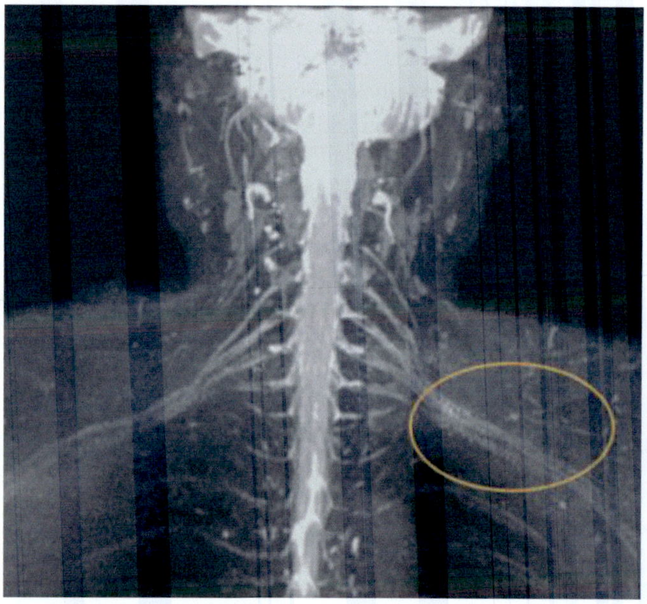

Fig. 14.2 MRI showed abnormal brachial plexus signals in the left clavicular fracture area

14.1.2 Experience of Diagnosis and Treatment

Clavicle fracture should be noted whether it is combined with brachial plexus or vascular injury. The brachial plexus, passing through the scalene triangle and the costoclavicular space, may be injured by a displaced clavicle fracture or an upper limb pull. Delayed injury caused by hypertrophic callus or clavicular bone impinging on the brachial plexus is rare [1–3]. Rowe [4] counted 690 cases of clavicle fracture, and only two cases were complicated with delayed neurological and vascular symptoms. A clavicle fracture with delayed brachial plexus injury may occur weeks, months, or years after the fracture. Hypertrophic callus of clavicle fractures often compresses the medial brachial plexus bundle, which may also cause compression of the posterior brachial plexus bundle. Once delayed brachial plexus palsy occurs, callus compression should be highly suspected, and three-dimensional CT reconstruction is helpful for definitive diagnosis. Once confirmed, brachial plexus exploration decompression, removal of callus, fracture reduction, and internal fixation should be performed as soon as possible.

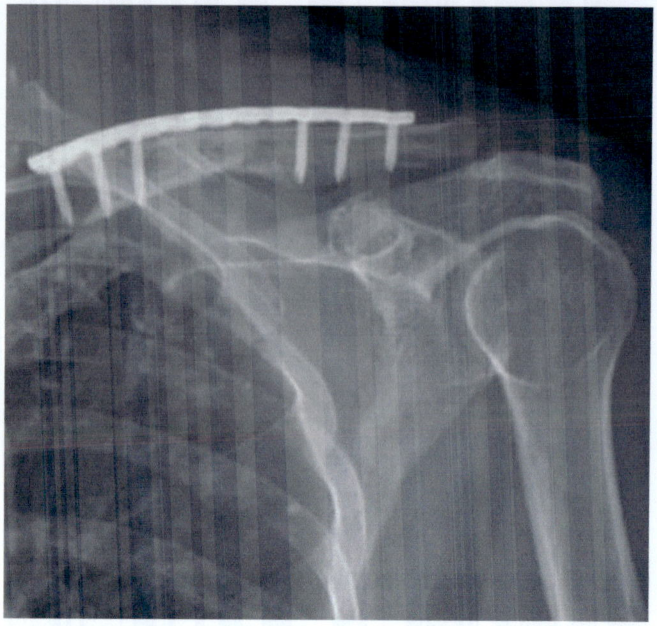

Fig. 14.3 Postoperative X-ray examination showed good alignment and alignment of the clavicle fracture

References

1. Karahanoglu E, Kasapoglu T, Ozdemirci S, et al. Risk factors for clavicle fracture concurrent with brachial plexus injury. Arch Gynecol Obstet, 2016, 293(4):783–787.
2. Saito T, Matusmura T, Takeshita K. Brachial plexus palsy after clavicle fracture: 3 cases. J Shoulder Elb Surg, 2020, 29(2):e60-e65.
3. Venkatramani H, Bhardwaj P, Raja S, et al. Floating shoulder injury resulting in delayed onset of infraclavicular brachial plexus palsy. J Hand Surg Asian Pac 2020, 25(4):499–503.
4. Rowe CR. An atlas of anatomy and treatment of midclavicular fractures. Clin Orthop Relat Res. 1968;58:29–42.

Misunderstandings and Countermeasures of Distal Clavicle Fracture

15

Chang-ming Huang, Yu-jie Liu, and Tian-hao Zhu

15.1 Overview of the Condition

15.1.1 Case I: Missed Diagnosis of Distal Clavicle Fracture

A 29-year-old male had fallen down while running 1 day ago with complaints of left shoulder pain and activity limitations, and plain AP X-ray confirmed the irregular cortical bone of left distal clavicle (Fig. 15.1), so treated with conservative therapy. After 5 days, he complaining of significantly increasing swelling and pain, with restriction of the left shoulder movement. On physical examination, the patient had a tender left shoulder with superficial ecchymoses and positive piano key sign. Three-dimensional CT reconstruction revealed a superiorly displacement of the proximal of distal clavicle fracture, so the surgical treatment was chosen (Fig. 15.2).

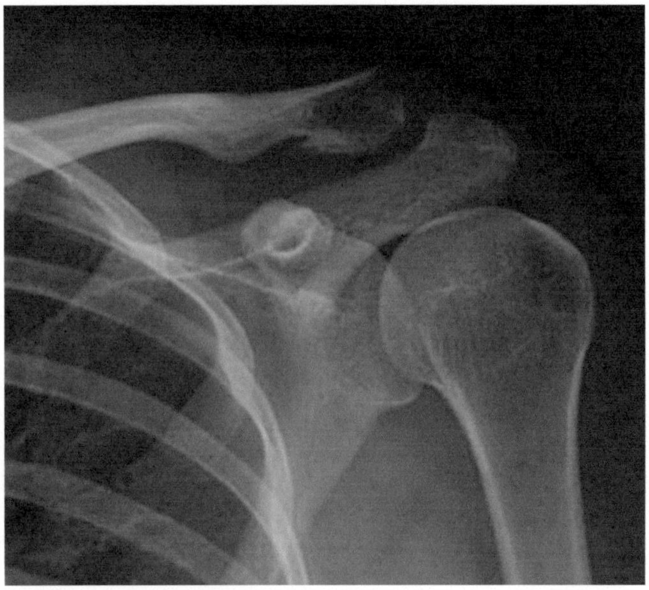

Fig. 15.1 Plain AP X-ray confirmed the irregular cortical bone of left distal clavicle

15.1.2 Case II: Failure of Conservative Treatment for Distal Clavicle Fracture

A 30-year-old male had fallen down while riding 7 days ago with complaints of left shoulder pain and activity limitations. Plain AP X-ray confirmed the left distal clavicle fracture without displacement (Fig. 15.3), the shoulder was then immobilized in a sling. After 1 week, the three-dimensional CT reconstruction revealed a displacement of the left distal clavicle fracture(Fig. 15.4). So the lateral clavicular plate and titanium cable fixation was chosen(Fig. 15.5).

15.1.3 Case III: Coracoid Process Was Cut after Titanium Cable Fixation of Distal Clavicle Fracture

A 39-year-old male had injury 2 days ago with complaints of right shoulder pain and activity limitations, and plain AP X-ray confirmed the right distal clavicle fracture (Fig. 15.6), the three-dimensional CT reconstruction revealed a displacement of the right distal clavicle fracture (Fig. 15.7). One year follow-up after the lateral clavicular plate and titanium cable fixation treatment (Fig. 15.8), the right shoulder joint regain good function, and X-ray and three-dimensional CT reconstruction revealed that the fracture union was achieved, but the coracoid process was cut (Fig. 15.9).

The original version of the chapter has been revised. A correction to this chapter can be found at https://doi.org/10.1007/978-981-96-2472-0_30

C.-m. Huang (✉) · T.-h. Zhu
Department of Orthopedics, The 73rd Group Army Hospital, Chenggong Hospital Affiliated to Xiamen University, Xiamen, China

Y.-j. Liu
Orthopaedics, Chinese PLA General Hospital, Beijing, China

Y.-j. Liu et al. (eds.), *Pitfalls in Diagnosis and Treatment of Shoulder Joint Diseases*,
https://doi.org/10.1007/978-981-96-2472-0_15

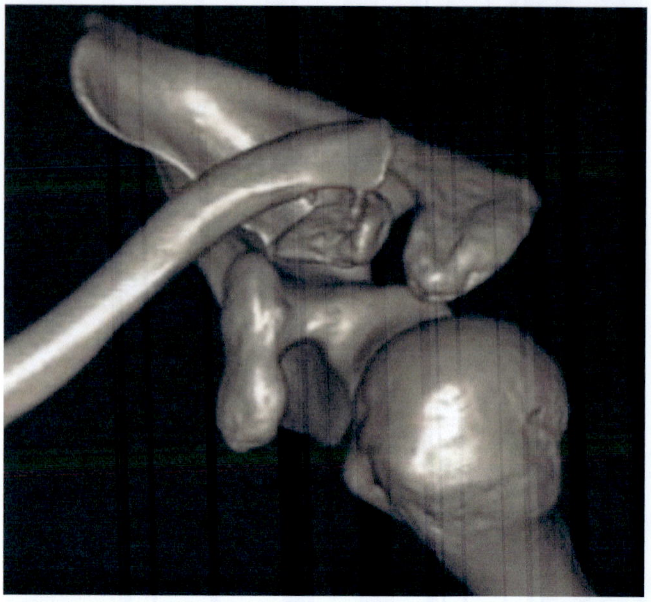

Fig. 15.2 Three-dimensional CT reconstruction revealed a superiorly displacement of the proximal of distal clavicle fracture of the left shoulder

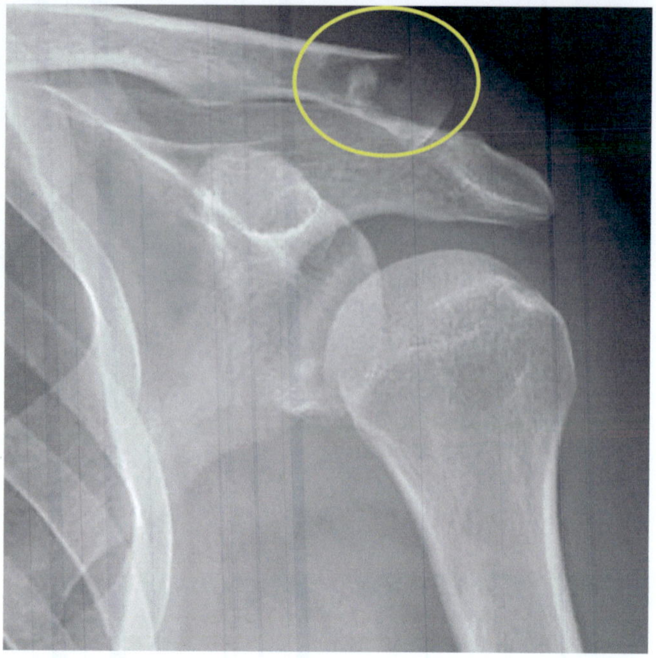

Fig. 15.3 Plain AP X-ray confirmed the left distal clavicle fracture without displacement

Fig. 15.4 The three-dimensional CT reconstruction revealed a displacement of the left distal clavicle fracture

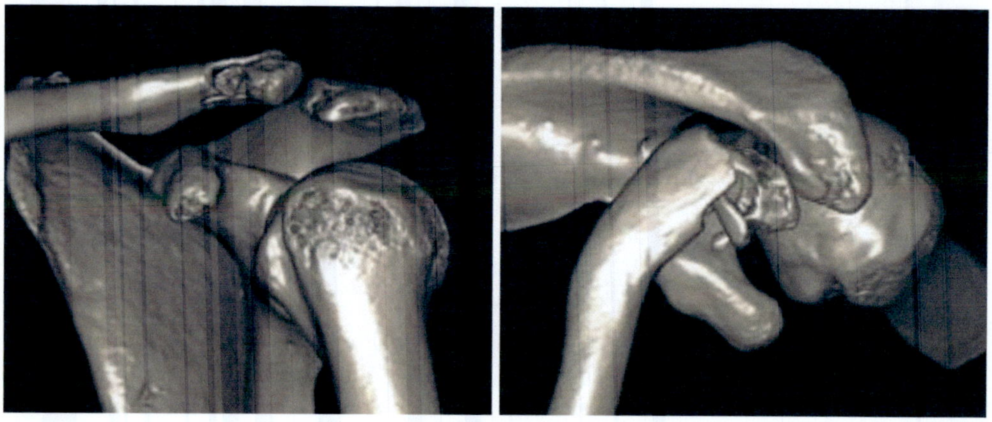

15.1.4 Case IV: Breakage of Titanium Cable after Titanium Cable Fixation of Distal Clavicle Fracture

A 39-year-old female had injury 1 days ago with complaints of left shoulder pain and activity limitations. X-ray and three-dimensional CT reconstruction revealed left lateral clavicle comminuted fracture (Fig. 15.10). After the plate and cerclage wires fixation treatment (Fig. 15.11), postoperative X-ray revealed that fracture reduction and position of internal fixtures are satisfactory (Fig. 15.12). Four months follow-up after surgery, X-ray revealed breakage of titanium cable, without displacement of fracture, and the fracture union was achieved (Fig. 15.13). The left shoulder joint regain normal function, after then, we performed internal fixation removal surgery (Fig. 15.14).

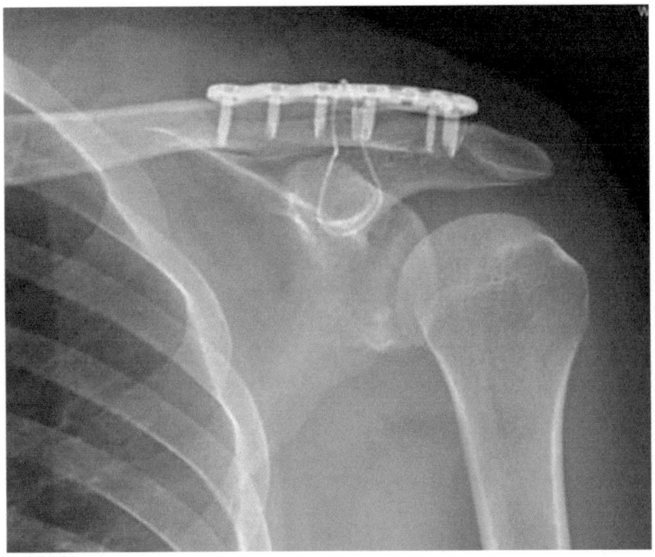

Fig. 15.5 Postoperative X-ray revealed the lateral clavicular plate and titanium cable fixation

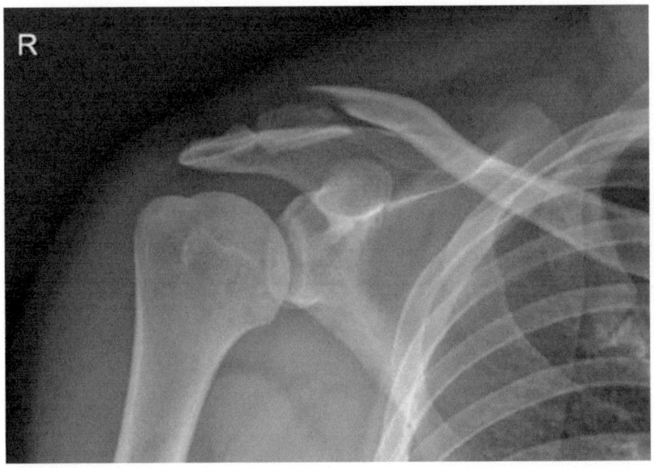

Fig. 15.6 Plain AP X-ray confirmed the right distal clavicle fracture

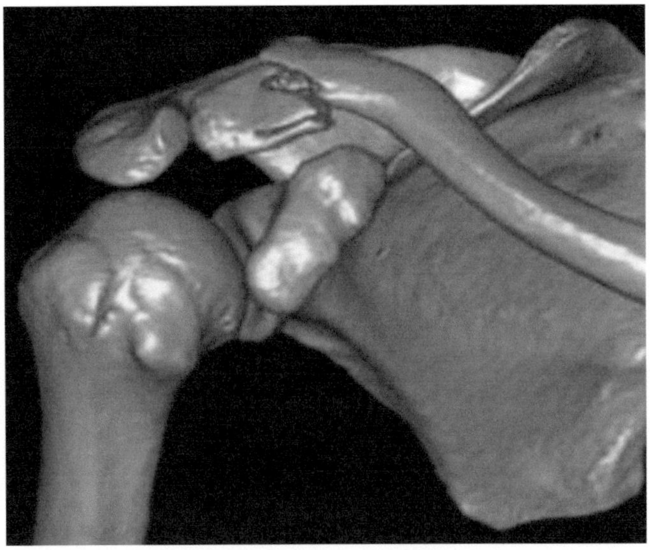

Fig. 15.7 The three-dimensional CT reconstruction revealed a displacement of the right distal clavicle fracture

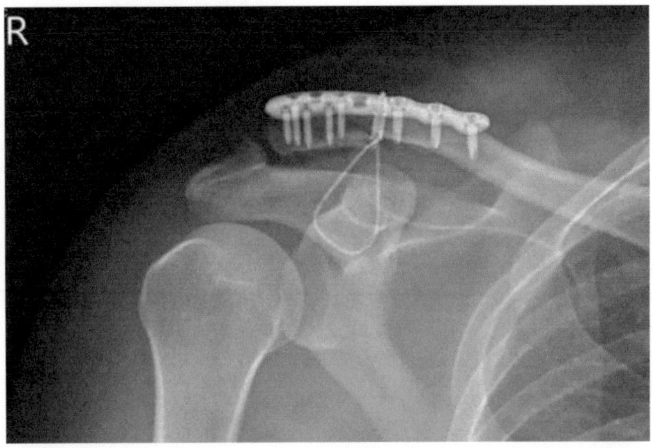

Fig. 15.8 Postoperative X-ray revealed anatomical reduction of fractures

15.1.5 Case V: Failure and Breakage of Titanium Cable After Titanium Cable Fixation for Distal Clavicle Fracture

A 47-year-old male had injury 1 month ago with complaints of left shoulder pain and activity limitations, was diagnosed with shoulder joint soft tissue injury, and chose conservative treatment, but ineffective. One month after the initial treatment, an outpatient X-ray revealed lateral clavicle comminuted fracture (Fig. 15.15). After hospitalization, clavicle fracture reduction with plate internal fixation and titanium cable coracoclavicular internal fixation surgery (Fig. 15.16). Four months after the plate and titanium cable fixation treatment, X-ray revealed breakage of titanium cable, and the fracture union was not achieved. Then we chose another surgery (Fig. 15.17)

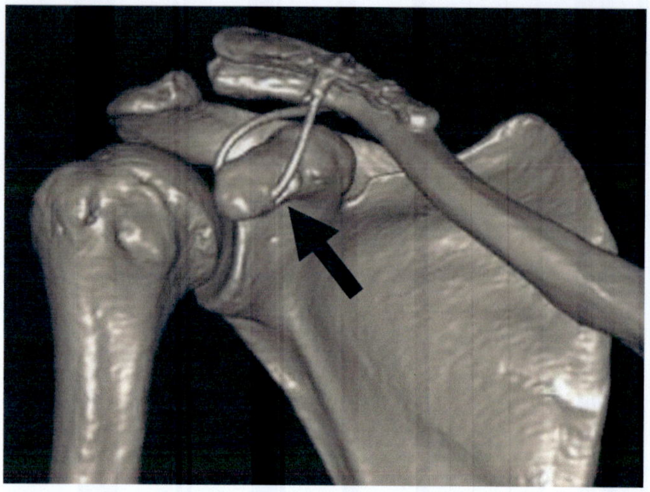

Fig. 15.9 Three-dimensional CT reconstruction revealed the fracture union was achieved, but the coracoid process was cut

Fig. 15.10 X-ray and three-dimensional CT reconstruction revealed left lateral clavicle comminuted fracture

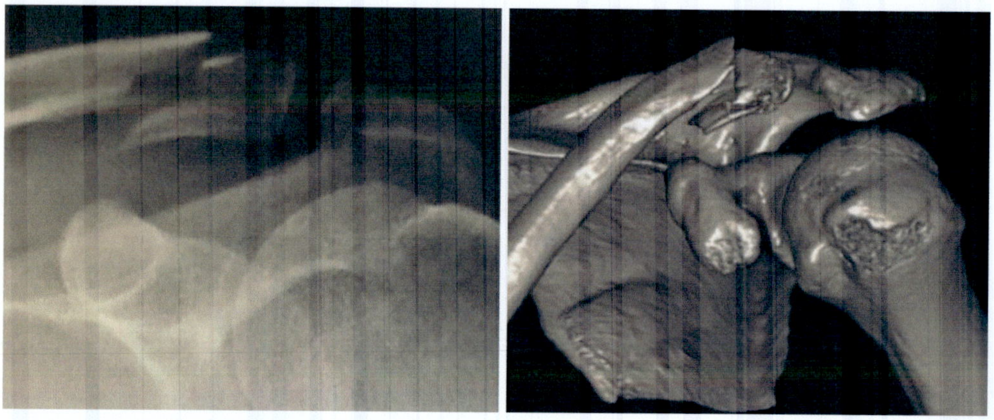

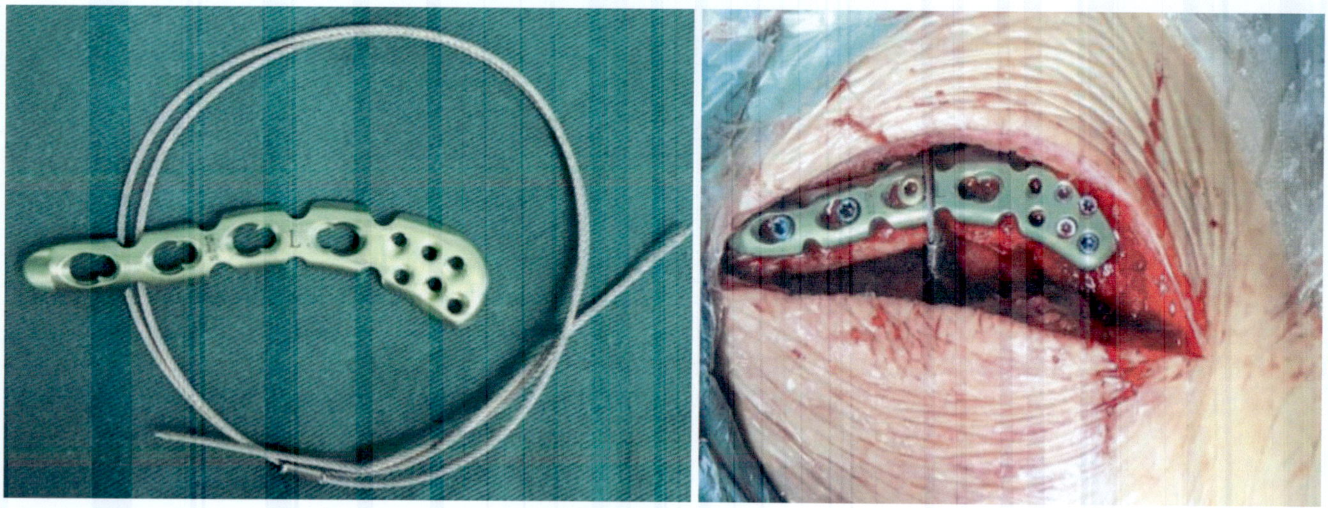

Fig. 15.11 Internal fixation materials and the situation after clavicle reduction and internal fixation

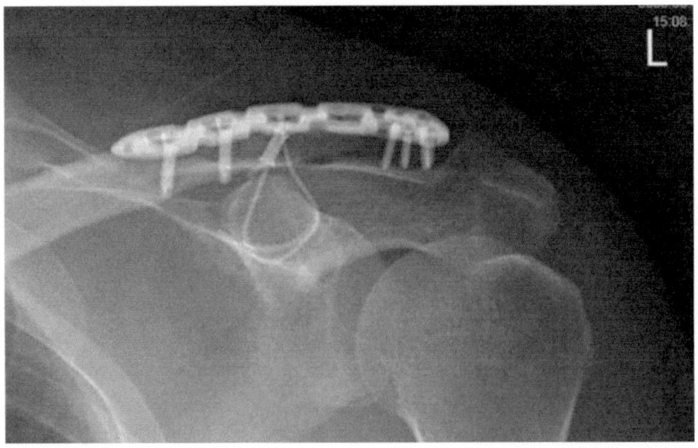

Fig. 15.12 Postoperative X-ray revealed fracture reduction and position of internal fixtures are satisfactory

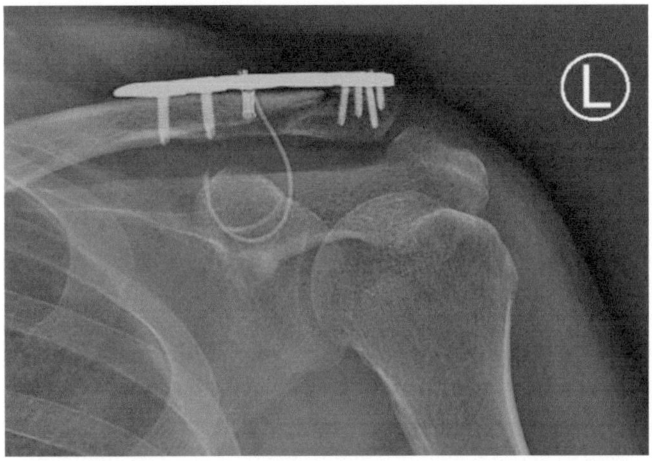

Fig. 15.13 Four months follow-up after surgery, X-ray revealed breakage of titanium cable, without displacement of fracture, and the fracture union was achieved

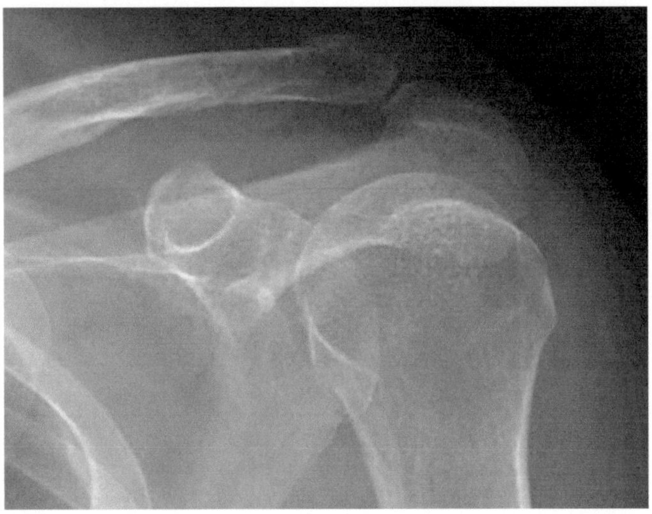

Fig. 15.14 One-year follow-up after surgery, we performed internal fixation removal surgery

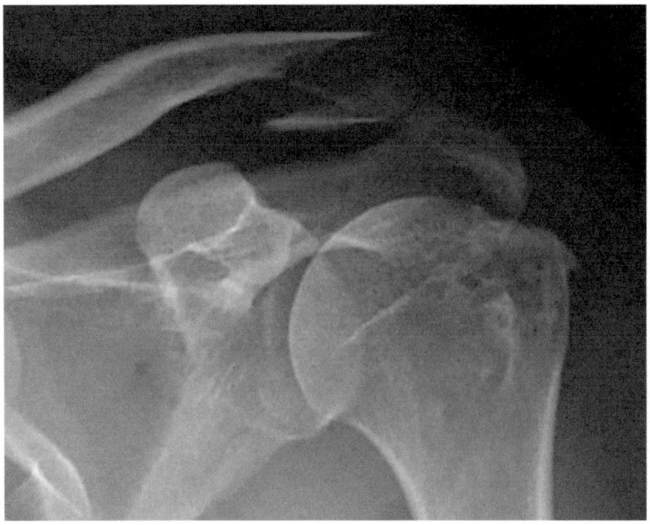

Fig. 15.15 Preoperative X-ray revealed lateral clavicle comminuted fracture

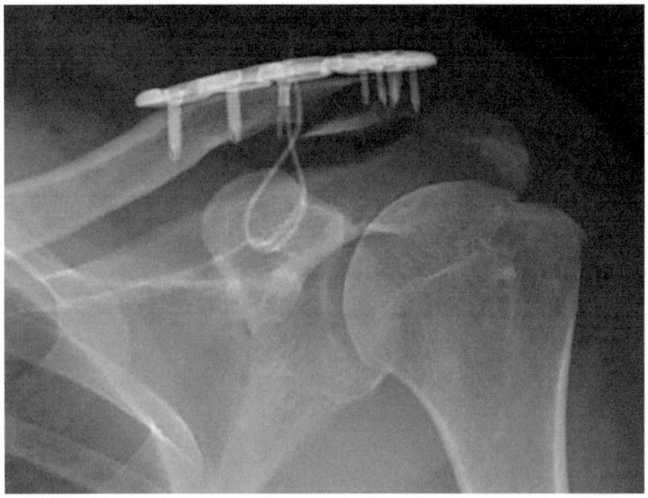

Fig. 15.16 Postoperative X-ray revealed a displacement of the distal clavicle fracture fragment

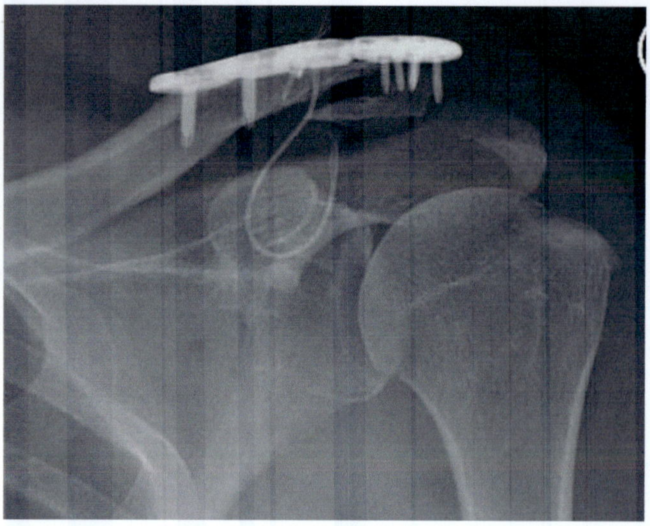

Fig. 15.17 Four months after the surgery, X-ray revealed breakage of titanium cable, and displacement of the distal clavicle fracture fragment

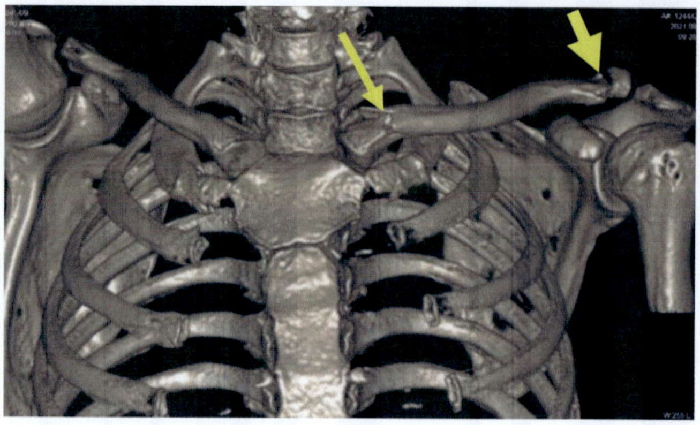

Fig. 15.18 The three-dimensional CT reconstruction revealed the left medial clavicle fracture and distal clavicle fracture

15.2 Misunderstandings and Countermeasures of Distal Clavicle Fracture

The distal clavicle fracture fragment is small, medial fracture fragment always move posterior, resulting in overlapping of fracture fragments, so a plain AP X-ray always missed diagnosis. When fracture is suspected, make sure the three-dimensional CT reconstruction was performed, it can clear diagnosis the distal clavicle fracture and rare bipolar fracture of clavicle (Fig. 15.18).

The distal clavicle fracture is accounting for 12–15% of all clavicular fractures [1, 2], and nonunion rate was 30% [3, 4]. Neer [5, 6] classified distal clavicle fractures into five types (Fig. 15.19): Type IIB is distal clavicle fracture, which results in loss of stability of the coracoclavicular ligament. The proximal end of a clavicle fracture is pulled upward and backward by the sternocleidomastoid and trapezius muscles, while the distal end is pulled downward and inward by the weight of the limb or the pectoralis major, pectoralis minor and latissimus dorsi muscles. When fracture is close to the acromioclavicular joint, proximal fracture is pulled by trapezius muscle, causing fracture displacement when conservative treatment is chosen. Lateral fracture fragments always move posterior, so a plain AP X-ray always missed diagnosis. The three-dimensional CT reconstruction can help to clarify fracture displacement and avoid missed diagnosis and delayed treatment.

We are not only consider classification of the distal clavicle fracture but also need pay attention to the injury of acromioclavicular ligament and coracoclavicular ligament. Old fractures should be treated with fresh treatment and then anatomical reduction and internal fixation with plates to avoid bone nonunion or internal fixation failure. The distal clavicle are mostly comminuted fracture. If plate and screw fixation is adopted, the screws must penetrate the contralateral bone cortex to avoid being driven into the fracture gap, which may affecting healing. Although titanium cable fixation between the coracoid and the clavicle can compensate for the damage of the acromioclavicular and coracoclavicular ligaments, premature activity of the affected limb before fracture healing will lead to micromotion of the titanium cable between the coracoid and the clavicle and friction against the coracoid process, which may result in coracoid process avulsion fractures or titanium cable rupture. Therefore, it is very necessary to pay attention to the immobilization of the affected shoulder in the early postoperative period, use external fixations to immobilize the affected limb, and avoid the interference of sagging gravity on the fracture.

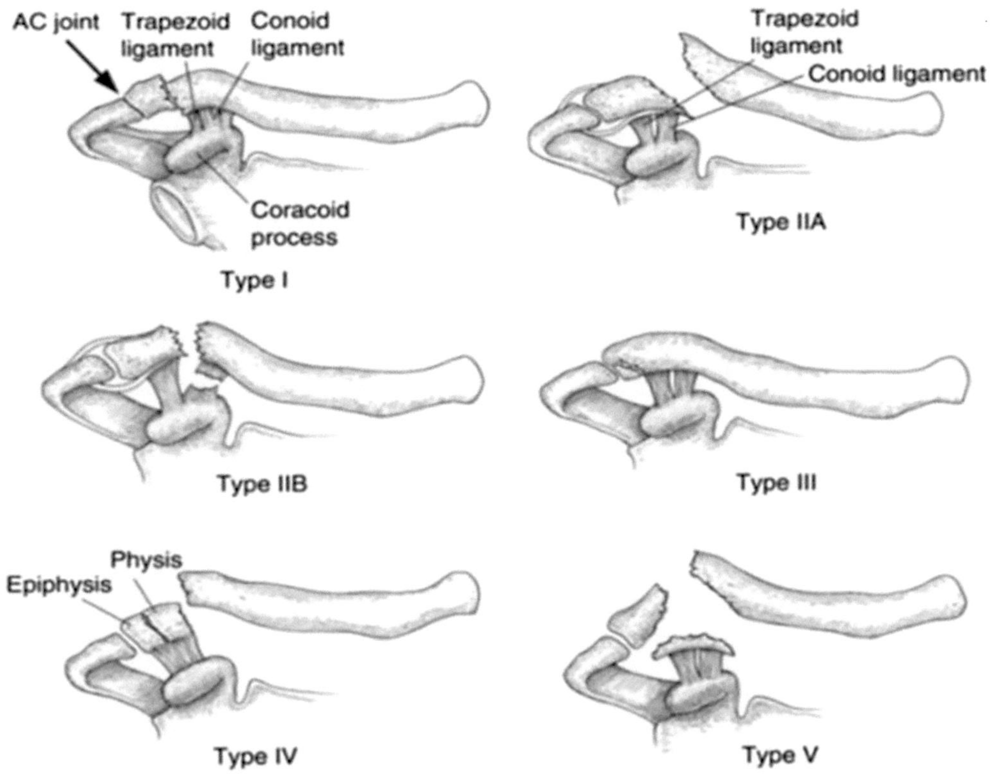

Fig. 15.19 Neer classification of the distal clavicle fracture. Source: Reprinted from the original figure

References

1. Nordqvist A, Petersson C. The incidence of fractures of the clavicle. Clin Orthop Relat Res. 1994;300:127–32.
2. Herscovici D Jr, Sanders R, DiPasquale T, et al. Injuries of the shoulder girdle. Clin Orthop Relat Res. 1995;318:54–60.
3. Robinson CM, Cairns DA. Primary nonoperative treatment of displaced lateral fractures of the clavicle. J Bone Joint Surg Am. 2004;86(4):778–82.
4. Edwards DJ, Kavanagh TG, Flannery MC. Fractures of the distal clavicle: a case for fixation. Injury. 1992;23(1):44–6.
5. Neer CS II. Fracture of the distal clavicle with detachment of the coracoclavicular ligaments in adults. J Trauma. 1963;3:99–110.
6. Neer CS II. Fractures of the distal third of the clavicle. Clin Orthop Relat Res. 1968;58:43–50.

16 Errors and Countermeasures in Suspension Fixation of Distal Bone Fracture with Coracoclavian Loop Plate

Chang-ming Huang, Yang-pan Fu, and Yu-jie Liu

16.1 Introduction

The use of plate or coracoclavicular loop plate suspension fixation for distal clavicle fractures is a commonly used surgical method by scholars both domestically and internationally [1, 2], but postoperative loop rupture is relatively rare. The reason for loop rupture may be related to early excessive exercise. Although the loop has good mechanical properties, repeated micromovements and wear can easily cause loop fracture.

There is still controversy over how to treat distal clavicle fractures. Clavicular hook plates have unique complications, and it is recommended to use them as little as possible. They should only be used as substitutes when combined with coracoid process fractures, or coracoid process loop plate fixation fails. The clavicle hook plate fixation is used for the treatment of acromioclavicular joint fractures and dislocations. Due to the slight movement of the acromion, the hook plate wears down the bone beneath the acromion, and some even experience acromion fractures. Therefore, the plate and screw should be removed as soon as possible after the fracture healing.

16.2 Overview of Disease Diagnosis and Treatment

The patient is a 55-year-old male with left shoulder trauma for 3 h. The diagnosis is a fracture of the distal left clavicle (Fig. 16.1). After admission, patients underwent distal clavicle fracture plate internal fixation and arthroscopic-assisted coracoclavian loop plate suspension fixation surgery (Fig. 16.2). Due to dysfunction of the right hand, the patient used the left hand for daily life after surgery. At 6 weeks post-surgery, there was pain in the left shoulder with a stepped protrusion. A follow-up X-ray showed displacement of the distal clavicle fracture (Fig. 16.3).

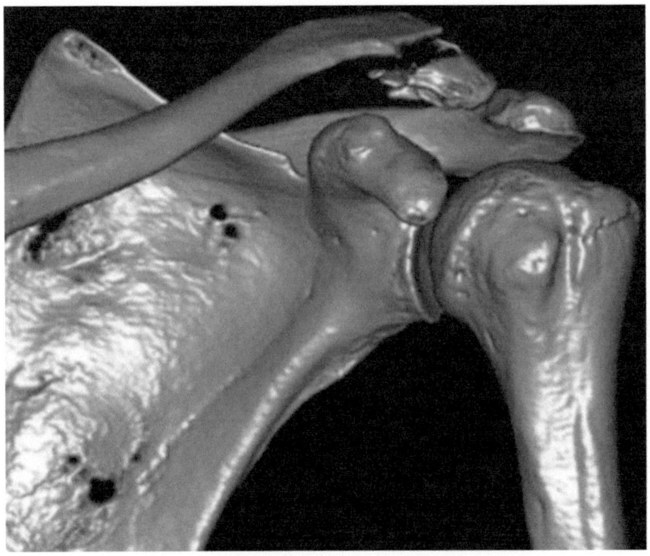

Fig. 16.1 CT three-dimensional reconstruction shows a comminuted fracture of the distal left clavicle with proximal displacement backward and upward

Hospitalized for revision surgery, intraoperative exploration revealed a ruptured loop of the plate (Fig. 16.4), which was then fixed with a hook plate (Fig. 16.5). The postoperative X-ray showed that the hook plate was firmly fixed (Fig. 16.6). The left shoulder joint function recovered well, and the distal clavicle fracture healed (Fig. 16.7). One year later, the patient was admitted to the hospital and underwent clavicle hook plate removal surgery (Fig. 16.8). During the surgery, arthroscopic exploration of the shoulder revealed that the clavicle hook plate caused groove-like bone wear on the shoulder peak (Fig. 16.9).

C.-m. Huang (✉) · Y.-p. Fu
Department of Orthopedics, The 73rd Group Army Hospital, Chenggong Hospital Affiliated to Xiamen University, Xiamen, China

Y.-j. Liu
Orthopaedics, Chinese PLA General Hospital, Beijing, China

Y.-j. Liu et al. (eds.), *Pitfalls in Diagnosis and Treatment of Shoulder Joint Diseases*,
https://doi.org/10.1007/978-981-96-2472-0_16

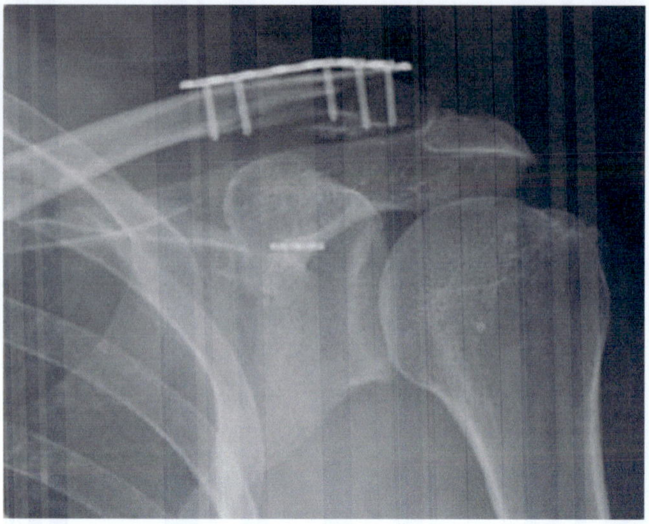

Fig. 16.2 Postoperative X-ray showing the middle screw located in the fracture gap

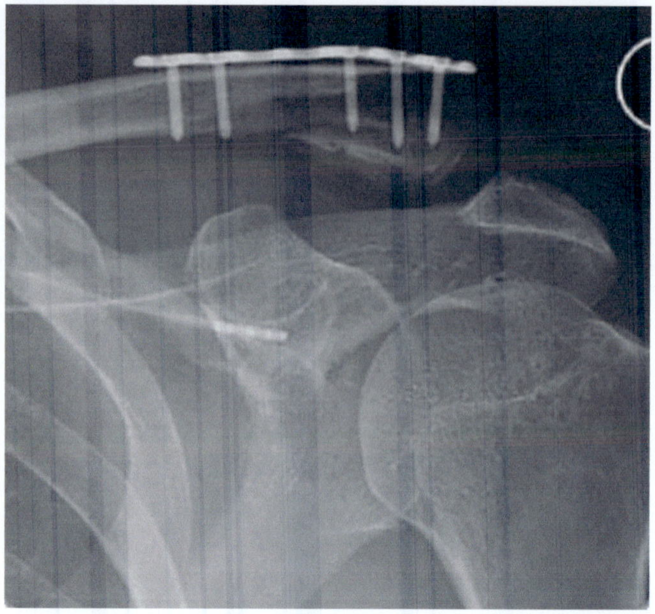

Fig. 16.3 X-ray shows fracture displacement at 6 weeks post-surgery

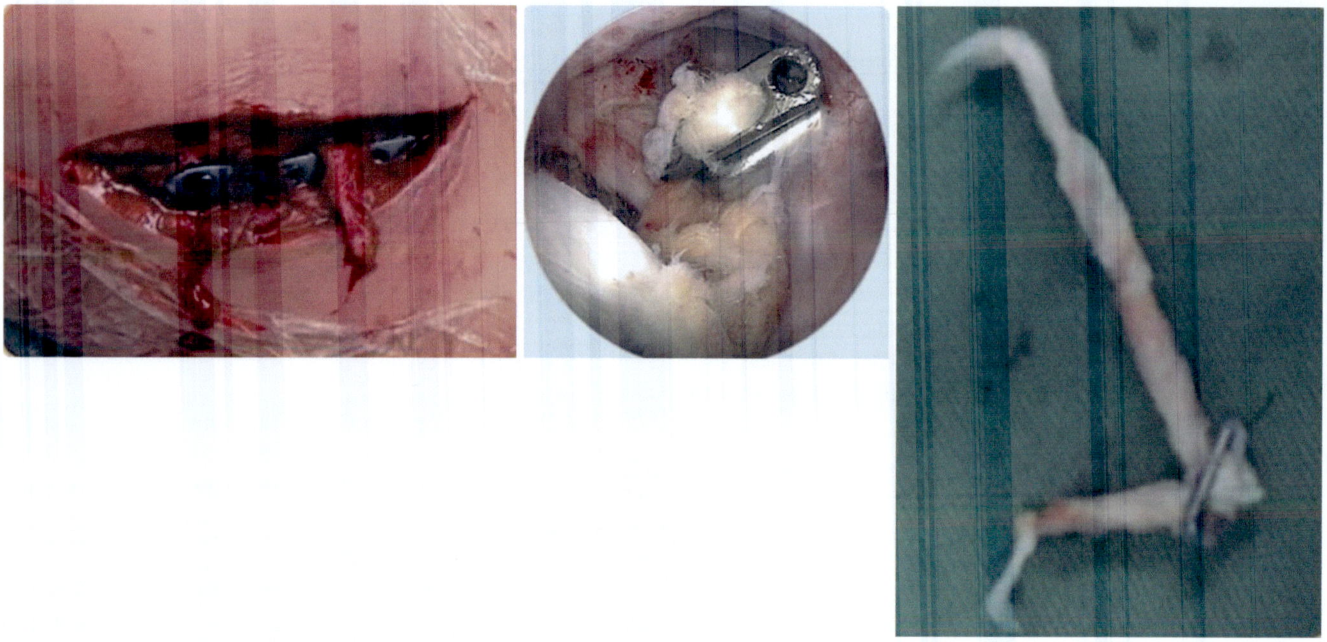

Fig. 16.4 Plate loop severance

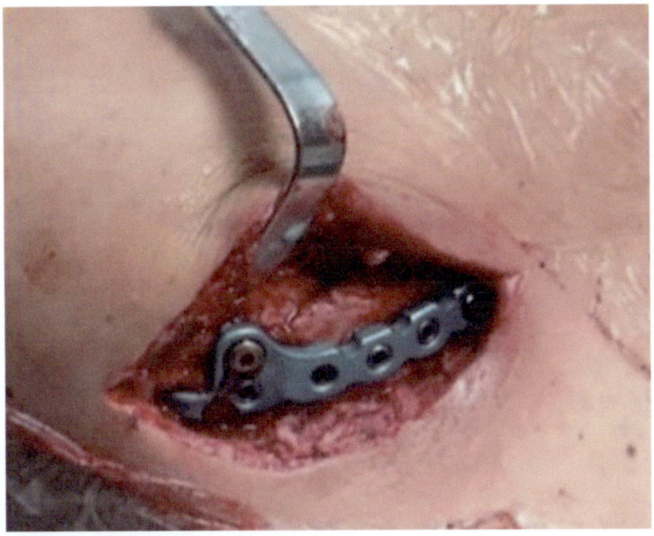

Fig. 16.5 Fixed with hook plates

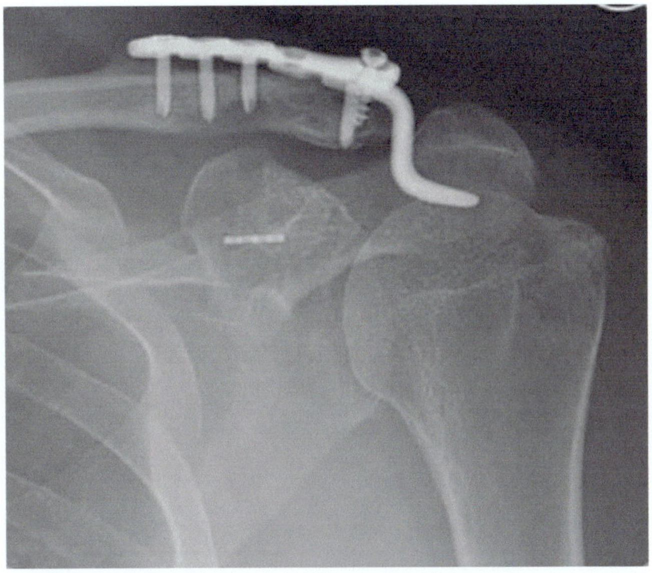

Fig. 16.7 Fracture healing 1 year after revision surgery

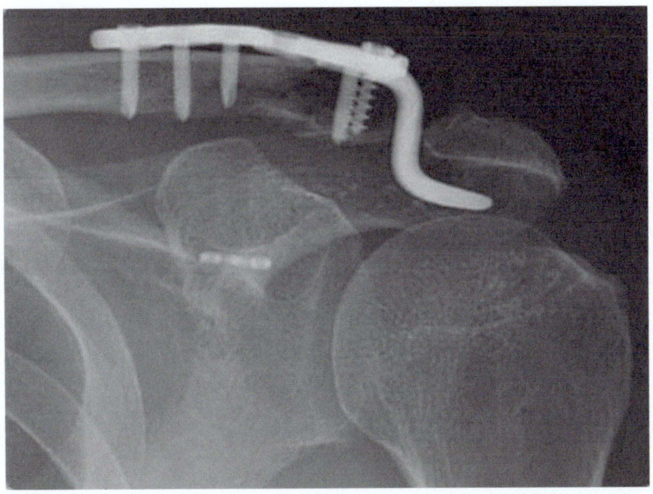

Fig. 16.6 X-ray images after revision surgery showing fracture reduction

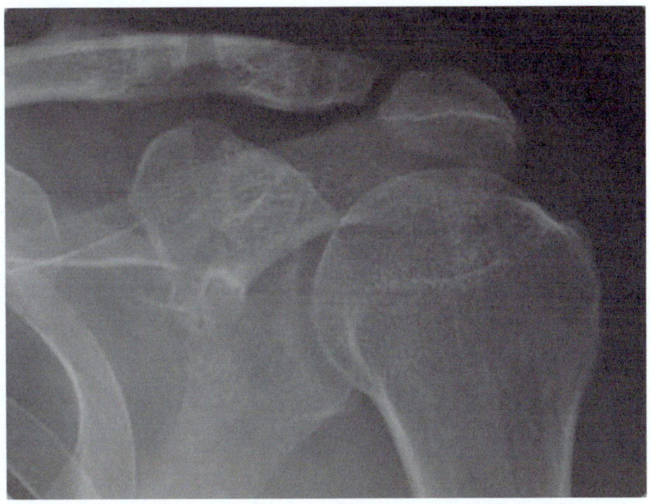

Fig. 16.8 X-ray film shows good fracture healing after removal of internal fixation

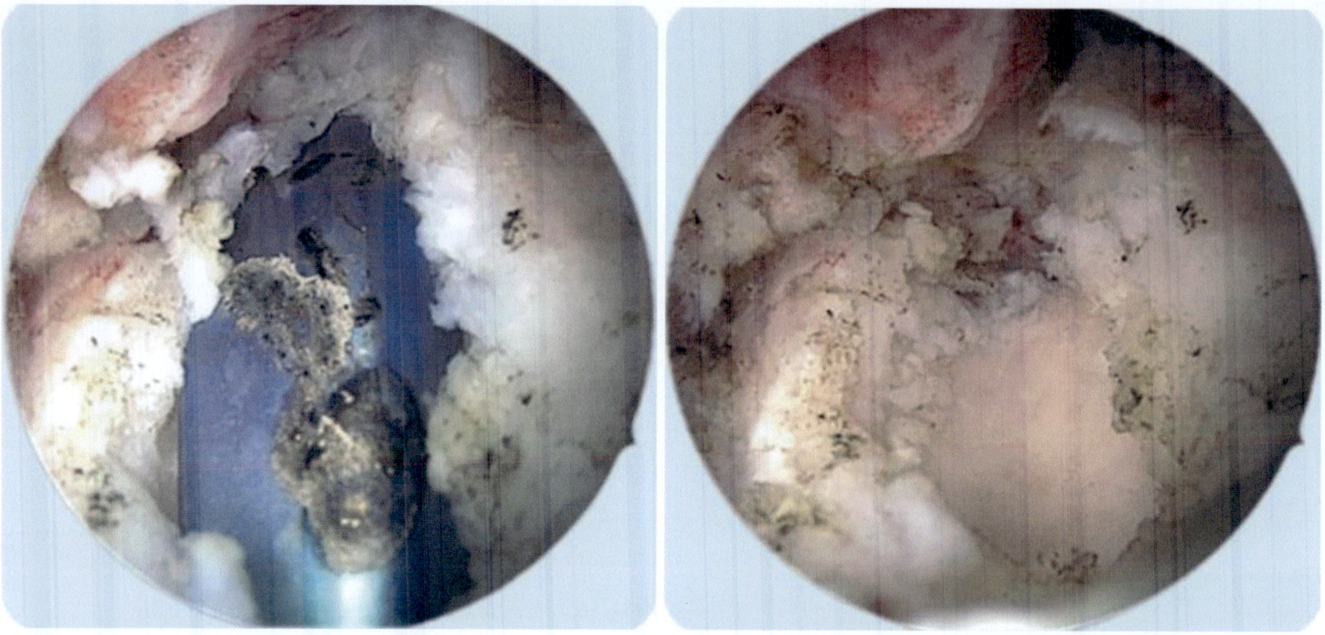

Fig. 16.9 Arthroscopic exploration of the shoulder reveals groove-like bone wear on the shoulder peak caused by clavicle hook plate

16.3 Errors and Countermeasures in Suspension Fixation of Distal Clavicle Fracture with Coracoclavian Loop Plate

It is important to establish a tunnel between the clavicle and coracoid process for distal clavicle fractures (Fig. 16.10) using loop plate fixation or coracoid interlocking fixation. The rupture of the clavicle and coracoid process tunnel is often the cause of surgical failure. During surgery, it is important to use the aiming device reasonably and pay attention to the direction of the tunnel [3]. Repeated drilling can easily cause the bone tunnel of the clavicle coronoid process to expand, leading to coronoid process fractures or dislocation of the loop plate fixation failure (Fig. 16.11). Therefore, using arthroscopic assisted double fixation between the coracoid process and clavicle can improve fracture healing rate and reduce complications.

In summary, the use of plate or coracoclavicular loop plate suspension fixation for distal clavicle fractures is a commonly used surgical method by scholars both domestically and internationally. Postoperative loop rupture is relatively rare, and the reason may be related to early excessive movement. The clavicle hook plate has unique complications, and it is recommended to use it as little as possible.

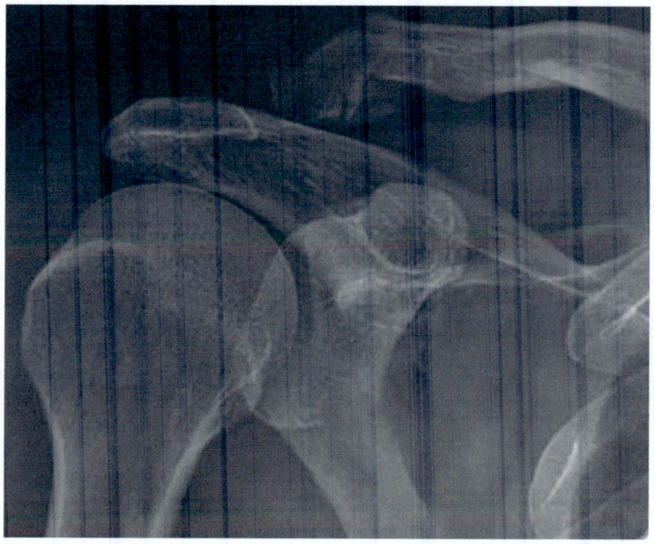

Fig. 16.10 X-ray showing right distal clavicle fracture

It should only be used as a substitute when combined with coracoid process fractures or coracoid process loop plate fixation failure. Arthroscopic assisted double fixation of the coracoid process and clavicle can improve fracture healing rate and reduce complications.

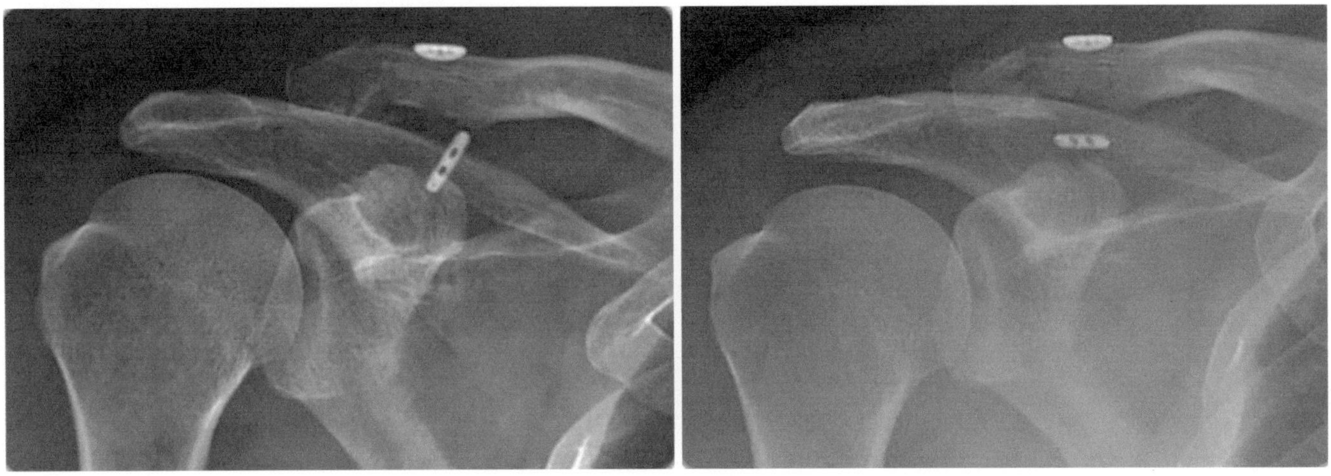

Fig. 16.11 Postoperative X-ray showing plate protruding from the lateral loop of the coronoid process outside the tunnel

References

1. Kraus N, Stein V, Gerhardt C, et al. Arthroscopically assisted stabilization of displaced lateral clavicle fractures with coracoclavicular instability. Arch Orthop Trauma Surg, 2015, 13(5 9):1283–1290.
2. Sajid S, Fawdington R, Sinha M. Locking plates for displaced fractures of the lateral end of clavicle: potential pitfalls. Int J Shoulder Surg, 2012, 6(4):126–129.
3. Joel VF, David C, Elifho O, et al. Biomechanical evaluation of effect of coracoid tunnel placement on load to failure of fixation during repair of acromioclavicular joint dislocations. Arthroscopy, 2012, 28(9): 1230–1236.

Part VII

Fracture and Dislocation of the Acromioclavicular Joint: A Guide and Summary

Chang-ming Huang

Guides

This part focuses on four aspects of content.

1. Through the introduction of misdiagnosis and missed diagnosis cases of dislocation of the acromioclavicular joint and thoracoclavicular joint, analyze the reasons for misdiagnosis and missed diagnosis of dislocation of the acromioclavicular joint and thoracoclavicular joint and propose diagnosis and treatment strategies.
2. Analyze the possible complications of using hook plate fixation for dislocation of the acromioclavicular joint and explain the complications based on the case, proposing surgical methods and strategies to reduce complications.
3. Based on the cases of complications caused by dislocation of the acromioclavicular joint and coracoclavicular fixation, this article elaborates on the causes of complications such as clavicle fractures and tunnel enlargement in coracoclavicular fixation. Double fixation or double bundle reconstruction techniques are proposed to reduce postoperative complications.
4. A variation of the pectoralis minor tendon was found during arthroscopic fixation of acromioclavicular joint dislocation with intercoracoclavicular loop plate. Combined with relevant literature review, the incidence and classification of variations in the pectoralis minor tendon were analyzed, as well as how to use the pectoralis minor tendon to strengthen the reconstruction of the coracoclavicular ligament.

Summary

Misdiagnosis and missed diagnosis of dislocation of the acromioclavicular and thoracoclavicular joints are not uncommon, especially in Rockwood III type of dislocation of the acromioclavicular joint and posterior dislocation of the thoracoclavicular joint. For Rockwood III acromioclavicular joint dislocation, it is easy to miss diagnosis in clinical practice, such as obvious tenderness and mild floating sensation at the acromioclavicular joint. If the dislocation is not detected by routine X-ray examination, additional X-rays should be taken in the crossed adduction position of the upper arm or in the stress position of both hands lifting heavy objects, which can help clarify the diagnosis and avoid missed diagnosis. Posterior dislocation of the sternoclavicular joint is difficult to detect on X-ray examination, while three-dimensional CT

C.-m. Huang
Department of Orthopedics, The 73rd Group Army Hospital,
Chenggong Hospital Affiliated to Xiamen University, Xiamen, China

reconstruction of the sternoclavicular and acromioclavicular joints can help clarify the diagnosis. The best treatment method for posterior dislocation of the sternoclavicular joint is open reduction, anchor nail suture repair, and reconstruction of the sternoclavicular joint capsule and ligament.

Dislocation of the acromioclavicular joint is fixed with hook steel plates, and complications during and after surgery are not uncommon. The main complications include steel plate dislocation, steel plate fracture and loosening, proximal clavicle fracture, subacromial bursitis, acromion impact, acromion bone wear, bone resorption, rotator cuff injury, and re-dislocation after removing the steel plate. Interclavicular fixation can avoid complications of hook plate fixation.

The complications of coracoclavicular fixation surgery for dislocation of the acromioclavicular joint are not uncommon, mainly including fixation failure, clavicle fracture, tunnel enlargement, and coracoid process fracture. Double fixation technique or double bundle anatomical reconstruction of the coracoclavicular ligament can reduce surgical complications of acromioclavicular joint dislocation. Double bundle anatomical reconstruction of the coracoclavicular ligament can reduce the position and stress imbalance of the coracoclavicular ligament, which is more in line with biomechanical characteristics.

The variation of the pectoralis minor tendon is not uncommon and can be divided into three types. Type I: The entire pectoralis minor tendon passes through the coracoid process and terminates at the glenoid lip or coracoacromial ligament; Type II: Part of the tendon is attached to the coracoid process, while the other part is attached to the coracoacromial ligament, supraspinatus muscle, or glenoid humeral joint capsule; Type III: The pectoralis minor muscle has no tendons, only abnormal attachment at the muscle insertion point, attached to the joint capsule and humeral tuberosity, not just on the coronoid process. If variations in the pectoralis minor tendon are found after acromioclavicular joint surgery, displacement of the pectoralis minor tendon can be used to strengthen the coracoclavicular ligament.

Misdiagnosis and Countermeasures of Acromioclavicular Joint and Sternoclavicular Joint Dislocation

17

Chang-ming Huang, Yu-jie Liu, and Yang-pan Fu

17.1 Introduction

Fracture and dislocation of sternoclavicular joint and medial clavicular bone are rare, accounting for 1.2~4% of shoulder joint injuries, while dislocations of sternoclavicular joint only account for 1% of total dislocations [1, 2]. Anterior dislocation of the sternoclavicular joint is significantly more than posterior dislocation, with a ratio of 20:1. The literature on posterior dislocation is mostly reported on individual cases, which is prone to misdiagnosis and missed diagnosis [3]. The sternoclavicular joint is the only joint connecting the upper limb to the trunk. It consists of the medial end of the clavicle, the clavicular trace of the sternal manubrium and the adjacent surface of the first costal cartilage .The complete ossification of the medial clavicular ossification center occurs at the age of 18–20 years and is not complete until the age of 23–25 years [4]. Due to the special anatomical characteristics, the injury of sternoclavicular joint in adolescents is often accompanied by medial clavicular fracture and posterior dislocation of sternoclavicular joint. The sternoclavicular joint is the most unstable joint in the whole body [4]. The articular surface of the medial end of the clavicle is inclined, 50% of the articular surface is in contact with the articular surface of the sternum, and there is a cartilage disc between the two articular surfaces. Despite this instability, sternoclavicular joint is rarely dislocated, and its stability is mainly protected by anterior and posterior sternoclavicular ligaments, costoclavicular ligaments, and interclavicular ligaments [4, 5]. Posterior dislocation of sternoclavicular joint often occurs in motor vehicle accidents, indirect violence is rare. Direct force acts on the anterior medial clavicle, pushing the clavicle behind the sternum into the mediastinum. Forward shoulder compression and rotation can lead to posterior dislocation of ipsilateral sternoclavicular joint [6]. If the violence is increased, it may cause dislocation of ipsoclavicular joint, which is prone to clinical misdiagnosis and missed diagnosis [7].

C.-m. Huang (✉) · Y.-p. Fu
Department of Orthopedics, The 73rd Group Army Hospital, Chenggong Hospital Affiliated to Xiamen University, Xiamen, China

Y.-j. Liu
Orthopaedics, Chinese PLA General Hospital, Beijing, China

17.2 Overview of the Diagnosis and Treatment Process

17.2.1 Case 1: Acromioclavicular Dislocation

The patient is a 65-year-old male who experienced right shoulder joint pain and limited mobility due to a fall for 5 days. Physical examination: Swelling of the right acromioclavicular joint, limited upper limb abduction and lifting activity, tenderness and floating sensation in the acromioclavicular joint (Fig. 17.1), and protrusion of the outer edge of the clavicle during right upper arm adduction (Fig. 17.2). No fractures or dislocations were found on the X-ray of the right shoulder joint in the A-P position (Fig. 17.3a), while the X-ray of the shoulder joint in the adduction position of the right upper arm showed dislocation of the right acromioclavicular joint (Fig. 17.3b, c).

17.2.2 Case 2: Dislocation of the Sternoclavicular Joint

The patient is a 56-year-old male who collided with a car while riding an electric bicycle. He experiences pain in the left shoulder joint and chest, as well as limited upper limb mobility for 2 weeks. Physical examination showed mild swelling and tenderness in the left acromioclavicular joint, with no feeling of emptiness in the acromioclavicular joint. The right side of the sternocleidomastoid muscle is clear,

Y.-j. Liu et al. (eds.), *Pitfalls in Diagnosis and Treatment of Shoulder Joint Diseases*,
https://doi.org/10.1007/978-981-96-2472-0_17

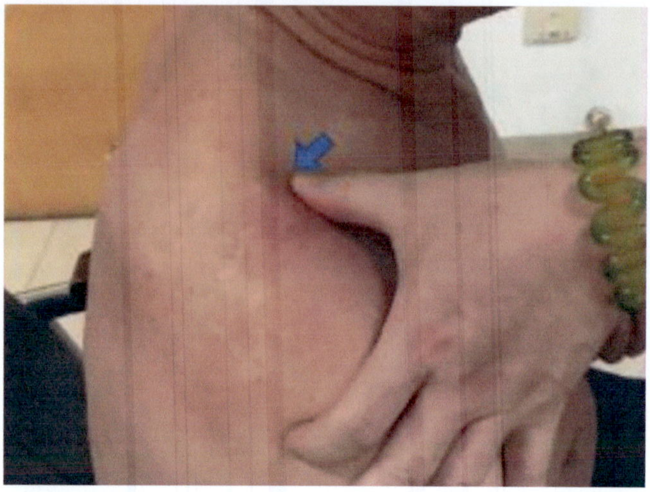

Fig. 17.1 Right acromioclavicular joint tenderness with floating sensation

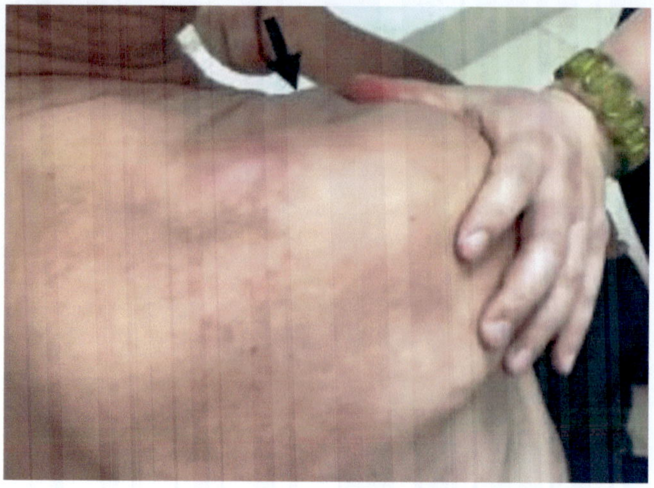

Fig. 17.2 Right upper arm adduction position, clavicle outer edge protrusion

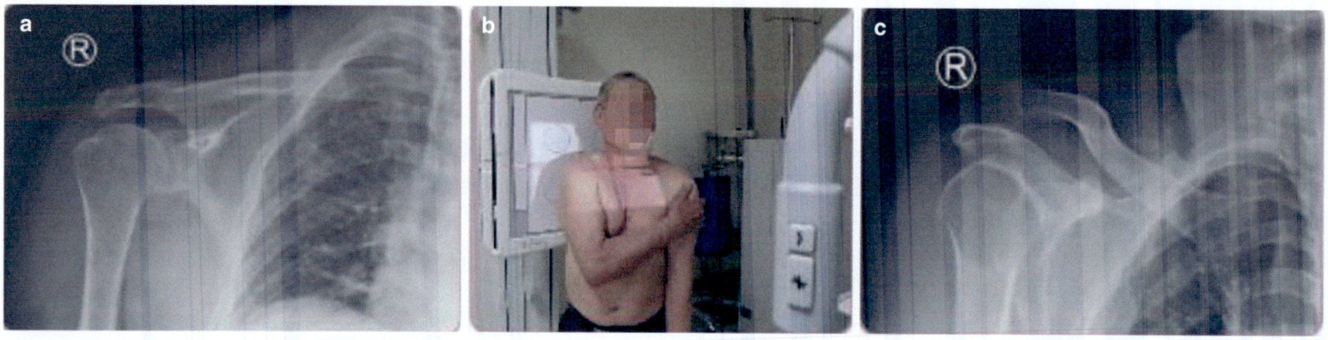

Fig. 17.3 X-ray examination of acromioclavicular joint dislocation. (**a**) There was no abnormality in the X-ray of shoulder joint; (**b**) Right upper arm adduction X-ray examination position; (**c**) Right upper arm adduction X-ray shows dislocation of the acromioclavicular joint

Fig. 17.4 The right side of the sternocleidomastoid muscle is clear, and the left side is concave

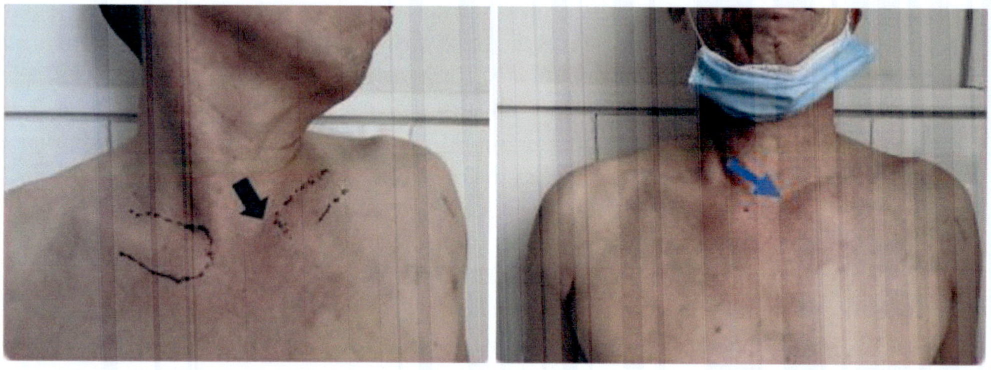

with a depression on the left side (Fig. 17.4), and limited shoulder joint abduction and upward movement (Fig. 17.5). The X-ray film shows no abnormalities in the clavicle and sternoclavicular joint (Fig. 17.6). CT three-dimensional reconstruction shows posterior dislocation of the left sternoclavicular joint (Fig. 17.7).

Under general anesthesia, an open surgical exploration was performed, and left sternoclavicular joint dislocation was found. The clavicle was lifted upward with tissue forceps, and the inner edge of the clavicle was pried to reposition the sternoclavicular joint (Fig. 17.8). Implant 2 anchor screws into the sternum, drill the clavicle to obtain the bone canal, thread the suture into the canal separately, and tie the suture in an 8-shaped knot to fix the sternoclavicular joint (Fig. 17.9), and the capsule of the sternoclavicular joint was sutured and repaired.

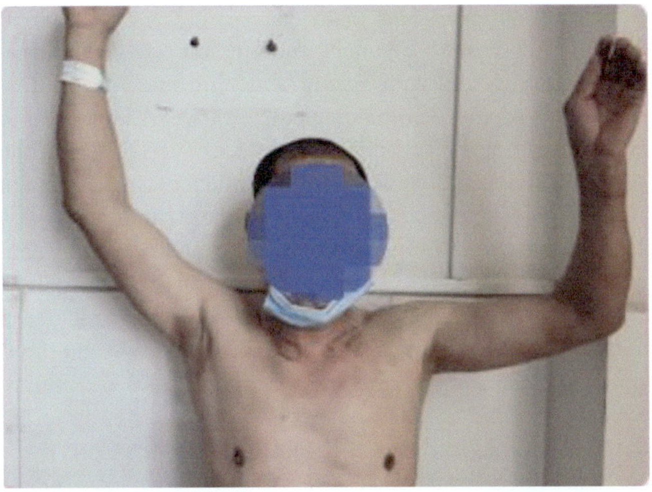

Fig. 17.5 Limited left shoulder joint abduction and lifting activity

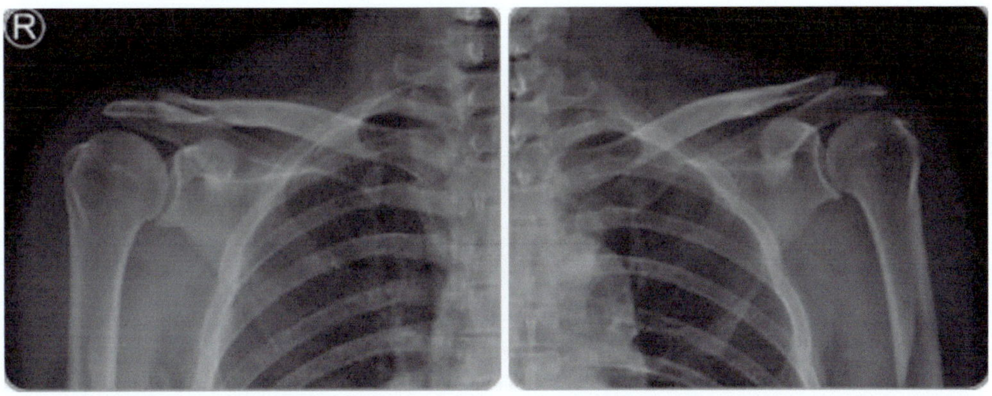

Fig. 17.6 Bilateral shoulder X-rays show no abnormalities in the shoulder and sternoclavicular joints

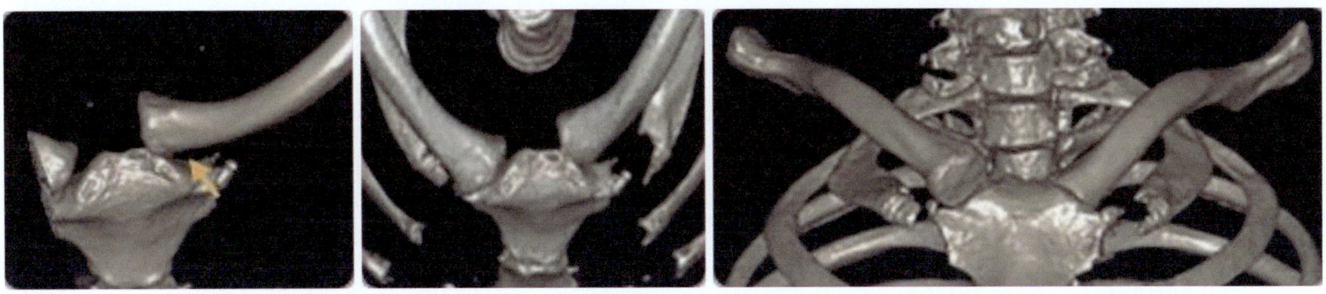

Fig. 17.7 CT 3D reconstruction showing posterior dislocation of the left sternoclavicular joint

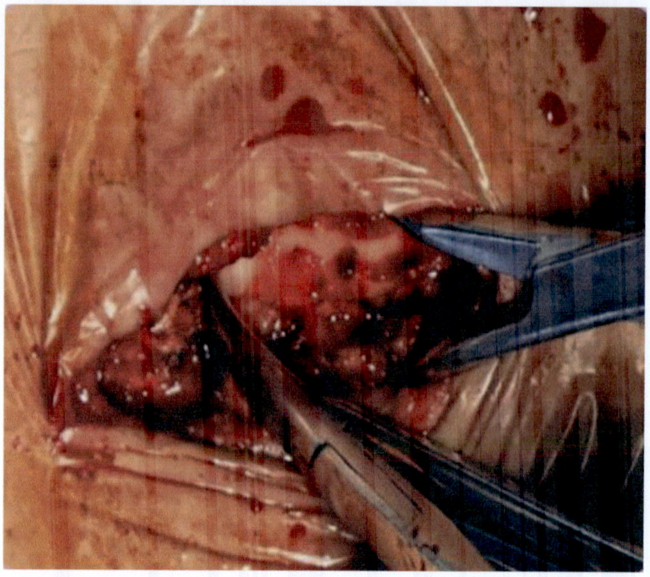

Fig. 17.8 Pry the sternoclavicular joint and use tissue forceps to pull the clavicle upward to reposition the sternoclavicular joint

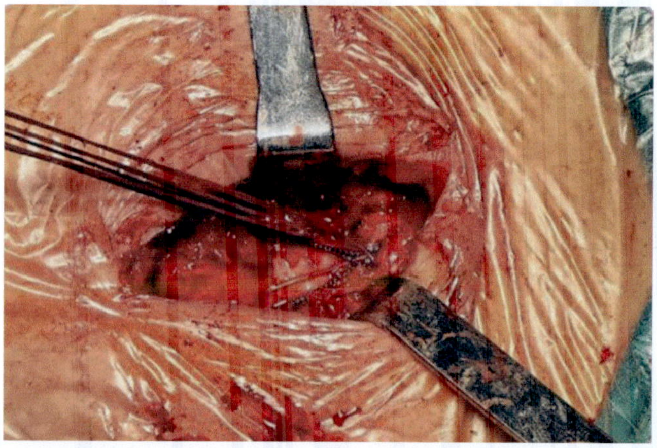

Fig. 17.9 Using suture anchor screws to fix the sternoclavicular joint and joint capsule

17.3 Analysis of the Reasons for Missed Diagnosis of Dislocation of the Acromioclavicular and Thoracoclavicular Joints

Rockwood [8] classified dislocation of the acromioclavicular joint into six types: Type I partial tear of the acromioclavicular ligament, but still intact, intact coracoclavian ligament, stable acromioclavicular joint, and normal X-ray. Type II: Shoulder clavicular ligament rupture, coracoclavian ligament injury, X-ray shows mild widening and longitudinal separation of the acromioclavicular joint space, and mild enlargement of the coracoclavian space. Type III: Both the acromioclavicular ligament and the coracoclavian ligament are broken. The attachment points of the deltoid and trapezius muscles were torn, and the distal clavicle was unstable in both horizontal and vertical planes. X-ray images showed significant displacement of the distal clavicle and an increase of 25–100% in the coracoclavian space. Type IV: Both the acromioclavicular and coracoclavian ligaments are ruptured, the fascia of the deltoid and trapezius muscles is ruptured, the clavicle moves backward, penetrates the trapezius muscle, and undergoes displacement, resulting in an elevation of the acromioclavicular joint. The X-ray shows an increase in the coracoclavian space, while the axillary X-ray shows a posterior displacement of the distal clavicle. Type V: Both the acromioclavicular and coracoclavian ligaments are ruptured, and the fascia of the deltoid and trapezius muscles is ruptured. The distal clavicle is unstable in both horizontal and vertical planes, but the displacement of the distal clavicle is more severe. X-ray shows an increase of 100–300% in the coracoclavicular space. Type VI: Both the acromioclavicular and coracoclavian ligaments are broken, and the distal clavicle is displaced to the coronoid process or below the acromion, which may be accompanied by damage to the brachial plexus or blood vessels. The X-ray film shows that the distal clavicle is located below the acromion or coronoid process, and the coracoclavicular space is smaller than the normal side (Fig. 17.10).

Rockwood III dislocation of the acromioclavicular joint is prone to misdiagnosis in clinical practice. When there is significant tenderness and mild floating sensation at the acromioclavicular joint, and no dislocation is detected by routine X-ray examination, an additional X-ray should be taken in the crossed adduction position of the upper arm or in the stress position of the double shoulder joint when lifting heavy objects with both hands (Fig. 17.11) to help clarify the diagnosis and avoid misdiagnosis.

Patients with posterior dislocation of the sternoclavicular joint usually complain of pain behind the sternum or in the clavicle area, some of which can radiate to the neck and even to the contralateral upper arm [9]. If the mediastinum, trachea, esophagus, or blood vessels are compressed, symptoms such as difficulty breathing, swallowing, and blood circulation disorders may occur. In clinical physical examination, only local swelling and tenderness are observed,

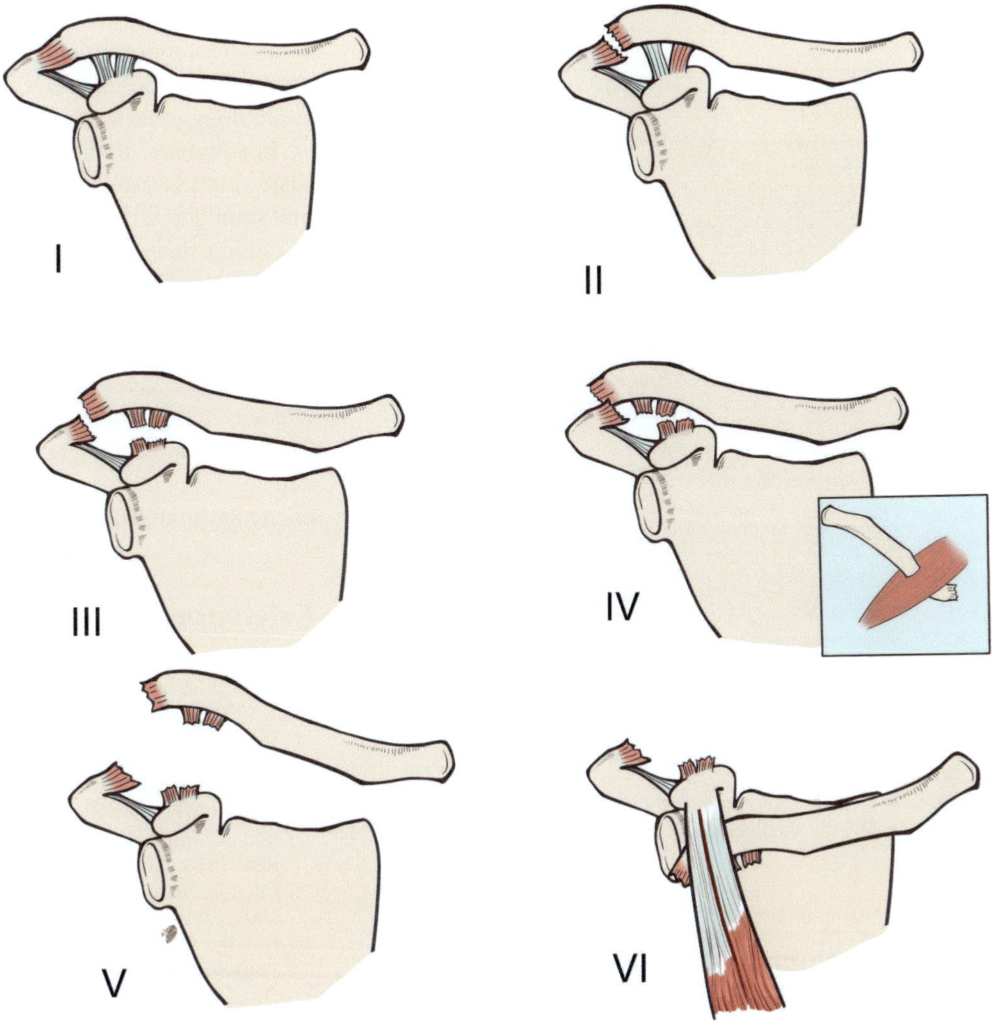

Fig. 17.10 Classification diagram of Rockwood acromioclavicular joint dislocation

making it difficult to feel the emptiness of the sternoclavicular joint, and local deformities are rare.

Conventional standard X-ray examinations are not easy to detect, and if there is a high suspicion of dislocation, special angle X-ray films (Rockwood and Heinig positions) need to be cast at 40° of the sternum stem [9, 10]. CT three-dimensional reconstruction is crucial for diagnosing posterior dislocation of the sternoclavicular joint. MRI is used to evaluate the relationship between ligament injury and dislocation and mediastinal tissue.

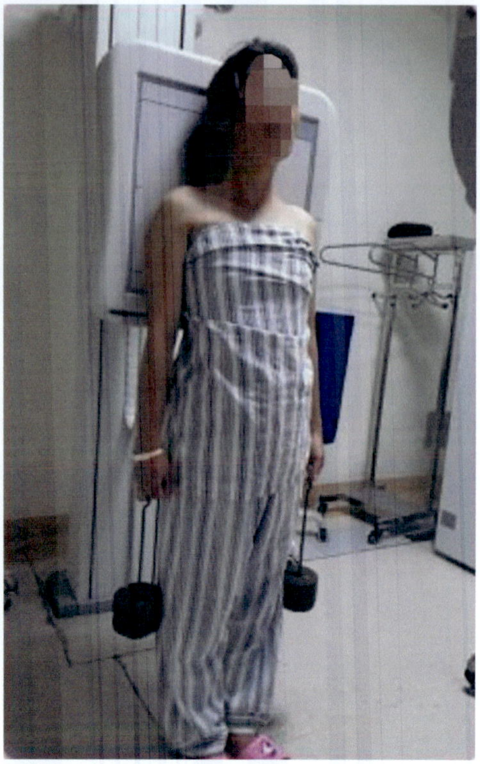

Fig. 17.11 X-rays taken from the weight-bearing position of both upper limbs and the shoulder joint in A–P position

17.4 Treatment of Posterior Dislocation of the Sternoclavicular Joint

Due to the important tissue structure in the rear, the reduction of thoracoclavicular joint dislocation must be performed in the presence of a cardiothoracic surgeon [8, 11]. Manual reduction is prone to dislocation, making it difficult to maintain normal anatomical relationships. If the esophagus, trachea, cervical and thoracic blood vessels, and nerves are compressed, serious complications may occur, requiring surgical treatment [11].

The sternoclavicular ligament is extremely important for maintaining joint stability. Special attention should be paid to repairing and reconstructing the structure of the sternoclavicular ligament and restoring the normal anatomy and function of the shoulder joint during surgical treatment of dislocation of the sternoclavicular joint and peripheral fractures.

The use of Kirschner wire tension band steel wire fixation may result in Kirschner wire movement, which poses a risk of damaging posterior blood vessels, nerves, and entering the thoracic cavity. Due to the fact that the sternoclavicular joint is a micromotion joint, steel plate fixation may cause the steel plate to loosen or even break. The suture anchor repair technology is currently receiving much attention [6, 12].

In summary, Rockwood III type acromioclavicular joint dislocation is prone to misdiagnosis. Cross arm adduction and shoulder X-rays in the upright position or shoulder joint X-rays in the weight-bearing position of both upper limbs are beneficial for diagnosis. Posterior dislocation of the sternoclavicular joint is rare and difficult to detect on X-ray examination. To avoid misdiagnosis and missed diagnosis, CT three-dimensional reconstruction of the sternoclavicular and acromioclavicular joints can help clarify the diagnosis. The best treatment method currently is to use open reduction and anchor nail suture to repair and reconstruct the thoracoclavicular joint capsule and ligament.

References

1. Medvecky MJ, Zuckerman JD. Sternoclavicular joint injuries and disorders. Instr Course Lect. 2000;49:397–406.
2. Rudzki JR, Matava MJ, Paletta GA. Complications of treatment of acromioclavicular and sternoclavicular joint injuries. Clin Sports Med. 2003;22(2):387–405.
3. Brinker MR, Bartz RL, Reardon PR, et al. A method for open reduction and internal fixation of the unstable posterior sternoclavicular joint dislocation. J Orthop Trauma. 1997;11(5):378–81.
4. Cope R. Dislocations of the sternoclavicular joint. Skeletal Radiol. 1993;22(4):233–8.
5. Hidalgo Ovejero AM, Garcia Mata S, Sanchez Villares JJ, et al. Posterior sternoclavicular dislocation, report of two cases. Acta Orthop Belg. 2003;69(2):188–92.
6. Morell DJ, Thyagarajan DS. Sternoclavicular joint dislocation and its management: a review of the literature. World J Orthop. 2016;7(4):244–50.
7. Ao R, Zhu Y, Zhou J, et al. Locking plate for treating traumatic sternoclavicular joint dislocation: a case series. BMC Musculoskelet Disord. 2018;19(1):7.
8. Rockwood CA. Dislocations of the sternoclavicular joint. In: Evan EB, editor. American Academy of Orthopaedic Surgeons instructional course lectures, vol. 24. St. Louis: CV Mosby; 1975. p. 144–59.
9. Salgado RA, Ghysen D. Post-traumatic posterior sternoclavicular dislocation: case report and review of the literature. Emerg Rad. 2002;9(6):323–5.
10. Heinig CF. Retrosternal dislocation of the clavicle: early recognition, X-ray diagnosis and management. J Bone Joint Surg Am. 1968;50(4):830.
11. Waters PM, Bae DS, Kadiyala RK. Short-term outcomes after surgical treatment of traumatic posterior sternoclavicular fracture-dislocations in children and adolescents. J Pediatr Orthop. 2003;23(4):464–9.
12. Widodo W, Fahrudhin M, Kamala F. Joint reconstruction using sternocleidomastoid tendon autograft as a treatment for traumatic posterior dislocation of sternoclavicular joint: a case report. Trauma Case Rep. 2018;18:8–16.

18 Complications and Countermeasures of Hook Steel Plate Fixation Surgery for Dislocation of the Acromioclavicular Joint

Chang-ming Huang, Yu-jie Liu, and Yang-pan Fu

18.1 Introduction

Dislocation of acromioclavicular joint is often caused by direct violence. Rockwood [1] divided the dislocation of acromioclavicular joint into six types: type I and type II injuries, coracoclavicular ligament is not completely broken (i.e., acromioclavicular joint subluxation), which can be treated by manual reduction and external fixation. After 4 weeks of surgery, external fixation is removed and functional exercise begins, achieving good therapeutic effects. Nonsurgical treatment can be attempted first for type III injuries, and surgical treatment can be performed after failure [2, 3]. Injuries above type III should be treated with surgery to facilitate early functional recovery.

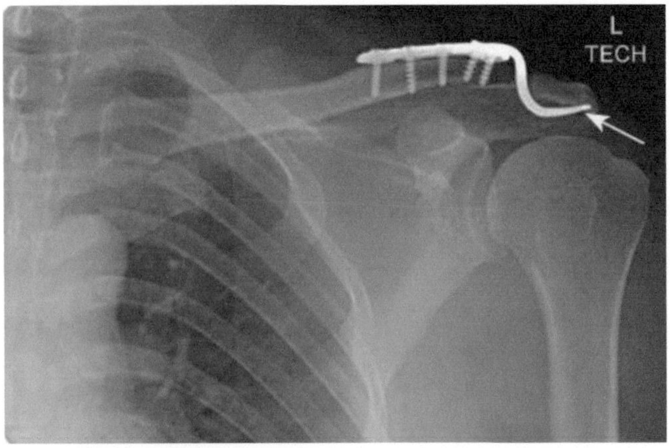

Fig. 18.1 Left shoulder joint anterior X-ray showing wear of hook plate and shoulder peak

18.2 Overview of the Diagnosis and Treatment Process

Patient is a 56-year-old male. The left acromioclavicular joint was dislocated after a fall. The incision healed in the first stage by open reduction hook plate fixation. Postoperative shoulder joint movement was limited, and the pain was unbearable, and it affected sleep. Shoulder joint radiographs showed subacromial bone surface wear (Fig. 18.1), and CT three-dimensional reconstruction showed a good reduction of the acromioclavicular joint (Fig. 18.2).

Five months after surgery, arthroscopic cleaning and removal of hook plates were performed. During the surgery, it was found that there was hypertrophic scar around the hook steel plate (Fig. 18.3), and the bone wear under the acromion was groove-like defect (Fig. 18.4). The hook steel plate was removed, and the postoperative X-ray showed that the position of the left acromioclavicular joint was normal (Fig. 18.5).

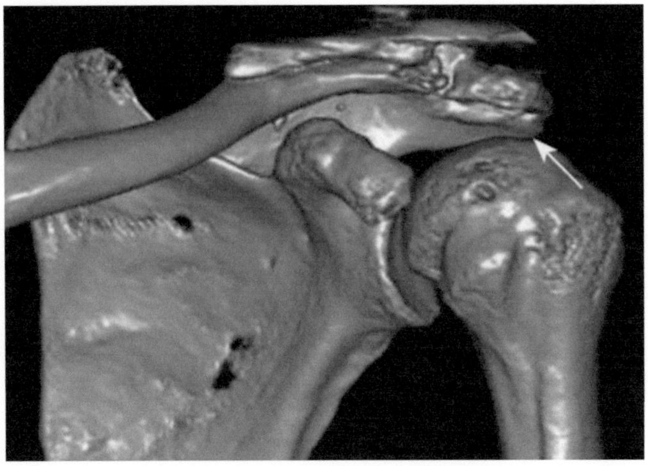

Fig. 18.2 3D CT reconstruction of the left shoulder joint shows good reduction of the left acromioclavicular joint

C.-m. Huang (✉) · Y.-p. Fu
Department of Orthopedics, The 73rd Group Army Hospital, Chenggong Hospital Affiliated to Xiamen University, Xiamen, China

Y.-j. Liu
Orthopaedics, Chinese PLA General Hospital, Beijing, China

Y.-j. Liu et al. (eds.), *Pitfalls in Diagnosis and Treatment of Shoulder Joint Diseases*, https://doi.org/10.1007/978-981-96-2472-0_18

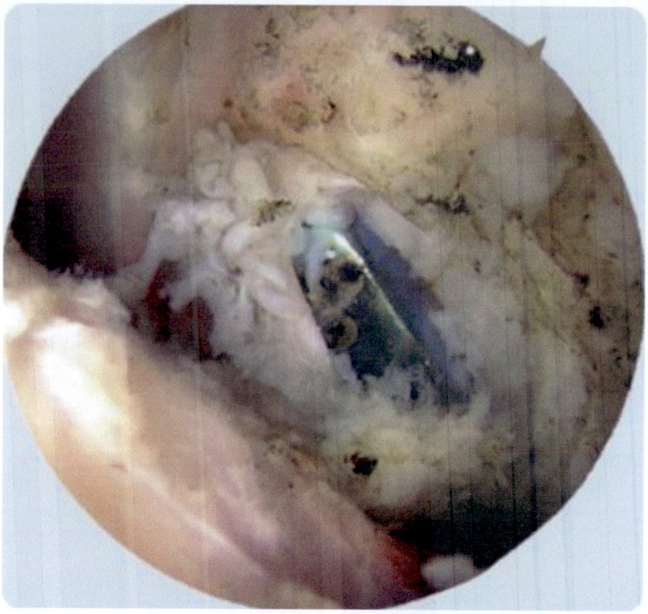

Fig. 18.3 Subacromial scar hyperplasia wrapped around hook steel plate

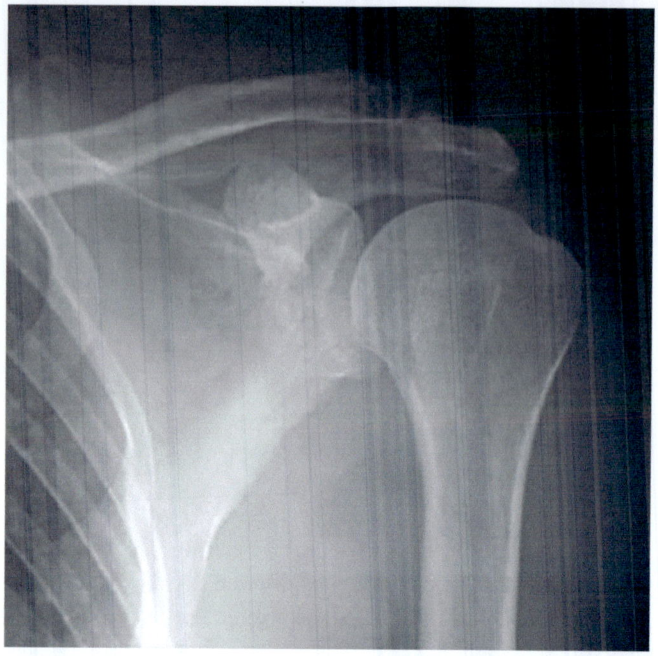

Fig. 18.5 Postoperative X-ray showing normal position of left acromioclavicular joint

Fig. 18.4 Groove-shaped bone defects in the hooked steel plate under the shoulder peak due to wear and tear

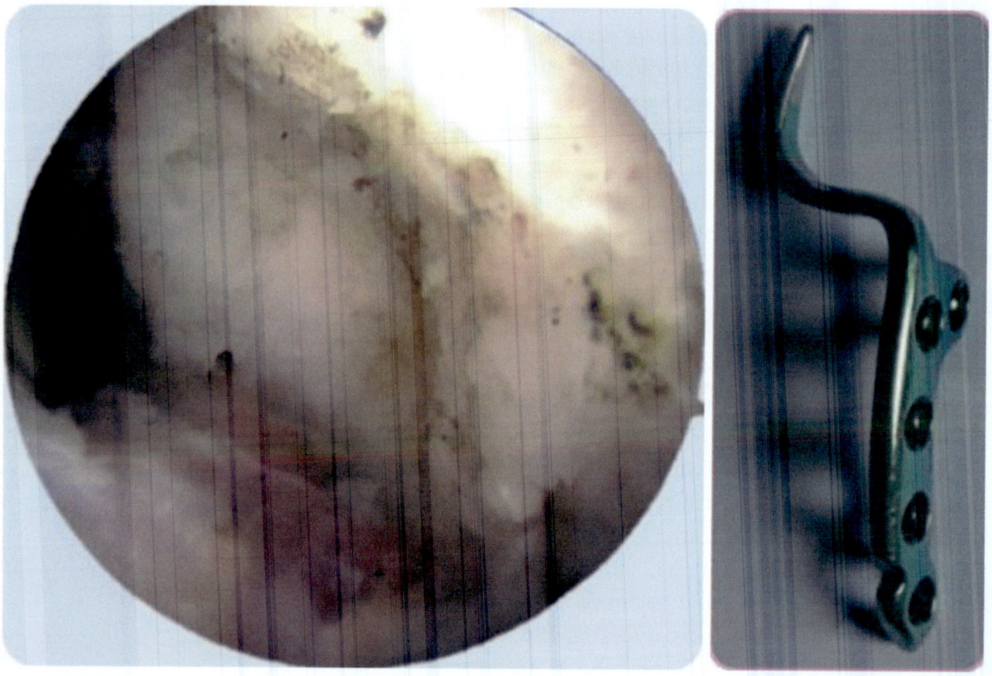

Four months after discharge, when carrying the child, the patient experienced pain and deformity in the left shoulder again. The X-ray of the left shoulder joint showed dislocation of the left acromioclavicular joint (Fig. 18.6). Upon admission, patients underwent arthroscopic reduction of the acromioclavicular joint and internal fixation of the coracoclavian suspension loop steel plate, as well as reconstruction of the semitendinosus tendon coracoclavian ligament (Fig. 18.7). The postoperative X-ray showed good reduction of the left acromioclavicular joint (Fig. 18.8), and the shoulder joint function returned to normal.

Fixation of acromioclavicular joint with hook plate was a common surgical method in the past. Clavicular joint provides relatively stable biomechanics, and hook plate treatment for acute acromioclavicular joint dislocation is one of the conventional options. With the deepening of the research on hook plate fixation, the common complications of hook plate fixation were clinically found to be dislocation of hook plate (Fig. 18.9), impingement of the greater tubercle of acromion humerus caused by hook plate length (Fig. 18.10), fracture and loose fixation of hook plate, and fracture of the proximal clavicle (Fig. 18.11). Hook plate fixation can be

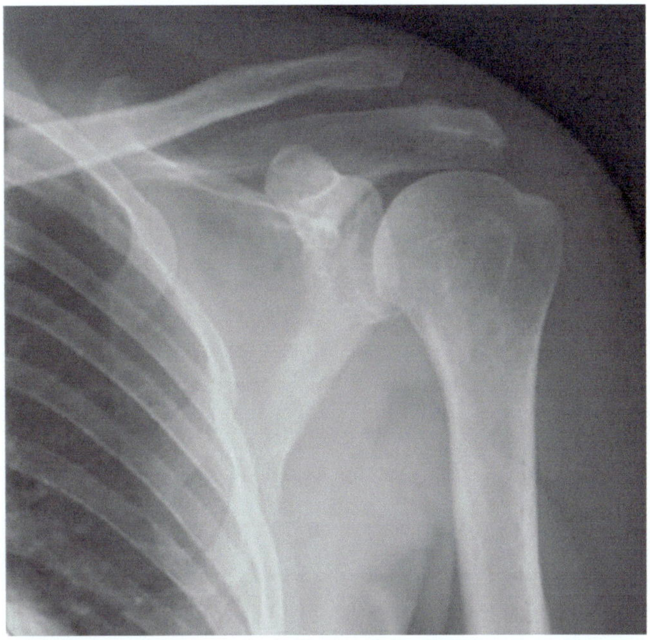

Fig. 18.6 Postoperative X-ray of the left shoulder joint at 4 months shows dislocation of the left acromioclavicular joint hook steel plate after removal

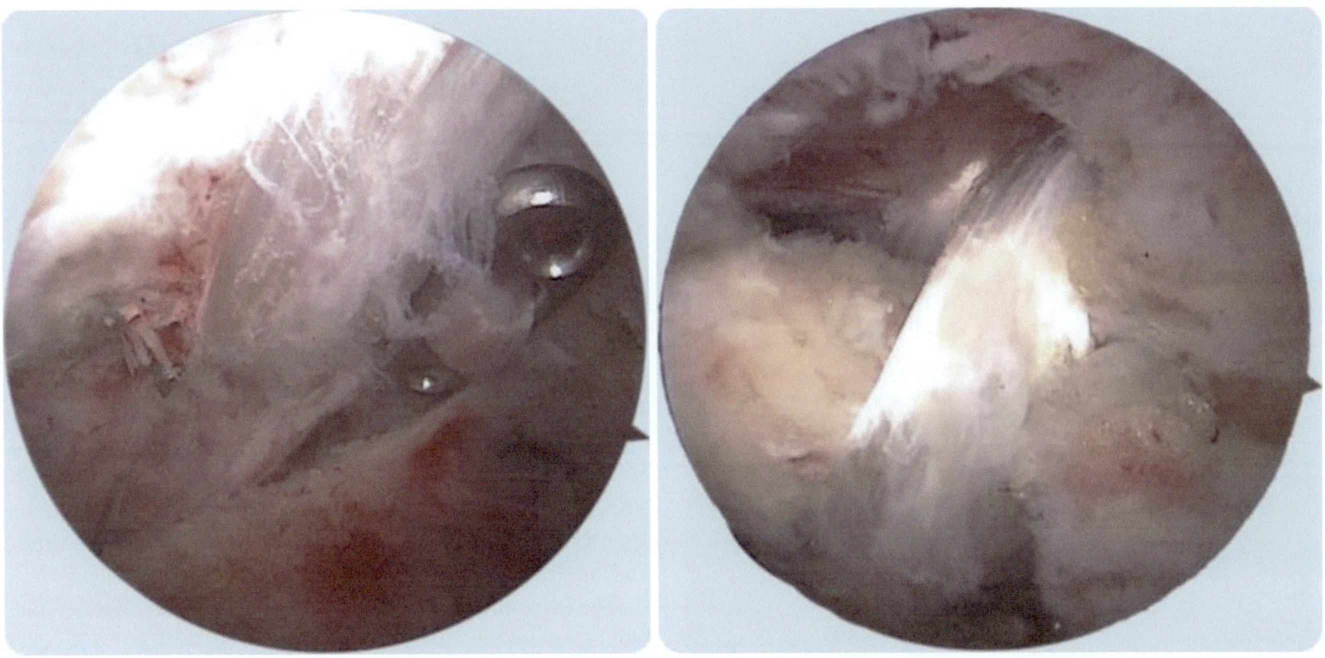

Fig. 18.7 Arthroscopic display of steel plate suspension fixation in the coracoclavian loop, with tendon reconstruction of the coracoclavian ligament

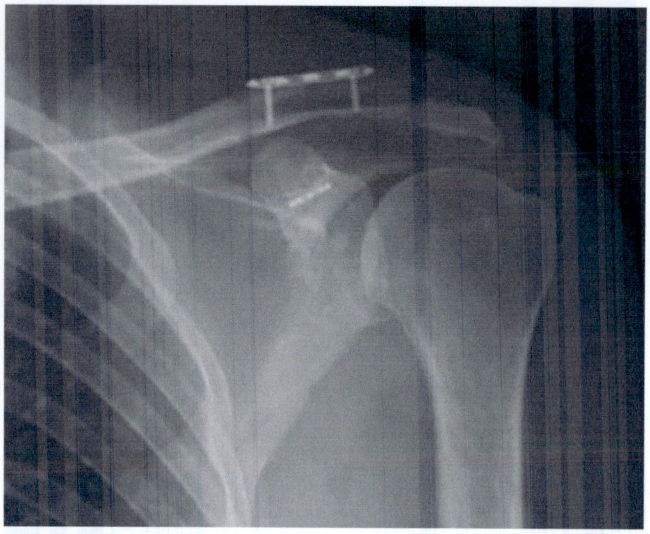

Fig. 18.8 After reoperation, the left shoulder joint in the upright position X-ray shows good reduction of the left acromioclavicular joint

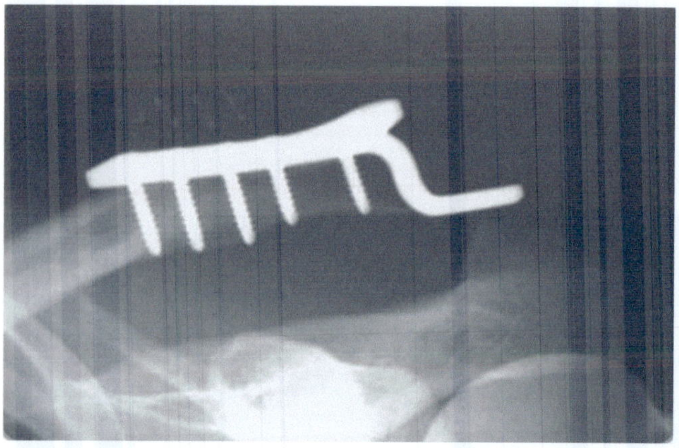

Fig. 18.9 Dislocation of hook steel plate

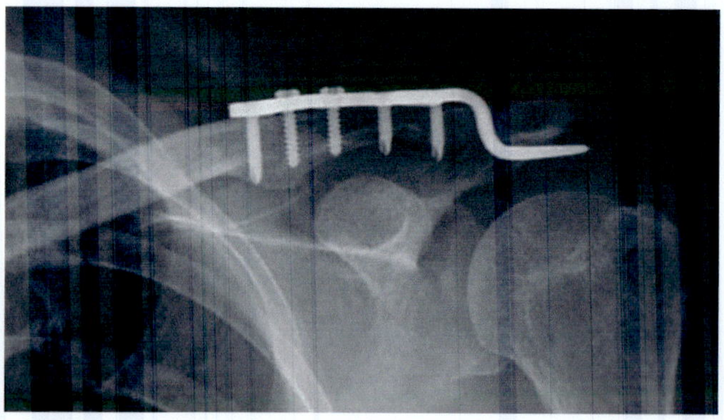

Fig. 18.10 Shoulder joint impact caused by hook length of steel plate hook

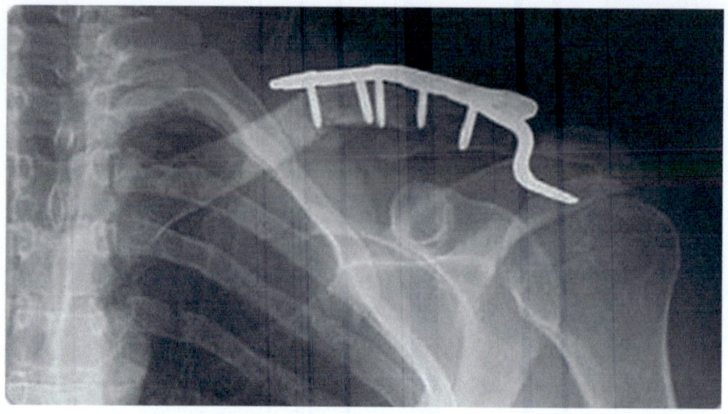

Fig. 18.11 Fracture of the clavicle end of the hook steel plate

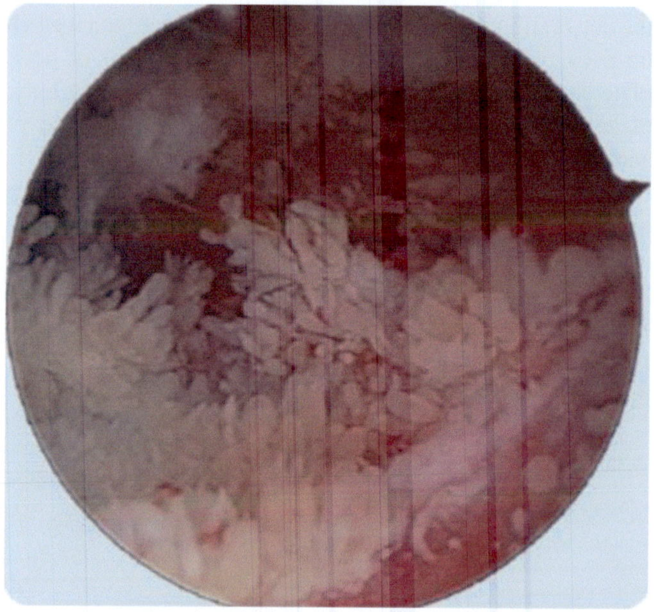

Fig. 18.12 Subacromial synovitis

associated with several complications, including subacromial synovitis (Fig. 18.12), acromial bone wear (Fig. 18.13), bone resorption (Fig. 18.14), and improper insertion of the hook into the supraspinatus muscle. These issues may subsequently result in further complications such as subacromial impingement and rotator cuff injury (Fig. 18.15).

The acromioclavicular joint belongs to micromotion fixation. Due to the different specifications of the hook steel plate (Fig. 18.16) and the height of the steel plate hook, the steel plate hook may cause wear and tear on the subacromial bone, resulting in wear debris, fractures, and synovitis. It is recommended to use it with caution in clinical practice.

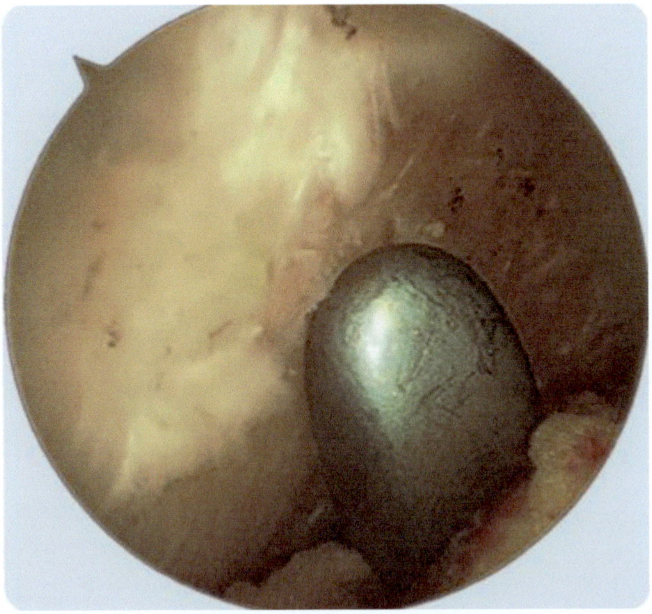

Fig. 18.13 Wear shoulder peak of hook steel plate hook

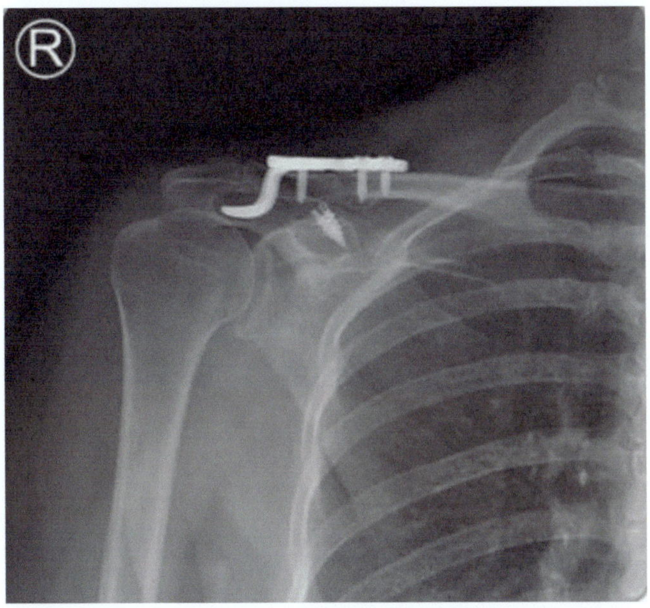

Fig. 18.14 Wear of hook steel plate hook shoulder peak bone

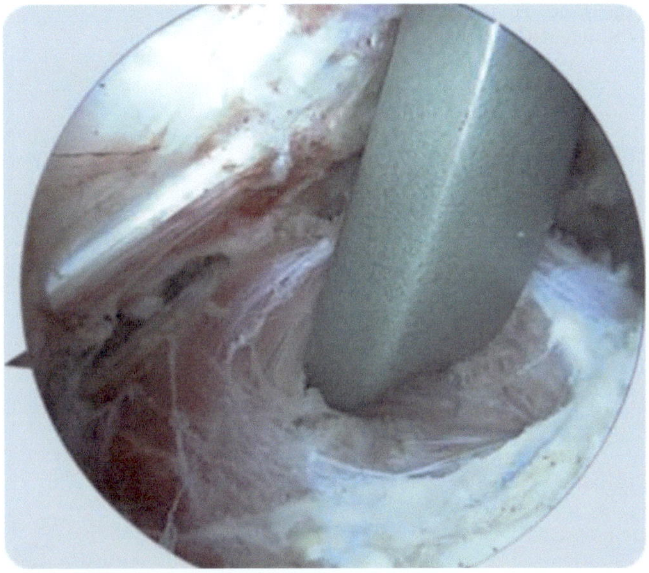

Fig. 18.15 Hook steel plate hook mistakenly inserted into the supraspinatus muscle

The acromioclavicular joint is divided into static stable structures and dynamic stable structures. The static stable structure includes the acromioclavicular ligament and the coracoclavian ligament, which are further divided into the conical ligament and the oblique ligament, both perpendicular to each other, forming a V-shaped structure. When using suspension fixation between the clavicle and coracoid process, two thick threads are used to wrap around the coracoid process and clavicle for fixation (Fig. 18.17), or suture anchor nails are used on the coracoid process for coracoid lock fixation (Fig. 18.18), or double fixation methods such as autologous tendon reconstruction of the coracoid lock ligament (Fig. 18.19) can be used for old dislocation to restore biomechanics and achieve good results. To avoid stress fractures at the clavicle drilling site, in addition to standardized drilling of clavicle holes, microsteel plates on the clavicle can be used for fixation (Figs. 18.20 and 18.21).

In summary, dislocation of the acromioclavicular joint is fixed with hook steel plates, and complications during and after surgery are not uncommon. The main complications

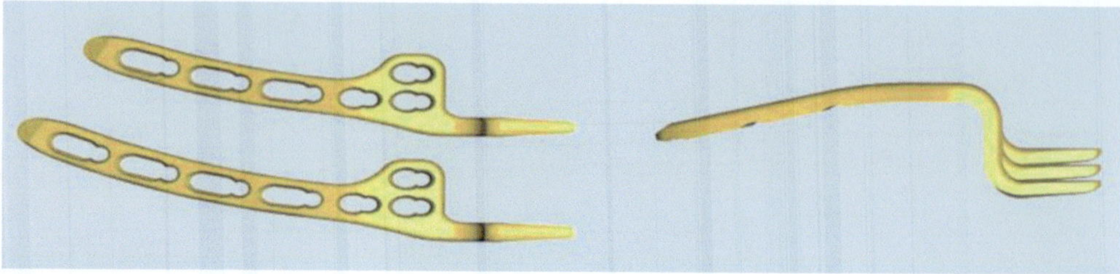

Fig. 18.16 Hook steel plates of different specifications

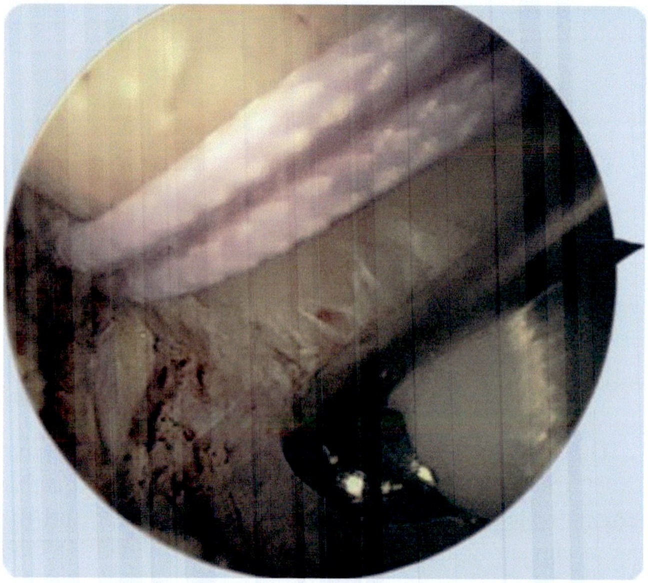

Fig. 18.17 Double fixation of suture and loop steel plate

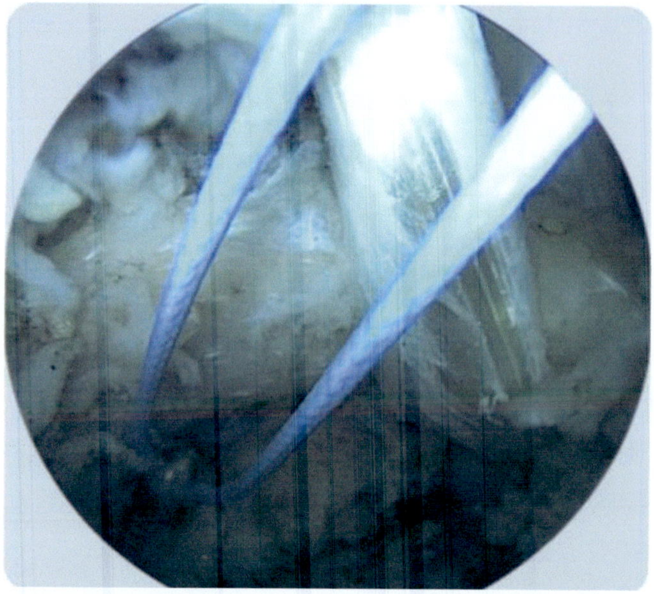

Fig. 18.19 Reconstruction of the tendon coracoclavian ligament using autologous muscle

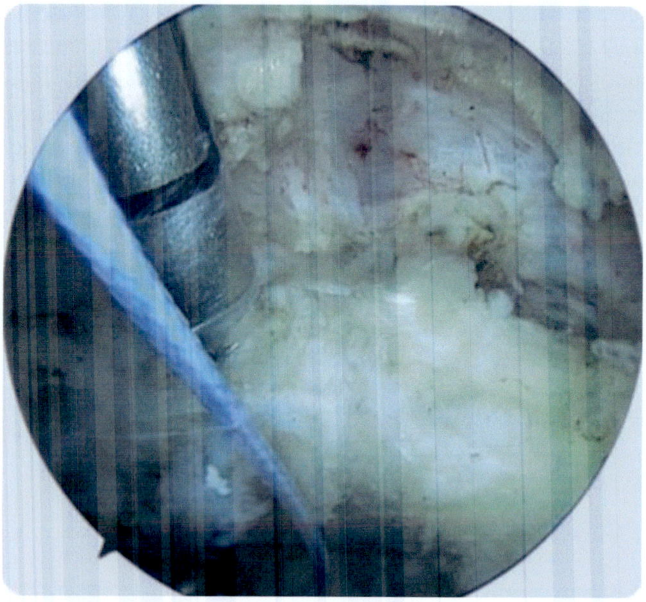

Fig. 18.18 Diagnosis and treatment of acromioclavicular joint dislocation using double fixation with anchor screws and loop steel plates

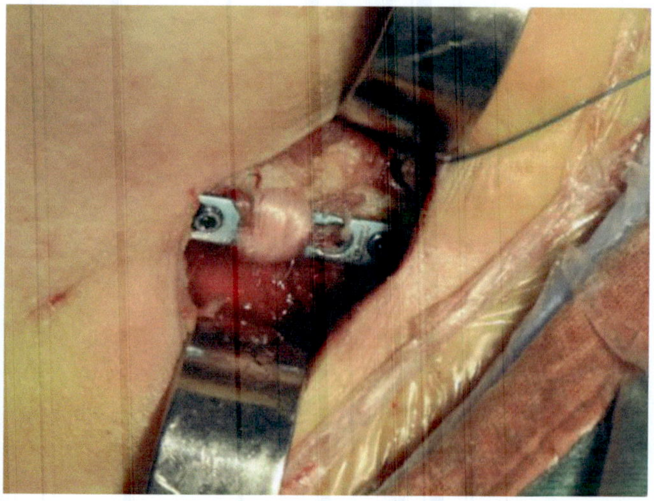

Fig. 18.20 Steel plate loop overlapping on microsteel plate

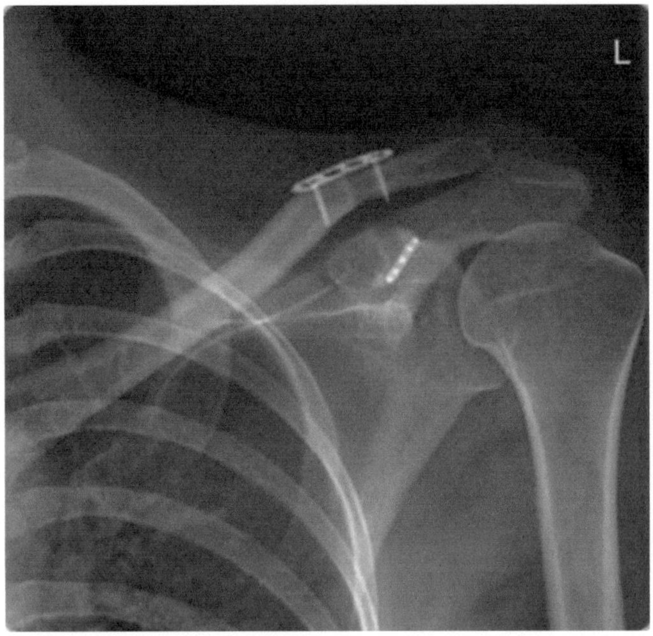

Fig. 18.21 Postoperative fixation with loop steel plate

include steel plate dislocation, steel plate fracture and loosening, proximal clavicle fracture, subacromial bursitis, acromion impact, acromion bone wear, bone resorption, rotator cuff injury, and re-dislocation after removing the steel plate. Interclavicular fixation can avoid complications associated with hook plate fixation.

References

1. Rockwood CA. Dislocations of the sternoclavicular joint. In: Evan EB, editor. American Academy of Orthopaedic Surgeons instructional course lectures, vol. 24. St. Louis: CV Mosby; 1975. p. 144–59.
2. Rollo J, Raghunath J, Porter K. Injuries of the acromioclavicular joint and current treatment options. Trauma. 2005;7(4):217–23.
3. Simovitch R, Sanders B, Ozbaydar M, et al. Acromioclavicular joint injuries: diagnosis and management. J Am Acad Orthop Surg. 2009;17(4):207–19.

Treatment Trap for Intercoracoclavicular Fixation of Plate for Acromioclavicular Dislocation Loop

19

Chang-ming Huang, Yu-jie Liu, and Yang-pan Fu

19.1 Introduction

Compared with clavicle hook steel plate fixation, minimally invasive loop steel plate suspension fixation under arthroscopy has unique advantages in treating acromioclavicular joint dislocation: it avoids the risk of complications such as large open surgical trauma, subacromial impact, shoulder wear and fracture, and rotator cuff injury. However, loop plate fixation surgery also carries the risk of postoperative loss of partial angle of the acromioclavicular joint, expansion of the clavicle tunnel, and even combined clavicle or coracoid process fractures.

19.2 Overview of the Diagnosis and Treatment Process

The patient is a 42-year-old female who experienced left shoulder joint pain and limited mobility due to a fall one day ago. The X-ray (Fig. 19.1) and CT three-dimensional reconstruction (Fig. 19.2) show dislocation of the left acromioclavicular joint with upward displacement of the distal clavicle. Arthroscopic-assisted descending loop steel plate fixation between the coracoid and clavicle was performed, and postoperative X-ray showed reduction of the left acromioclavicular joint (Fig. 19.3). Five months after surgery, X-rays showed that the clavicle tunnel had gradually expanded. During a heavy lifting, the left shoulder joint suddenly experienced severe pain, swelling, and limited mobility. The X-ray (Fig. 19.4) and CT three-dimensional reconstruction (Fig. 19.5) showed a fracture at the bone tunnel of the loop steel plate. After another surgery, the fracture was found at the clavicle tunnel opening (Fig. 19.6), and a revision surgery with clavicle plate internal fixation was performed (Fig. 19.7).

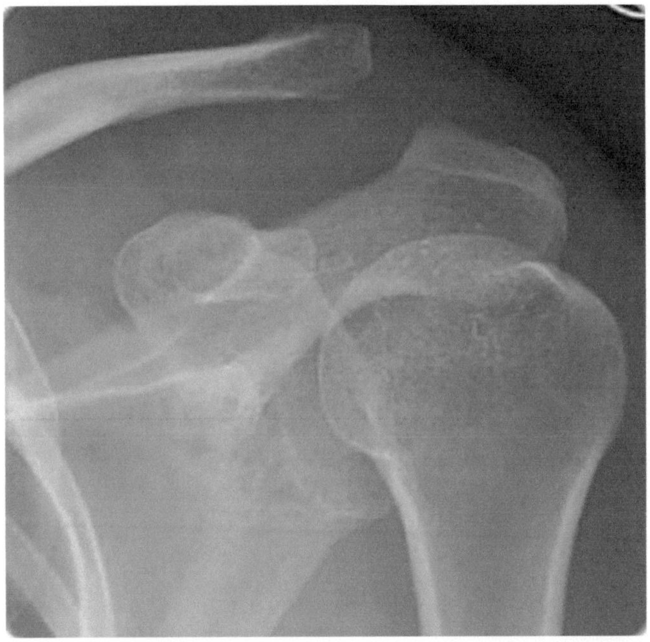

Fig. 19.1 Left shoulder joint X-ray showing dislocation of the left acromioclavicular joint

C.-m. Huang (✉) · Y.-p. Fu
Department of Orthopedics, The 73rd Group Army Hospital, Chenggong Hospital Affiliated to Xiamen University, Xiamen, China

Y.-j. Liu
Orthopaedics, Chinese PLA General Hospital, Beijing, China

Y.-j. Liu et al. (eds.), *Pitfalls in Diagnosis and Treatment of Shoulder Joint Diseases*, https://doi.org/10.1007/978-981-96-2472-0_19

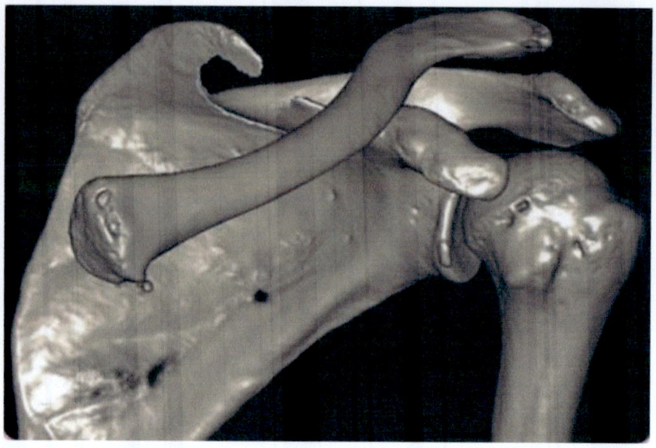

Fig. 19.2 CT 3D reconstruction shows dislocation of the left acromio-clavicular joint with posterior and upward displacement of the clavicle end

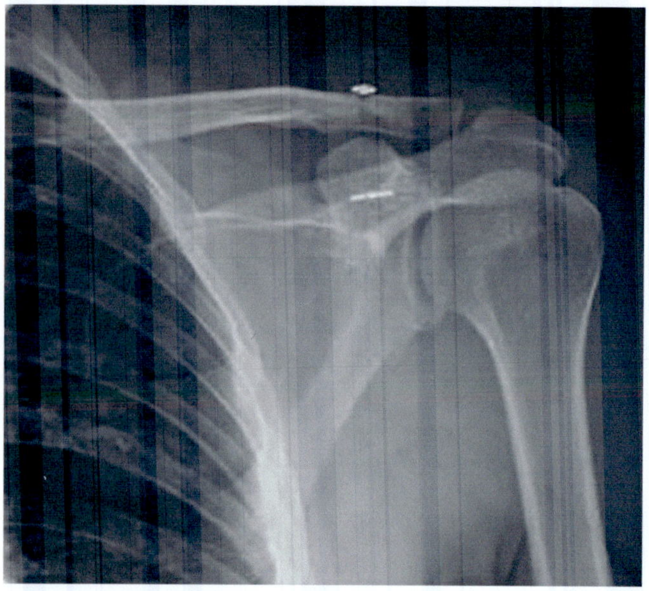

Fig. 19.3 X-ray film shows postoperative fixation of the beak and clavicle with the loop steel plate

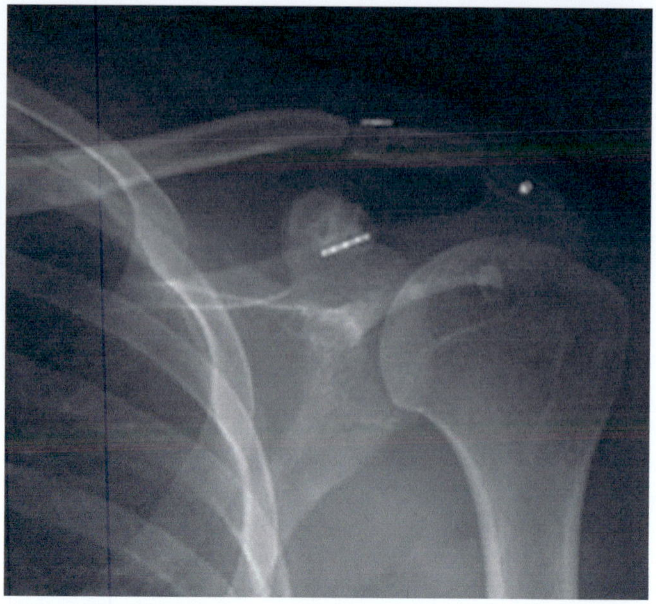

Fig. 19.4 X-ray shows clavicle fracture located at the clavicle tunnel

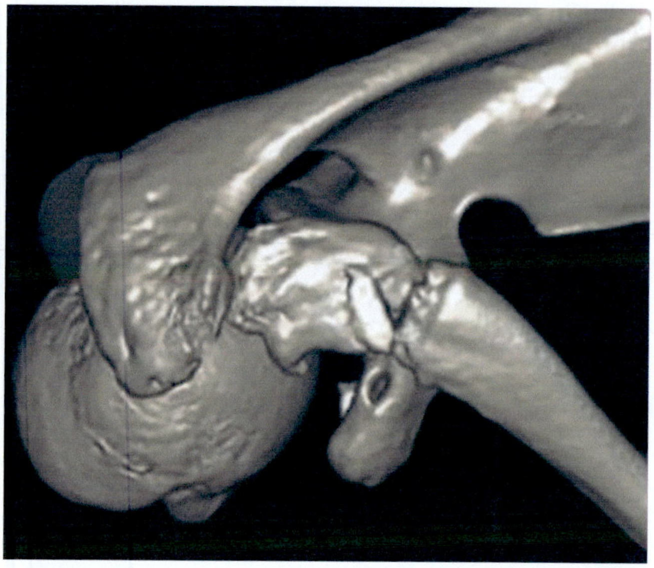

Fig. 19.5 CT 3D reconstruction showing fracture at the clavicle tunnel

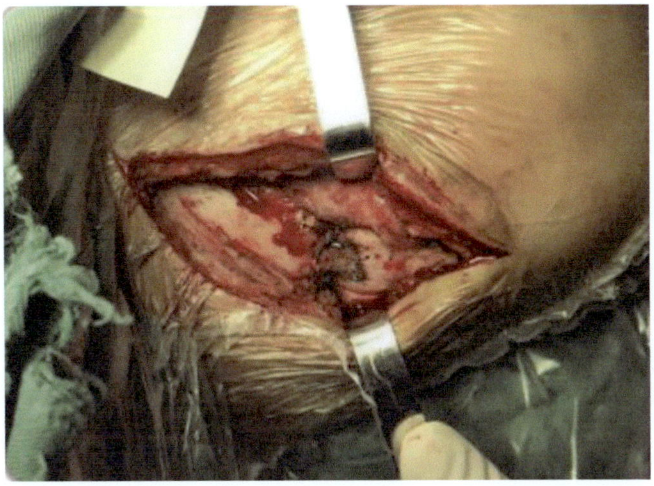

Fig. 19.6 Intraoperative discovery of fracture at the clavicle tunnel

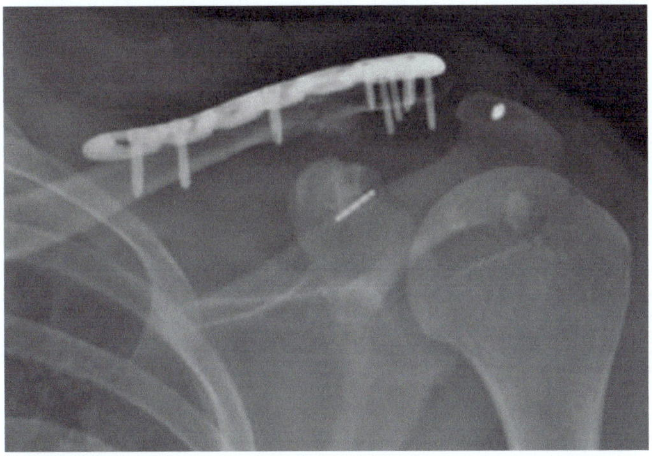

Fig. 19.7 X-ray of the left shoulder joint showing the postoperative situation of clavicle fracture after revision surgery

19.3 Strategies for the Treatment of Acromioclavicular Joint Dislocation with Loop Steel Plate and Coracoclavian Fixation

There are few reports in the literature on the expansion of the clavicle tunnel with clavicle fracture caused by fixation between the beak and the clavicle. Enlargement of the clavicle tunnel is an important risk factor for clavicle fractures. The reason is related to the location, direction, diameter of the drill bit, and osteoporosis of the tunnel being drilled. The diameter of the drill bit used to drill the bone tunnel is thicker, the wall of the clavicle tunnel becomes thinner, and with osteoporosis in the patient, stress is concentrated around the clavicle tunnel, making it prone to fractures when subjected to violence and stress.

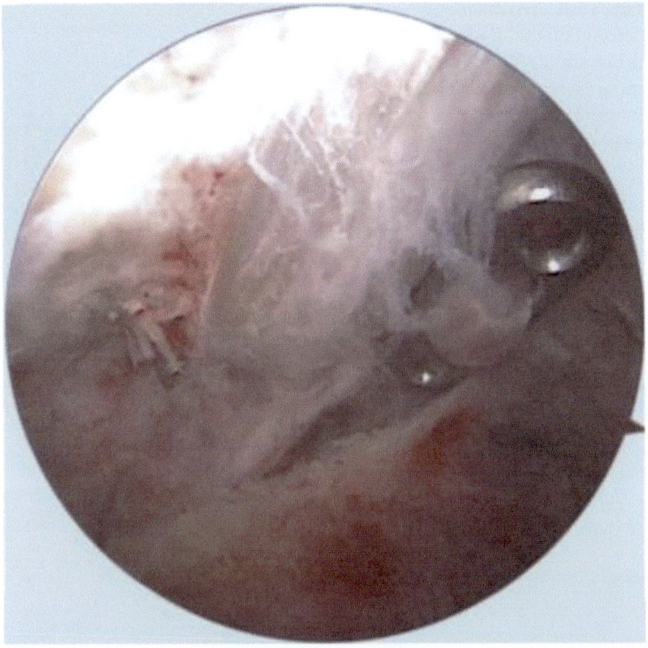

Fig. 19.8 Anatomical reconstruction of the coracoclavian ligament using shoulder lock joint loop steel plate and tendon transplantation

There are literature reports that long-term preservation of the loop inside the tunnel after surgery is a risk factor for fractures. The author observed that after surgery, the inner loop of the tunnel was selectively removed, and the tunnel could heal on its own, avoiding the occurrence of fractures. The non-anatomical fixation reconstruction between the beak and clavicle, with the loop swaying slightly inside the tunnel hole and causing a wiper effect, is an important factor causing the expansion of the clavicle tunnel [3–5]. Simple reconstruction of coracoclavicular ligament after tendon transplantation, tendon creep, and relaxation are important reasons for surgical failure. Therefore, it is recommended to reconstruct coracoclavicular ligaments by tendon transplantation, along with acromioclavicular joint loop plate fixation (Fig. 19.8).

The use of supraclavicular microplate traversing loops (Fig. 19.9) can disperse the stress of microplate loops, avoid coracoclavicular micromotion, reduce the wiper effect, and avoid bone tunnel enlargement and fracture. The postoperative stability is more precise than that of single reconstruction (Fig. 19.10), and the functional recovery is better (Fig. 19.11).

Double bundle anatomical reconstruction of the coracoclavian ligament can reduce complications caused by the position and stress imbalance of the coracoclavian ligament. Preoperative MRI examination of both shoulder joints, scanning the contralateral coracoclavian ligament (Fig. 19.12), with reference to their position during surgery, selecting the localization points of the oblique and conical ligaments in

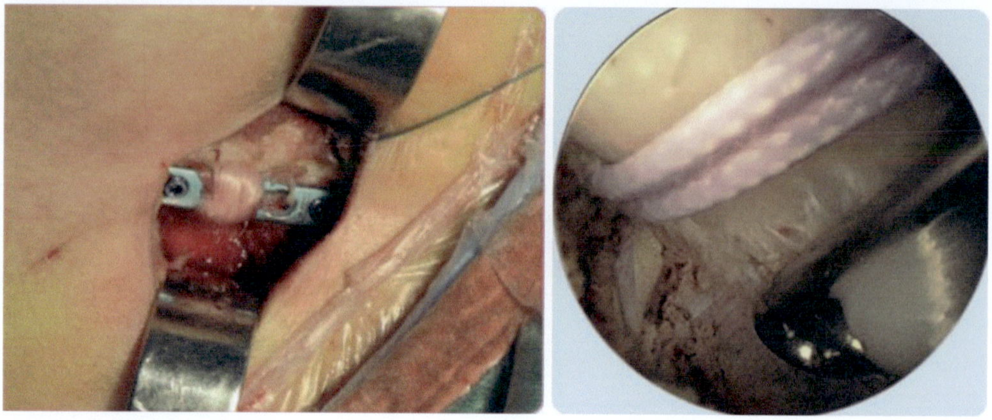

Fig. 19.9 Treatment of acromioclavicular joint dislocation with intraclavicular suspension and internal fixation using loop steel plates

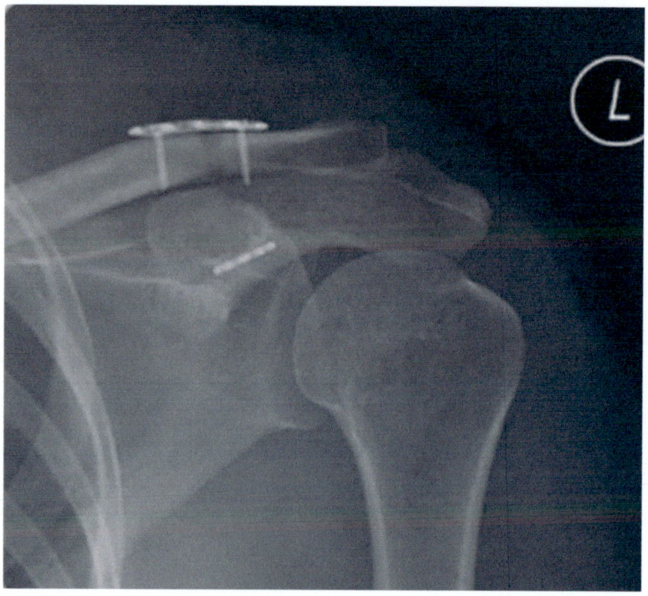

Fig. 19.10 X-ray shows the reconstruction of the coracoclavian ligament

the clavicle (Fig. 19.13). Following the reduction, the acromioclavicular joint was provisionally stabilized using a specialized aiming device (Fig. 19.14), and subsequently, the clavicle and coracoid tunnels were drilled under arthroscopic guidance (Fig. 19.15).

Under arthroscopic monitoring, the clavicle and coracoid process tunnels were drilled, and loop steel plates were implanted (Fig. 19.16). Microsteel plates were inserted into the loop ring for fixation. Postoperative X-ray (Fig. 19.17) and CT three-dimensional reconstruction (Fig. 19.18) showed good tunnel position and reduction of the acromioclavicular joint.

In summary, the complications of coracoclavicular fixation surgery for dislocation of the acromioclavicular joint are not uncommon, mainly including fixation failure, clavicle fracture, tunnel enlargement, and coracoid process fracture. Double fixation technique or double bundle anatomical reconstruction of the coracoclavian ligament can reduce surgical complications of acromioclavicular joint dislocation. Double bundle anatomical reconstruction of the coracoclavian ligament can reduce the position and stress imbalance of the coracoclavian ligament, which is more in line with biomechanical characteristics.

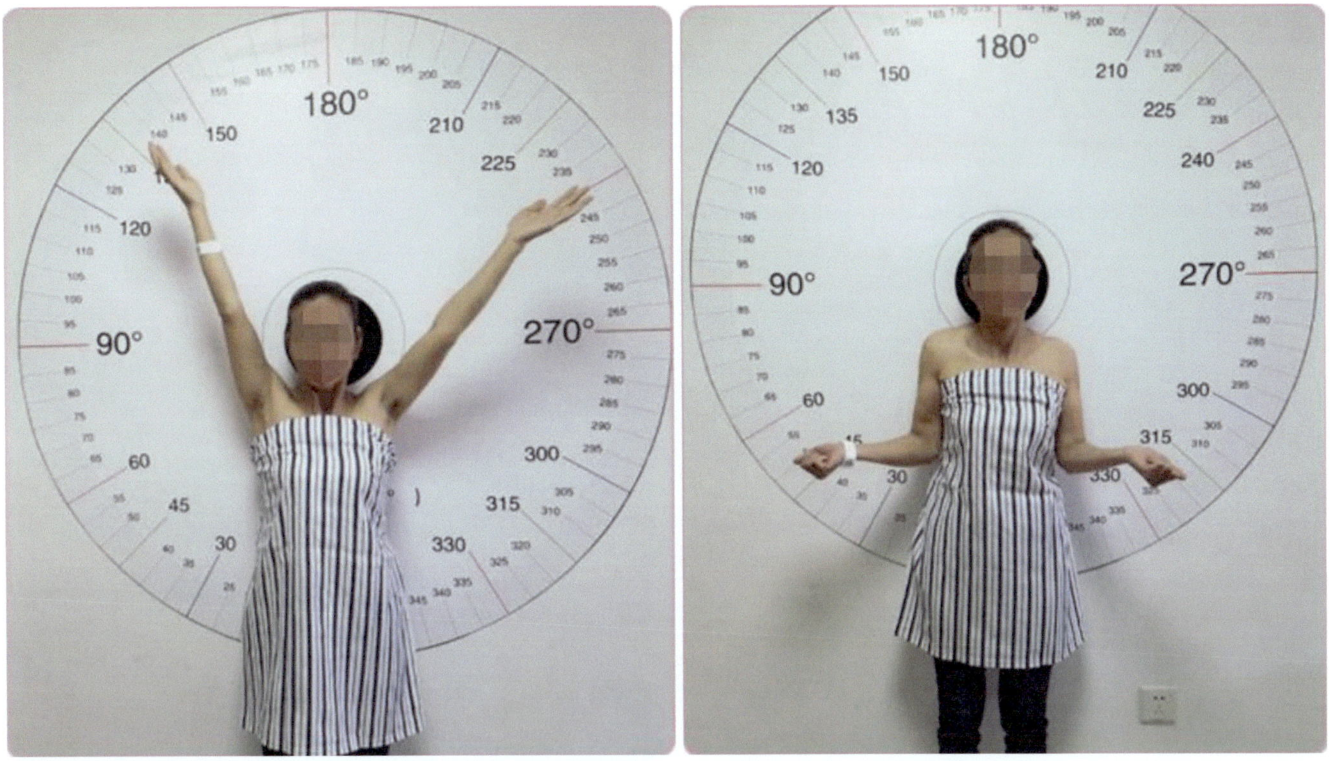

Fig. 19.11 Function is good 1 year after surgery

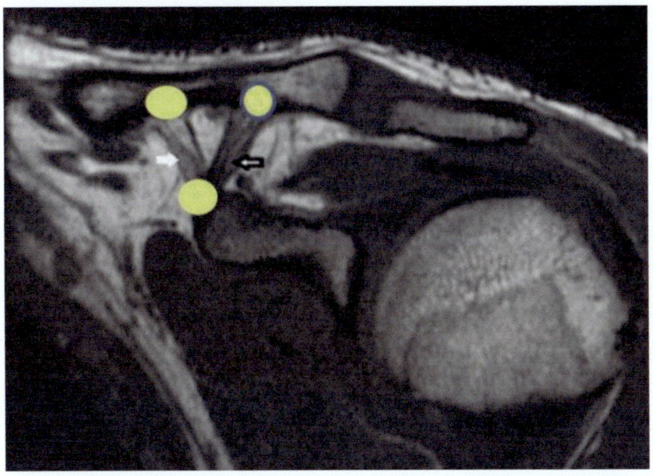

Fig. 19.12 MRI showing coracoclavian ligament

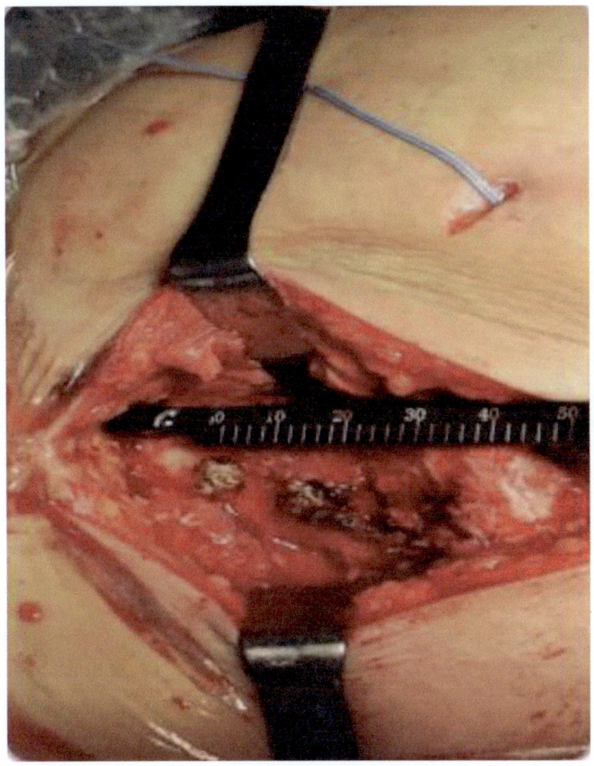

Fig. 19.13 Measurement and localization of the clavicle tunnel points of the oblique and conical ligaments

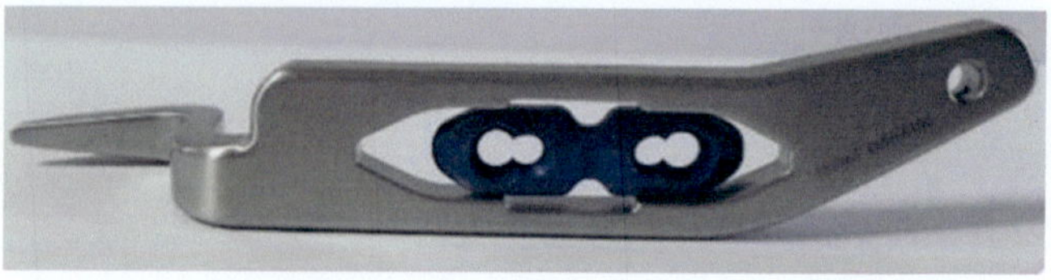

Fig. 19.14 Specially designed reducers and clavicle side microplates

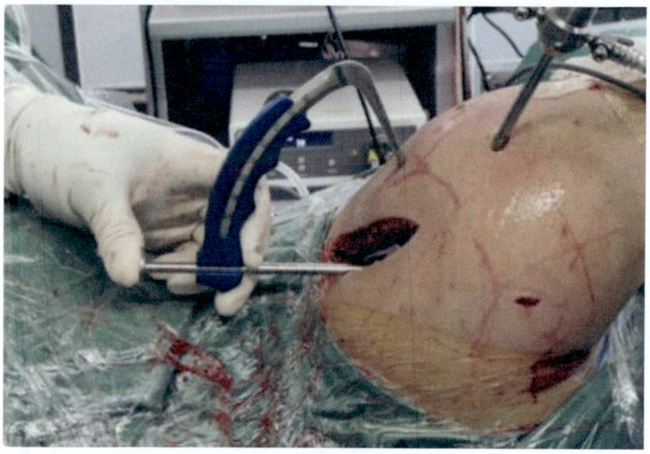

Fig. 19.15 Sight positioning, drilling the tunnel between the beak and lock

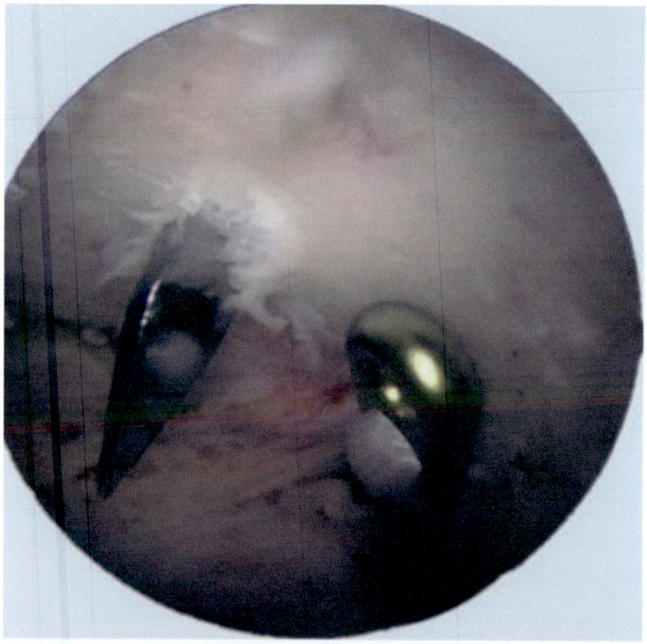

Fig. 19.16 Drilling of the coracoid process tunnel with arthroscopic assistance and implantation of loop steel plate

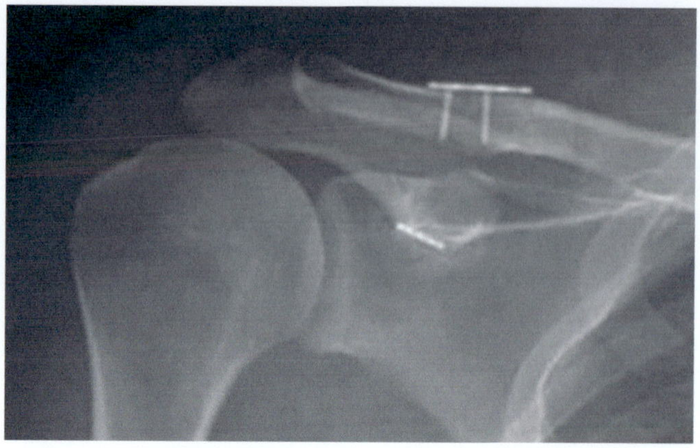

Fig. 19.17 Postoperative X-ray of the right shoulder joint shows good reduction of the acromioclavicular joint

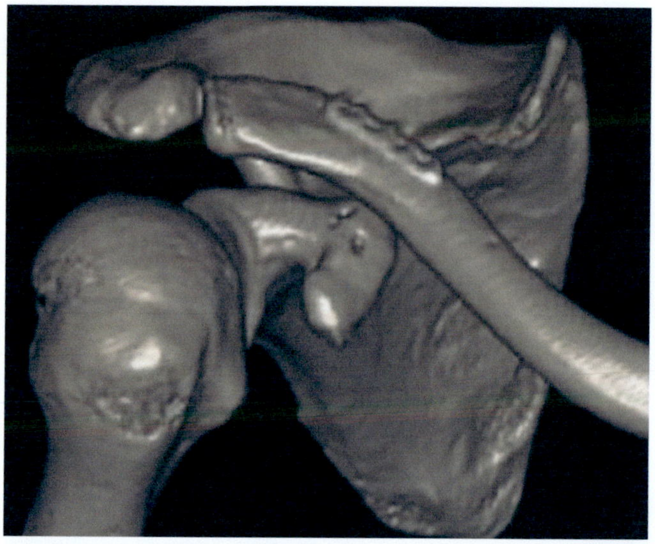

Fig. 19.18 Postoperative 3D CT reconstruction of the shoulder joint showing tunnel position and good reduction of the acromioclavicular joint

References

1. Thangaraju S, Tauber M, Habermeyer P, et al. Clavicle and coracoid process periprosthetic fractures as late postoperative complications in arthroscopically assisted acromioclavicular joint stabilization. Knee Surg Sports Traumatol Arthrosc. 2019;27(12):3797–802.
2. Sun LJ, Lu D, Tao ZY, et al. Analysis of risk factors for loss of reduction after acromioclavicular joint dislocation treated with the suture-button. J Orthop Sci. 2019;24(5):817–21.
3. Cook JB, Shaha JS, Rowles DJ, et al. Early failures with single clavicular transosseous coracoclavicular ligament reconstruction. J Shoulder Elbow Surg. 2012;21(12):1746–52.
4. Yoo JC, Choi NH, Kim SY, et al. Distal clavicle tunnel widening after coracoclavicular ligament reconstruction with semitendinosus tendon: a case report. J Shoulder Elbow Surg. 2006;15(2):256–9.
5. Singh B, Mohanlal P, Bawale R. Early failure of coracoclavicular ligament reconstruction using Tight Rope system. Acta Orthop Belg. 2016;82(1):119–23.

20 Reconstruction of the Coracoclavian Ligament by Transposition of the Pectoralis Minor Tendon Variant Insertion Point

Chang-ming Huang and Yang-pan Fu

20.1 Introduction

The pectoralis minor muscle originates from the third to fifth ribs, and the tendon terminates at the coracoid process of the scapula. The pectoralis minor muscle tendon terminates at the coracoacromial ligament, glenoid humeral joint margin, supraspinatus muscle tendon, humeral tuberosity, clavicle midpoint, glenoid humeral joint capsule, and the base of the coracoid process, which is rare and only occasionally found during autopsy.

In 1897, French anatomist Le Double reported that the incidence of variation in the pectoralis minor tendon was 15% [1]. There are three types of variations in the pectoralis minor tendon. Type I: The entire pectoralis minor tendon passes through the coracoid process and terminates at the glenoid lip or coracoacromial ligament; Type II: Part of the tendon is attached to the coracoid process, while the other part is attached to the coracoacromial ligament, supraspinatus muscle, or glenoid humeral joint capsule; Type III: The pectoralis minor muscle has no tendons, only abnormal attachment at the muscle insertion point, attached to the joint capsule and humeral tuberosity, not just to the coracoid process (Fig. 20.1). Weinstab [2] reported a 16% incidence of variation in the pectoralis minor tendon. The cadaver study by Lian et al. [3] reported a variation rate of 23.33% in the pectoralis minor tendon. Zhang [4] reported through anatomy that the incidence of variation in the pectoralis minor tendon was 19.38%, with a male to female ratio of 5:1, and the variants were symmetrical and consistent on both sides. Clinically, it is divided into single tendon type and double tendon type, and the double tendon type is further divided into two subtypes. Homsi et al. [5] reported using ultrasound examination that the incidence of variation in the pectoralis minor tendon was 9.57% and found no significant correlation between the variation and clinical symptoms. The incidence rate on the left side is 12.2%, and the incidence rate on

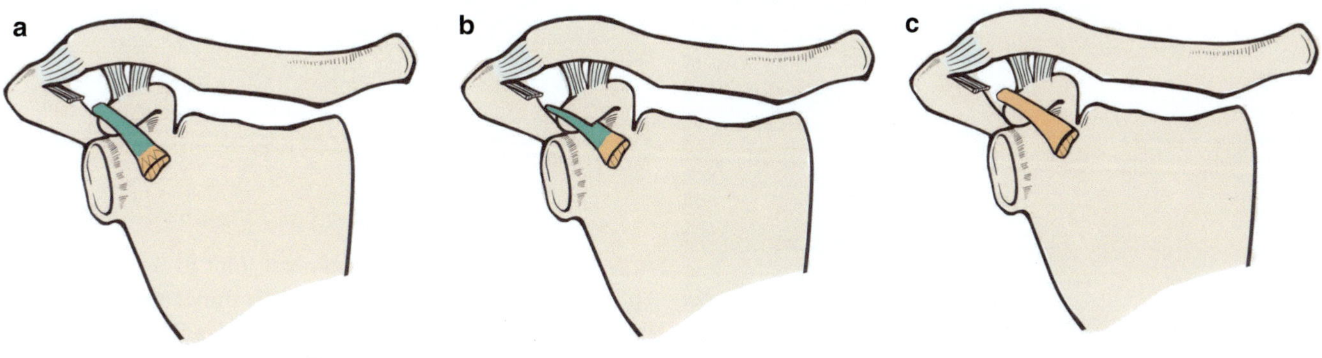

Fig. 20.1 Variant typing of pectoralis minor tendon: (**a**) Type I; (**b**) Type II; (**c**) Type III

C.-m. Huang (✉) · Y.-p. Fu
Department of Orthopedics, The 73rd Group Army Hospital, Chenggong Hospital Affiliated to Xiamen University, Xiamen, China

Y.-j. Liu et al. (eds.), *Pitfalls in Diagnosis and Treatment of Shoulder Joint Diseases*, https://doi.org/10.1007/978-981-96-2472-0_20

the right side is 6.9%. The male to female ratio is 1:2.6, and the incidence of variations in the pectoralis minor tendon detected under arthroscopy is 10–15%. Lee et al. [6] found through MRI examination of 335 patients that the incidence of variation in the pectoralis minor muscle tendon was 13.4% [7], with 1.5% of the pectoralis minor muscle passing through the coracoid process and terminating at the glenohumeral joint capsule.

20.2 Overview of the Diagnosis and Treatment Process

The patient was a 48-year-old male. Car accident injury caused left shoulder pain and limited mobility for 2 h. Physical examination: There was no redness or swelling in the left shoulder joint, tenderness at the acromioclavicular joint, distal clavicle raised, piano key sign (+), and limited rotation, external rotation, and upward movement of the shoulder joint. The X-ray film of the left shoulder joint (Fig. 20.2) and CT three-dimensional reconstruction showed dislocation of the left acromioclavicular joint (Rockwood III type) (Fig. 20.3).

Arthroscopic surgery was performed using general anesthesia, with the healthy side lying 30° backward and the affected limb flexing 15° forward and abduction 45° traction. Establish a conventional posterior approach and an anterior external superior approach. Explore for Bankart injuries, SLAP injuries, and rotator cuff injuries. Through the approach from the glenoid humeral joint to the rotator cuff space, it was found that the pectoralis minor muscle crossed over the coracoid process and stopped at the rotator cuff (Fig. 20.4). Carefully dissect the mutated pectoralis minor muscle, protect the coracoacromial ligament, expose and clean the surface of the coracoid process, and observe the pectoralis minor muscle tendon spanning over the coracoid process (Fig. 20.5). At the same time, determine the position of the anchor screw and the drilling tunnel of the coracoclavian ligament.

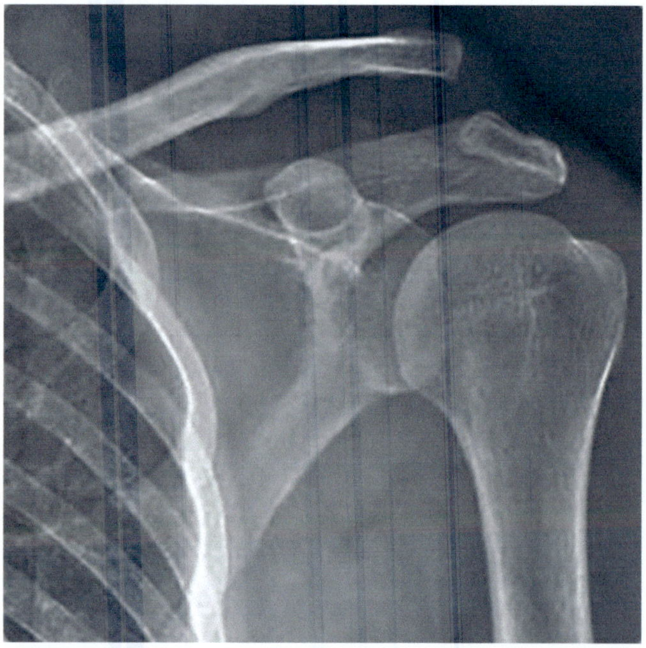

Fig. 20.2 Left shoulder joint anteroposterior X-ray showing dislocation of the acromioclavicular joint (Rockwood III type)

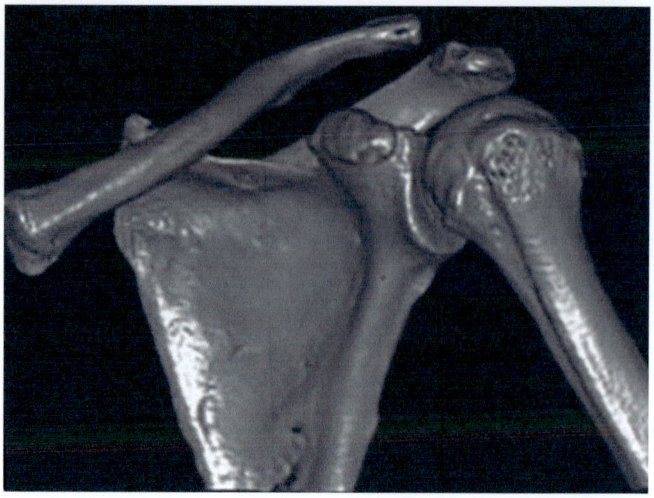

Fig. 20.3 CT three-dimensional reconstruction of the left shoulder joint showing Rockwood III dislocation of the acromioclavicular joint

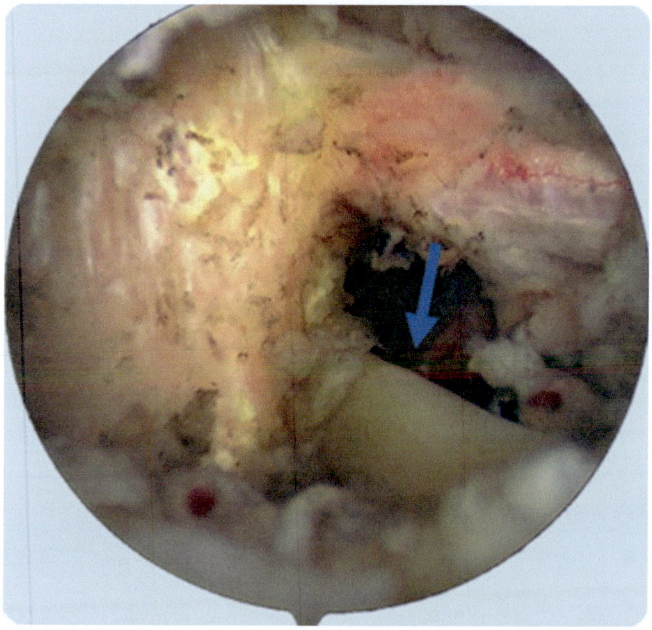

Fig. 20.4 Variant pectoralis minor muscle seen in the glenoid humeral joint (arrow)

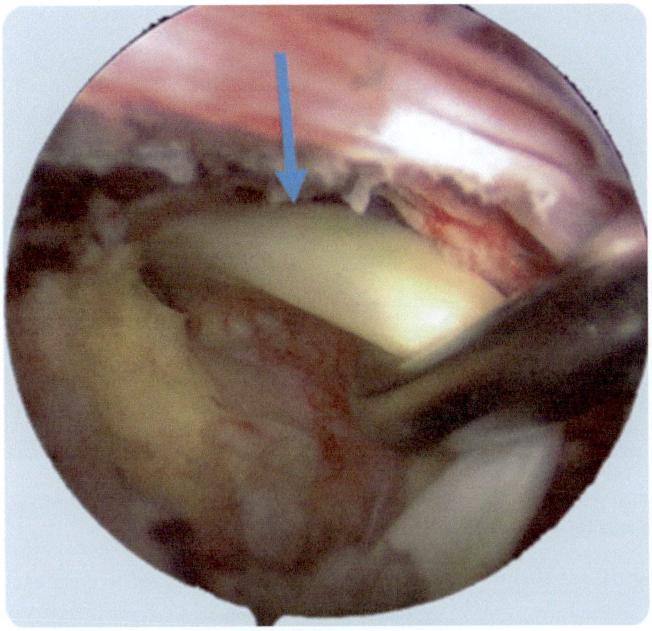

Fig. 20.5 The pectoralis minor tendon spanning over the coronoid process in the subacromial space (arrow)

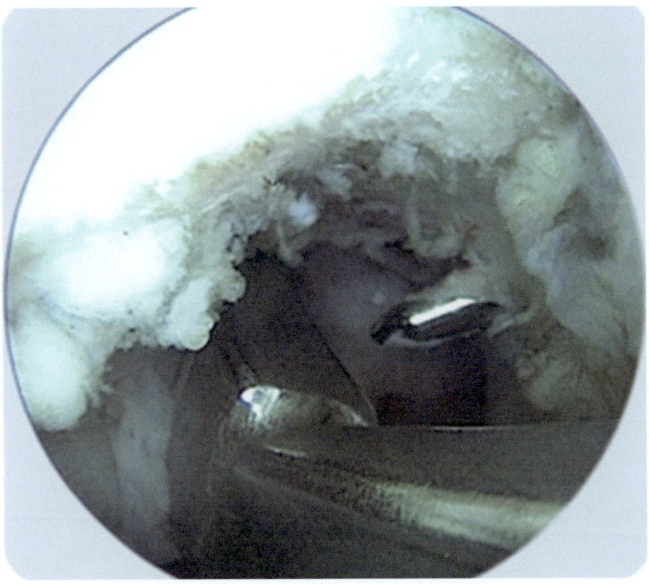

Fig. 20.6 Drilling a beak lock tunnel under the guidance of a guide

Create a coracoclavicular tunnel, insert a locator after the reduction of the acromioclavicular joint, drill a guide needle through the insertion point of the conical ligament of the clavicle, and drill through the clavicle and coracoid process respectively (Fig. 20.6). Use a hollow drill with a diameter of 4.5 mm to expand the tunnel, measure the length of the tunnel, introduce an Endobutton loop steel plate below the

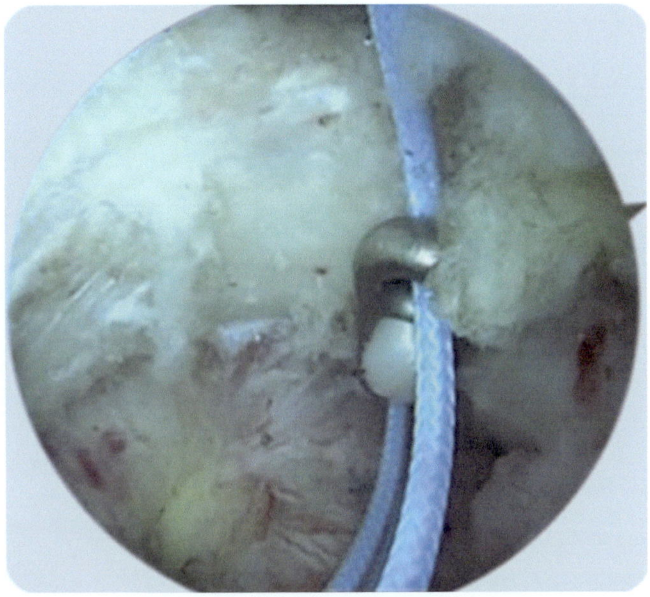

Fig. 20.7 Introduction of loop steel plate under arthroscopy

coracoid process (Fig. 20.7), and fix it with a miniature steel plate above the clavicle.

An anchor was implanted in the coracoid process, and the oblique ligament was fixed with sutures (Fig. 20.8). Postoperative radiographs of the left shoulder joint (Fig. 20.9) and three-dimensional CT reconstruction of the left shoulder showed reduction of the acromioclavicular joint (Fig. 20.10).

Variations in the pectoralis minor tendon may lead to limited external rotation of the shoulder joint. Vivek [8] reported a case of type I pectoralis minor tendon variation treated under arthroscopy. After 12 weeks, the patient regained full range of shoulder joint movement and strength, and bilateral shoulder joint symptoms completely disappeared one year after surgery. Alvaro [9] reported a 36-year-old male with type III acromioclavicular joint dislocation, which was fixed using the Tight Rope technique. During the surgery, it was found that variations in the pectoralis minor tendon had minimal clinical impact. Arthroscopic surgery must avoid potential complications. The variation of the pectoralis minor tendon and the complex anatomical structure below the acromion may prolong the surgical time or increase surgical complications. Goldman [10] believed that the absence of pectoralis minor muscle does not affect shoulder joint function, and the pectoralis minor muscle tendon can be used as a material for autologous transplantation and reconstruction. The author used the mutated pectoralis minor muscle tendon combined with loop steel plate to reconstruct the coracoclavian ligament in three cases of acromioclavicular joint dislocation with variation of pectoralis minor muscle tendon (Figs. 20.11 and 20.12) and achieved good results.

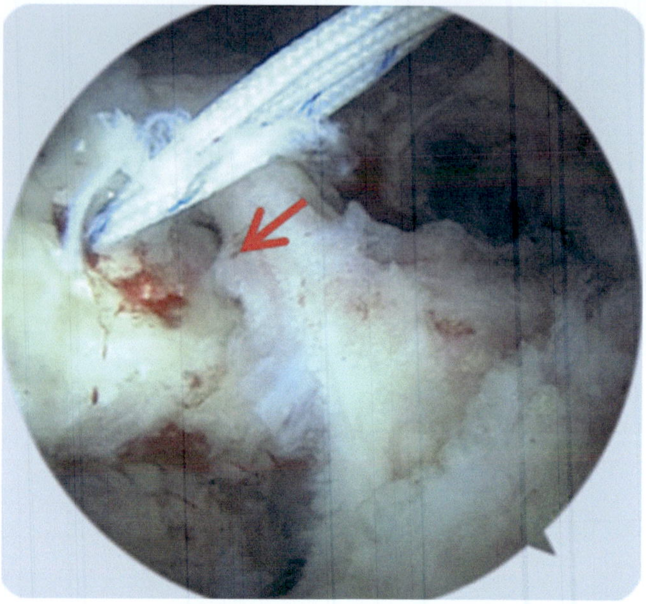

Fig. 20.8 Implantation of one anchor nail on the coracoid process, fixation of the oblique ligament with the tail line (arrow represents the pectoralis minor muscle)

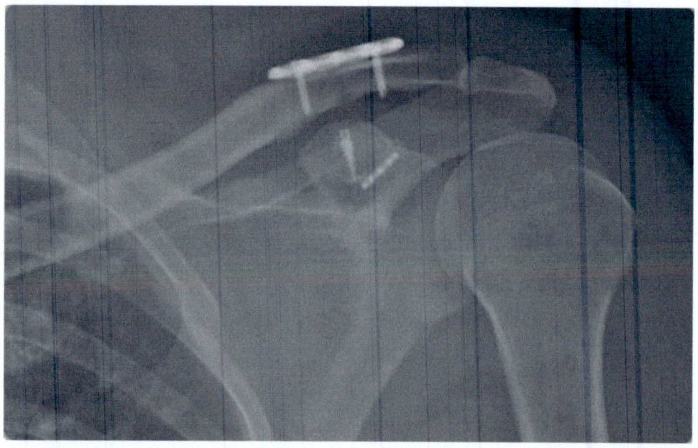

Fig. 20.9 Postoperative left shoulder X-ray showing reduction of the acromioclavicular joint

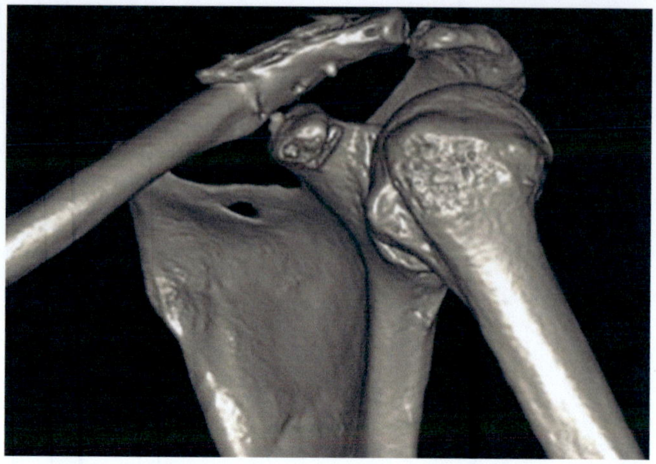

Fig. 20.10 Postoperative left shoulder CT three-dimensional reconstruction showing reduction of the acromioclavicular joint

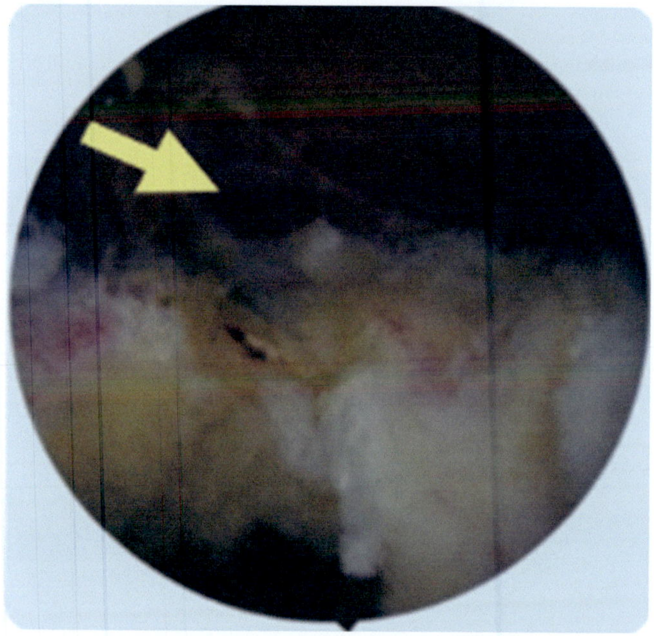

Fig. 20.11 Variation of pectoralis minor tendon in coracoid process (arrow)

In summary, the variation of the pectoralis minor tendon is not uncommon and can be divided into three types. Type I: The entire pectoralis minor tendon passes through the coracoid process and terminates at the glenoid lip or coracoacromial ligament; Type II: Part of the tendon is attached to the coracoid process, while the other part is attached to the coracoacromial ligament, supraspinatus muscle, or glenoid humeral joint capsule; Type III: The pectoralis minor muscle has no tendons, only abnormal attachment at the muscle insertion point, attached to the joint capsule and humeral tuberosity, not just on the coronoid process. If variations in the pectoralis minor tendon are found after acromioclavicular joint surgery, displacement of the pectoralis minor tendon can be used to strengthen the coracoclavian ligament.

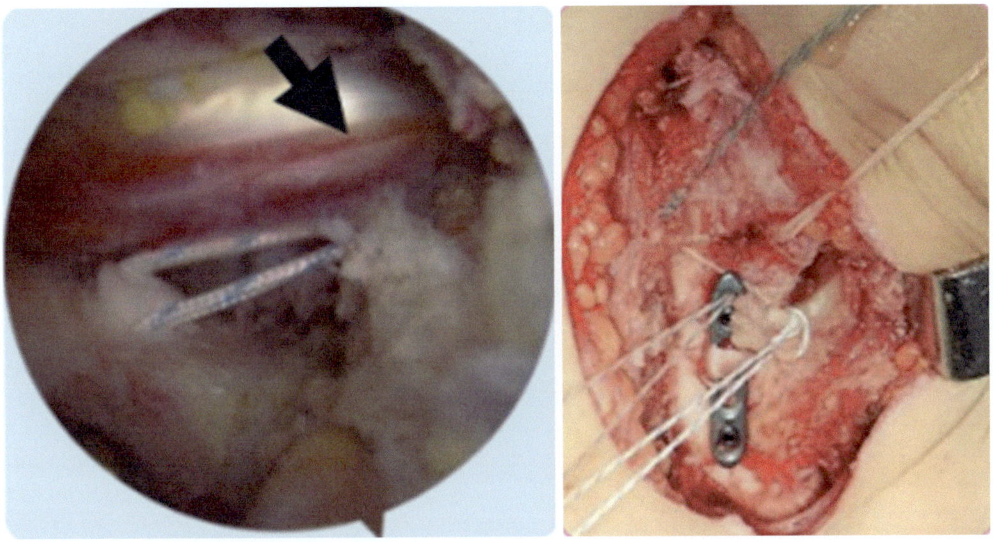

Fig. 20.12 Reconstruction of the coracoclavian ligament with transposition of the pectoralis minor muscle tendon and enhanced fixation with suture anchor screws

References

1. Le Double H. Traité des variations du système musculaire de l'homme, Tome 2. Paris: Scleicher Frères Ed; 1897. p. 516.
2. Weinstabl R, Hertz H, Firbas W. Zusammenhang des ligamentum coracoglenoidale mit dem musculus pectoralis minor. Cells Tissues Organs. 1986;125(2):126–31.
3. Lian JQ, Dong LL, Zhao YJ, et al. Anatomical study of the coracoid process in Mongolian male cadavers using the Latarjet procedure. J Orthop Surg Res. 2016;11(1):126.
4. 张增方，杜建春，张岩，等.胸小肌止点变异的解剖学研究.中华创伤骨科杂志. 2004;6(9):1080.
5. Homsi C, Rodrigues MB, Silva JJ, et al. Anomalous insertion of the pectoralis minor muscle: ultrasound findings. J Radiol. 2003;84(9):1007–11.
6. Lee SJ, Ha DH, Lee SM. Unusual variation of the rotator interval: insertional abnormality of the pectoralis minor tendon and absence of the coracohumeral ligament. Skeletal Radiol. 2010;39(12):1205–9.
7. Lee CB, Choi SJ, Ahn JH, et al. Ectopic insertion of the pectoralis minor tendon: interreader agreement and findings in the rotator interval on MRI. Korean J Radiol. 2014;15(6):764–70.
8. Vivek P, Sandesh M, Satish M, et al. A case of bilateral aberrant pectoralis minor insertion with absent coracohumeral ligament: clinical relevance and controversies. J Clin Orthop Trauma. 2016;7(1):76–9.
9. Alvaro MA, Carmen BA, Ignacio GG, et al. Arthroscopic stabilisation of an acute acromioclavicular dislocation grade III in a patient with ectopic insertion of the pectoralis minor: technical considerations. Knee Surg Sports Traumatol Arthrosc. 2016;24(7):2197–9.
10. Goldman E, Vasan C, Lopez-Cardona H, et al. Unilateral ectopic insertion of the pectoralis minor: clinical and functional significance. Morphologie. 2016;100(328):41–4.

Part VIII

Perioperative Pain and Infection of the Shoulder Joint: An Introduction and Summary

Jing Xue

Introduction

The management of perioperative infections and postoperative pain is a pervasive challenge in healthcare. It is imperative to meticulously address preoperative, intraoperative, and postoperative infection prevention strategies while effectively diagnosing and treating infections. By reducing the incidence of infections and alleviating patient discomfort, we can significantly enhance patient outcomes.

Corticosteroid injection is a therapeutic approach for managing rotator cuff tendinitis and impingement syndrome; however, it is important to acknowledge that corticosteroid injection into the subacromial space and joint may lead to adverse effects. This part aims to analyze and discuss the etiology and treatment of shoulder joint infection resulting from steroid injections for shoulder pain. Syphilitic shoulder arthritis, although uncommon, will be examined in terms of its diagnostic challenges, along with proposed differential diagnoses and corresponding measures. Additionally, this part will focus on exploring the causes, diagnosis, and treatment options for both rotator cuff pain and postoperative infections.

Summary

1. The incidence of infection resulting from corticosteroid injection for shoulder pain is not uncommon. It is crucial to strictly control the indications for its use. In case of infection, timely arthroscopic debridement should be performed to prevent serious consequences.
2. The timely diagnosis of syphilitic arthritis in the shoulder joint poses a challenge. An exclusive approach is required for differential diagnosis, distinguishing it from traumatic arthritis, villonodular synovitis, rheumatoid arthritis, suppurative arthritis, hemophilic arthritis, tuberculous arthritis, and Charcot's arthropathy.
3. There are numerous factors that influence postoperative pain following rotator cuff repair. It is imperative to assess and manage patients' anxiety levels, employ anti-anxiety medications judiciously, and adhere strictly to surgical indications. Diabetic patients should diligently control their blood glucose levels during the perioperative period. When suturing the rotator cuff, it is crucial to evaluate the tension in order to ensure optimal post-suturing tension without excessive strain. Patients with partial rotator cuff tears often present with concomitant shoulder periarthritis; therefore, meticulous attention should be given to fully releasing shoulder joint adhesions. In cases of tendinopathy of the long head of the biceps

J. Xue (✉)
Orthopaedics, Air Force Medical Center of Chinese PLA, Beijing, China

brachii muscle, options such as debridement, repair, or fixation can be considered. Perioperative shoulder pain can be managed using multimodal analgesia techniques, including preemptive analgesia and sequential analgesia. It is advisable to exercise caution when injecting glucocorticoids and sodium hyaluronate into the joint cavity and subacromial space after sleeve repair.

4. The infection rate after rotator cuff repair is relatively low. Once infection occurs, it will be catastrophic. There are many perioperative-related factors leading to infection after rotator cuff repair. Patients who received corticosteroid injection within 1 month before surgery had a higher incidence of postoperative infection. Diabetes mellitus increases the infection rate after rotator cuff repair. Gender and age were associated with postoperative infection. Smokers have a higher incidence of postoperative infection. Obesity is a risk factor for infection after shoulder arthroscopy. ***P. acnes*** is a non-sporulation gram-positive microaerobic bacteria, which often grows in the axillae. It is the main strain of postoperative infection of shoulder joint. It takes 14–17 days or more to cultivate ***P. acnes***. Rotator cuff injury infection mostly occurs about 6 weeks after surgery. Most patients have no obvious symptoms in the early stage, and there is no clear chief complaint, which is not easy to attract attention. When infection after rotator cuff reconstruction is suspected, arthrocentesis is helpful for diagnosis. Bacterial culture encompasses aerobic, anaerobic, acid-fast, and fungal cultures, serving as a definitive diagnostic method for identifying infections. Etiological diagnosis plays a pivotal role in guiding postoperative treatment. The optimal treatment for postoperative rotator cuff infection is early arthroscopic debridement, which effectively eliminates inflammatory synovium, necrotic tissue, fibrous cords, and scar adhesions to promote expedited joint function recovery after surgery.

Infection Following Corticosteroid Shoulder Injection

21

Yu-jie Liu, Wei Qi, and Chang-ming Huang

21.1 Overview of Diagnosis and Treatment

The patient was a 62-year-old lady. She suffered from pain in the left shoulder joint with limited abduction for more than 3 months. Conservative treatment such as physical therapy had no obvious effect. The patient had a history of diabetes for more than 5 years.

Physical examination showed atrophy of the muscles around the left shoulder joint, weakness in abduction and elevation, 60° active abduction, no significant limitation in passive movement, significant limitation in both internal and external rotation (Fig. 21.1), bear hug test (+), Neer sign (+), and acromial impact test (+). The patient was diagnosed with left rotator cuff lesion by MRI. The patient was treated with corticosteroid shoulder injections for three times within 3 months. After the last treatment, the patient developed fever, severe shoulder pain, severe swelling, and range of motion limitation of the shoulder was more obvious than before treatment.

Physical examination showed atrophy of the left deltoid muscle, swelling of the shoulder joint, and plump from the subacromial space to the subscapular angle (Fig. 21.2), with a feeling of fluctuation on palpation, tenderness (++) in the swelling area, and high skin temperature. The lifting, abduction, and rotation of the left shoulder joint were limited. Radiographs of the left shoulder showed osteoporosis and decreased density of the left humeral head (Fig. 21.3), narrowing of the left shoulder joint space, and uneven destruction of the humeral head (Fig. 21.4). MRI showed numerous hyperintense areas in the left shoulder joint cavity and periarticular soft tissue, as well as destruction of the left humeral head (Fig. 21.5).

Blood tests showed increased erythrocyte sedimentation rate, white blood cell count, and C-reactive protein. Aspiration of the shoulder joint cavity yielded 65 mL of yellow, viscous purulent fluid (Fig. 21.6).

During the arthroscopic operation, the humeral head and glenoid cartilage of shoulder joint were damaged and stripped, and the humeral head bone was exposed. The proliferative synovium and necrotic tissue were removed, and the negative pressure suction tube and perfusion irrigation tube were placed. The joint was washed through the tube for 1 week postoperatively, then the tube was closed. After the results of various examinations were normal, the tubes were extubated, and functional training was carried out according to the rehabilitation program.

Y.-j. Liu
Orthopaedics, Chinese PLA General Hospital, Beijing, China

W. Qi (✉)
Department of Orthopedics, The Fourth Medical Center, Chinese PLA General Hospital, Beijing, China

C.-m. Huang
Department of Orthopedics, The 73rd Group Army Hospital, Chenggong Hospital Affiliated to Xiamen University, Xiamen, China

Y.-j. Liu et al. (eds.), *Pitfalls in Diagnosis and Treatment of Shoulder Joint Diseases*, https://doi.org/10.1007/978-981-96-2472-0_21

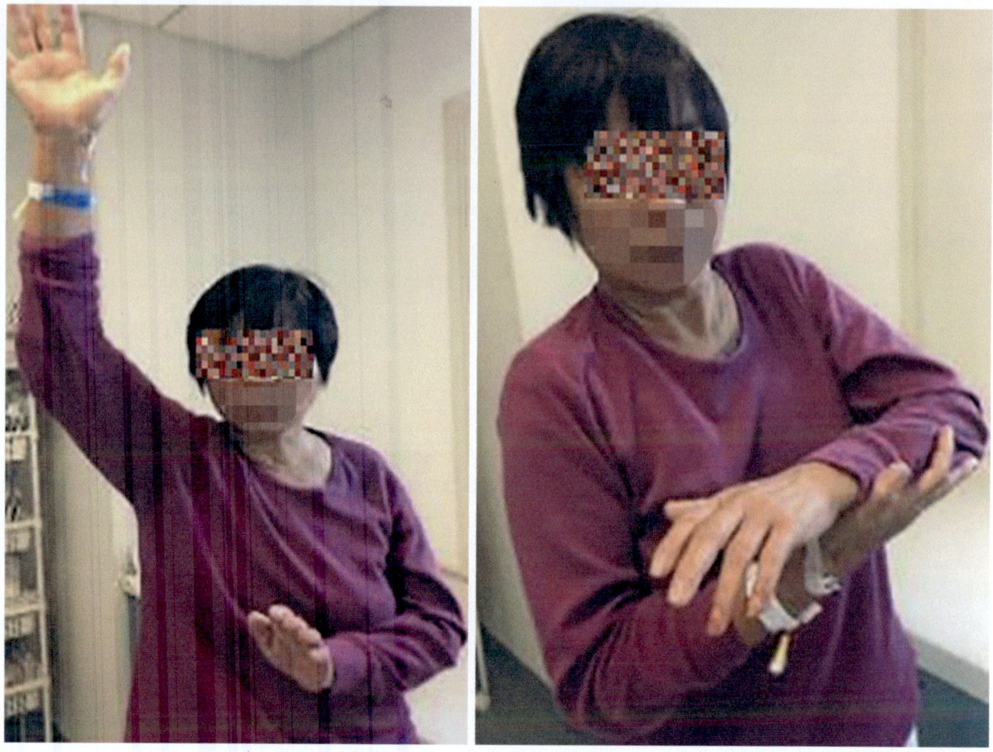

Fig. 21.1 Left rotator cuff lesion with limited joint movement

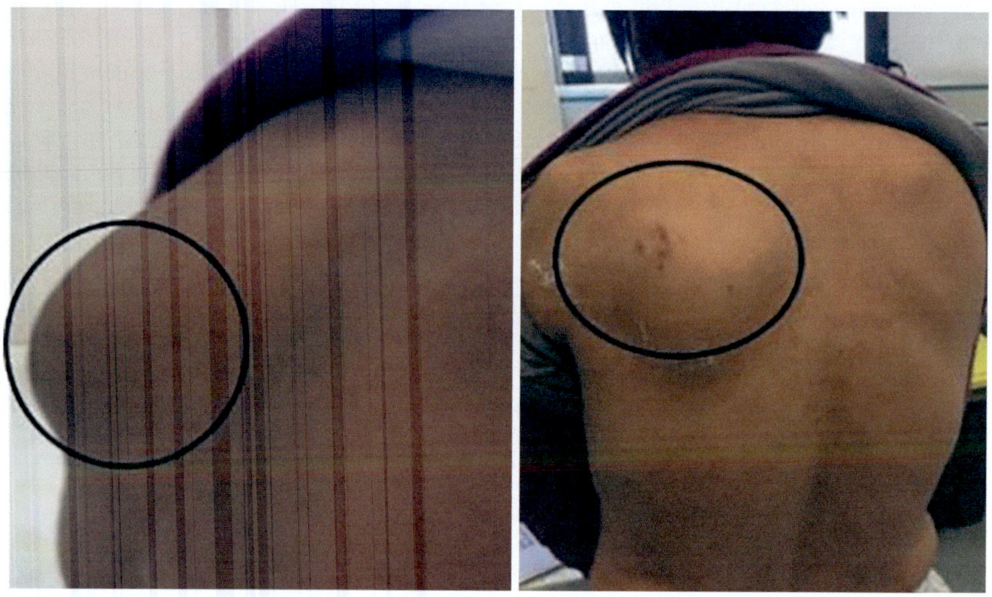

Fig. 21.2 Swelling of the posterior area of the left shoulder

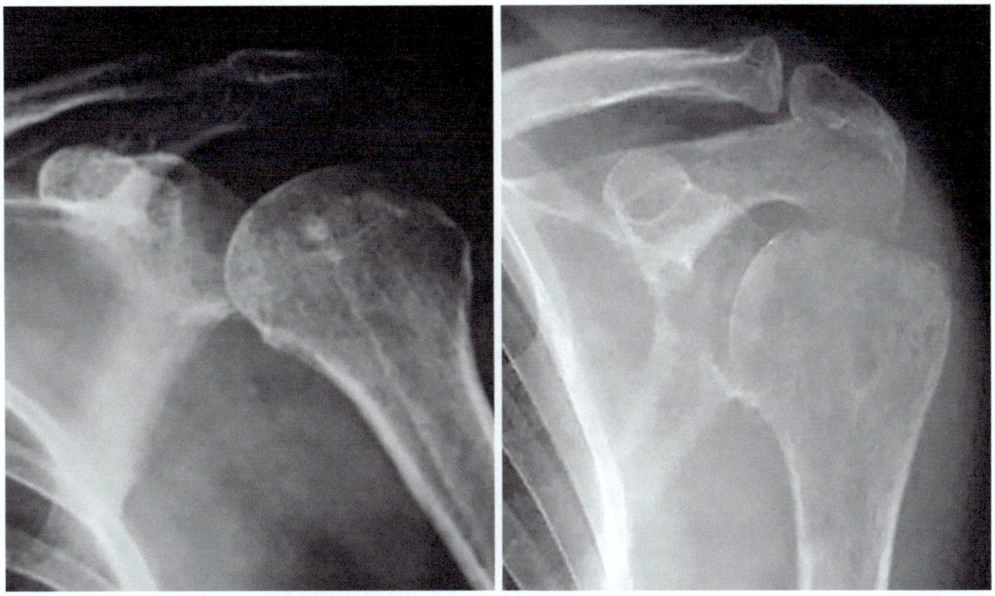

Fig. 21.3 X-ray shows osteoporosis, destruction of the humeral head

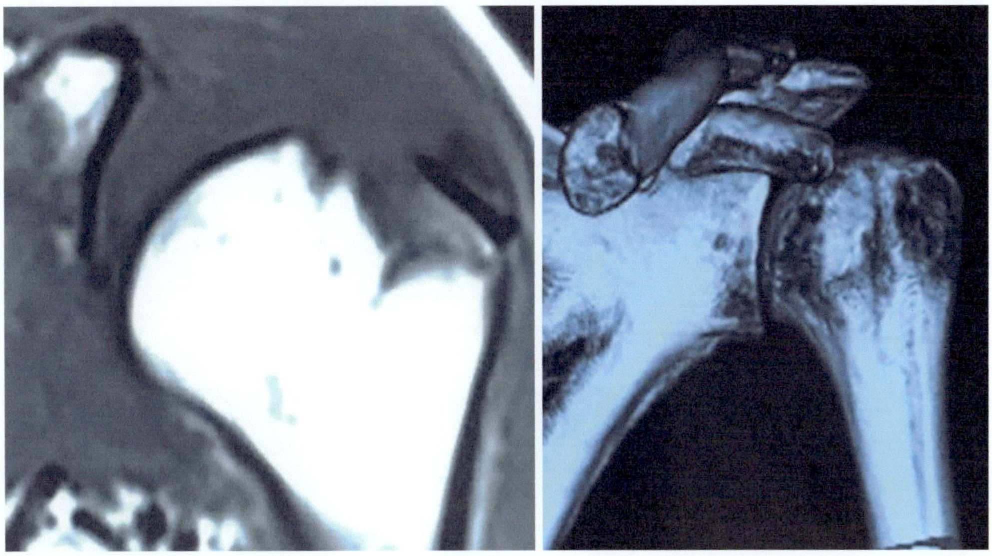

Fig. 21.4 CT of the left shoulder joint shows osteoporosis of the greater tuberosity of the humerus with uneven density

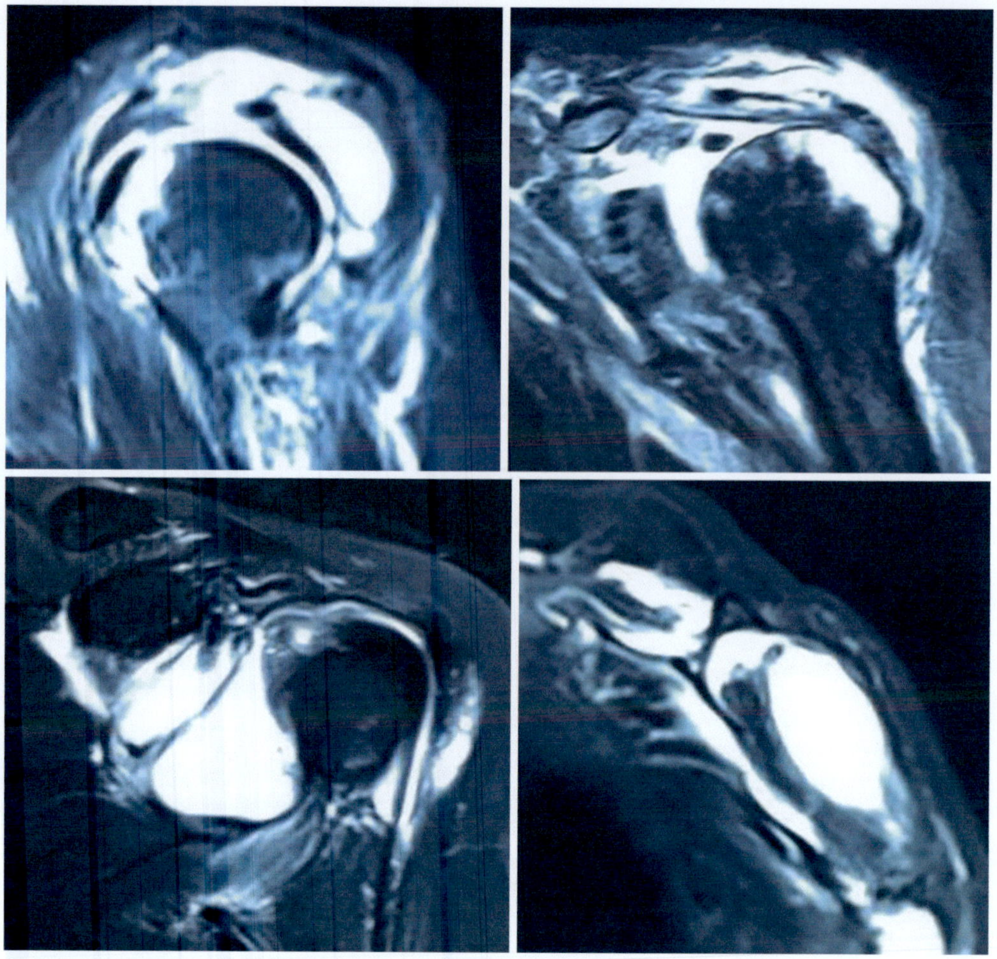

Fig. 21.5 MRI of the left shoulder shows numerous areas of hyperintensity within the joint, subacromial, and soft tissue

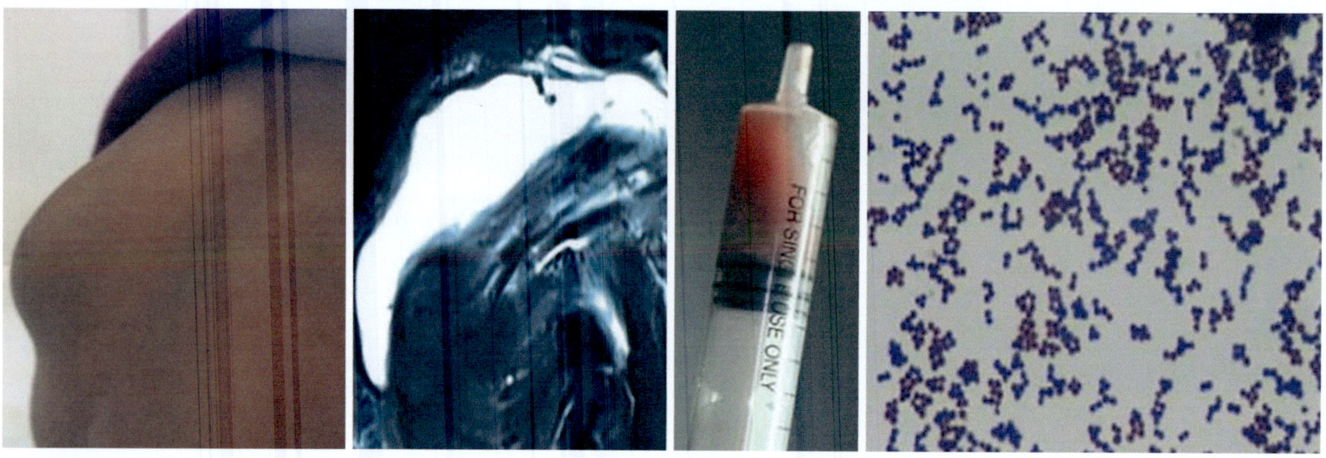

Fig. 21.6 Left subacromial puncture was performed to draw out jam-like purulent fluid; bacterial culture showed *Staphylococcus aureus*

21.2 Summary

Corticosteroid shoulder injection therapy has been shown to have short-term benefits for shoulder pain and is a treatment for rotator cuff tendinitis and impingement syndrome [1]. However, corticosteroid injections into the subacromial space and into the joint are not without side effects. Studies have shown that after local corticosteroid injection, histological changes with necrosis and disordered collagen fibers occur, which may lead to tendon weakening or rupture, while being harmful to glenohumeral cartilage [2, 3]. For patients with diabetes, immune abnormalities, and frailty, joint infection is prone to occur with corticosteroid shoulder injection therapy. Thompson et al. [4] reported a case of subacromial infection in a diabetic patient. Ward et al. [5] reported four cases of subacromial infection in immunocompromised hosts, three of them had glenohumeral septic arthritis. Roschmann et al. [6] reported a case of subacromial space fungal infection in an immunocompromised host. Sepkowitz et al. [7] reported a case of subacromial cryptococcal bursitis. Hiemstra et al. [8] reported that once subacromial space infection occurred after corticosteroid shoulder injection treatment, the consequences were disastrous, and two of the three patients were disabled due to the sequelae of subacromial space infection and could not work again. Therefore, doctors should be reminded to pay attention to the risk of subacromial injection. The intra-articular injection procedure must follow the principles of aseptic technique and use disposable syringes in aseptic packaging, which can reduce the incidence of intra-articular infection [9]. If shoulder swelling and pain aggravate after injection, infection should be considered. Joint aspiration and etiological examination are helpful for early diagnosis. Timely debridement, irrigation, and drainage under arthroscopy can achieve reliable results.

References

1. Coombes BK, Bisset L, Vicenzino B. Efficacy and safety of corticosteroid injections and other injections for management of tendinopathy: a systematic review of randomised controlled trials. Lancet. 2010;376(9754):1751–67.
2. Tillander B, Franzen LE, Karlsson MH, et al. Effect of steroid injections on the rotator cuff: an experimental study in rats. J Shoulder Elbow Surg. 1999;8(3):271–4.
3. Mankin HJ, Conger KA. The effect of cortisol on articular cartilage of rabbits. I. Effect of a single dose of cortisol on glycine-C-14 incorporation. Lab Invest. 1966;15(4):794–800.
4. Thompson GR, Manshady BM, Weiss JJ. Septic bursitis. JAMA. 1978;240(21):2280–1.
5. Ward WG, Eckardt JJ. Subacromial/subdeltoid bursa abscesses, an overlooked diagnosis. Clin Orthop. 1993;288:189–94.
6. Roschmann RA, Bell CL. Septic bursitis in immunocompromised patients. Am J Med. 1987;83(4):661–5.
7. Sepkowitz D, Maslow M, Farber M, et al. Cryptococcal bursitis. Ann Intern Med. 1988;108(1):154.
8. Hiemstra LA, MacDonald PB, Froese W. Subacromial infection following corticosteroid injection. J Shoulder Elbow Surg. 2003;12(1):91–3.
9. Seror P, Pluvinage P, D'Andre FL, et al. Frequency of sepsis after local corticosteroid injection (an inquiry on 1160000 injections in rheumatological private practice in France). Rheumatology. 1999;38(12):1272–4.

22 Diagnostic and Therapeutic Misconceptions in Syphilitic Arthritis of the Shoulder Joint

Feng Qu, Yu-jie Liu, and Jing Xue

22.1 Overview of Diagnosis and Treatment

A 61-year-old female patient presented with persistent pain and limited mobility in the right shoulder, enduring for over 10 months. Initially, the patient experienced pain and restricted movement in her shoulder after carrying heavy loads a year prior, with the symptoms progressively worsening, significantly impairing daily activities and sleep. An X-ray at a local hospital identified periarthritis of the shoulder, leading to nine sessions of intra-articular steroid injections.

The patient, a 61-year-old female, presented with pain in her right shoulder joint and restricted movement for more than 10 months. A year prior, the patient had experienced pain and limited mobility in the right shoulder due to carrying heavy burdens, with symptoms gradually worsening and severely impacting daily life and sleep. X-ray imaging at a local hospital diagnosed the condition as periarthritis of the shoulder, for which she was given nine sessions of intra-articular steroid injections. Subsequently, the patient developed fever, increased swelling, and intensified pain in the shoulder joint, with symptoms persisting despite systemic antibiotic treatment. Surgical intervention involving incision, drainage, and lavage was executed on the infected joint. Two weeks post-surgery, her body temperature stabilized, and symptoms gradually ameliorated following drainage tube removal. The patient has no history of trauma, cervical spine disease, fever, or night sweats.

Physical examination showed limited elevation, flexion, and extension in the right shoulder, with active abduction at 30°, flexion at 15°, external rotation at 30°, and internal rotation at 20° (Fig. 22.1). Notable findings included tenderness at the greater tuberosity of the humerus (+), positive anterior drawer test (+), Sulcus sign (+), and Hawkins sign (+) The right upper limb maintained normal sensory and motor functions.

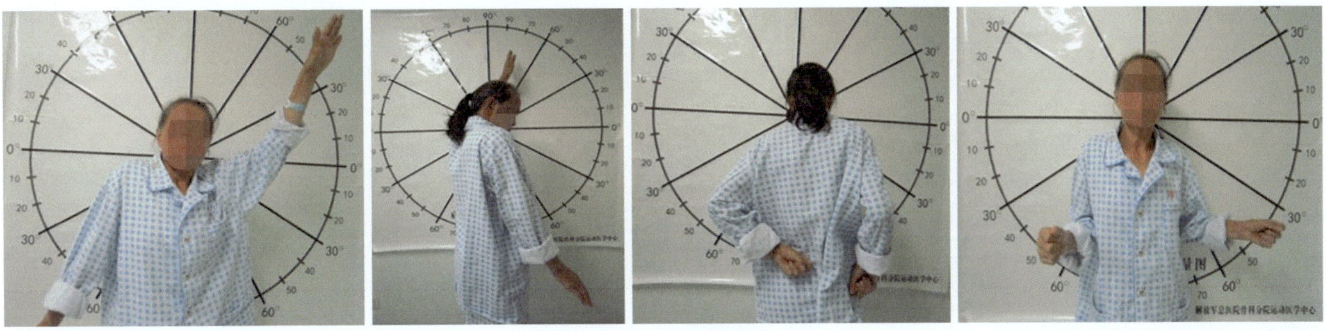

Fig. 22.1 Physical examination depicting restricted movement in the right shoulder joint

F. Qu (✉)
Beijing Chaoyang Hospital, Capital Medical University, Beijing, China

Y.-j. Liu
Orthopaedics, Chinese PLA General Hospital, Beijing, China

J. Xue
Orthopaedics, Air Force Medical Center of Chinese PLA, Beijing, China

Y.-j. Liu et al. (eds.), *Pitfalls in Diagnosis and Treatment of Shoulder Joint Diseases*, https://doi.org/10.1007/978-981-96-2472-0_22

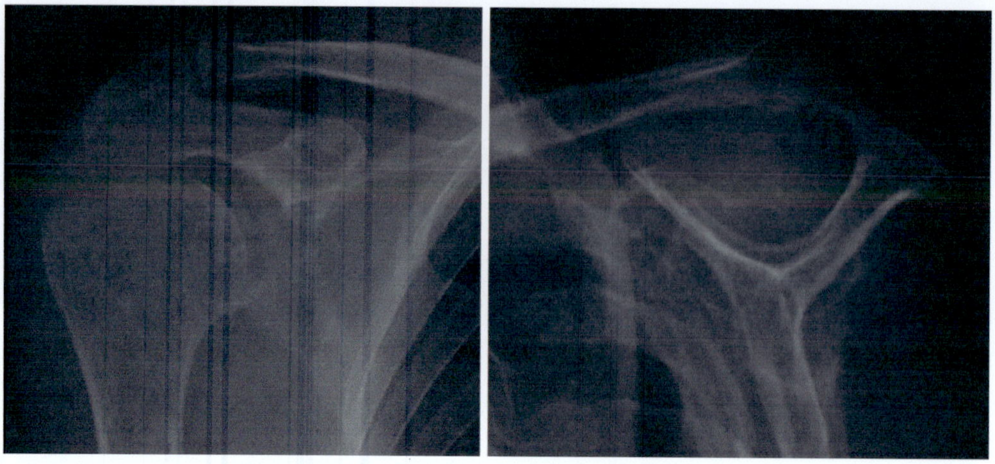

Fig. 22.2 X-ray depiction of reduced bone density, severe osteoporosis, and irregular destruction of the joint surfaces of the right shoulder

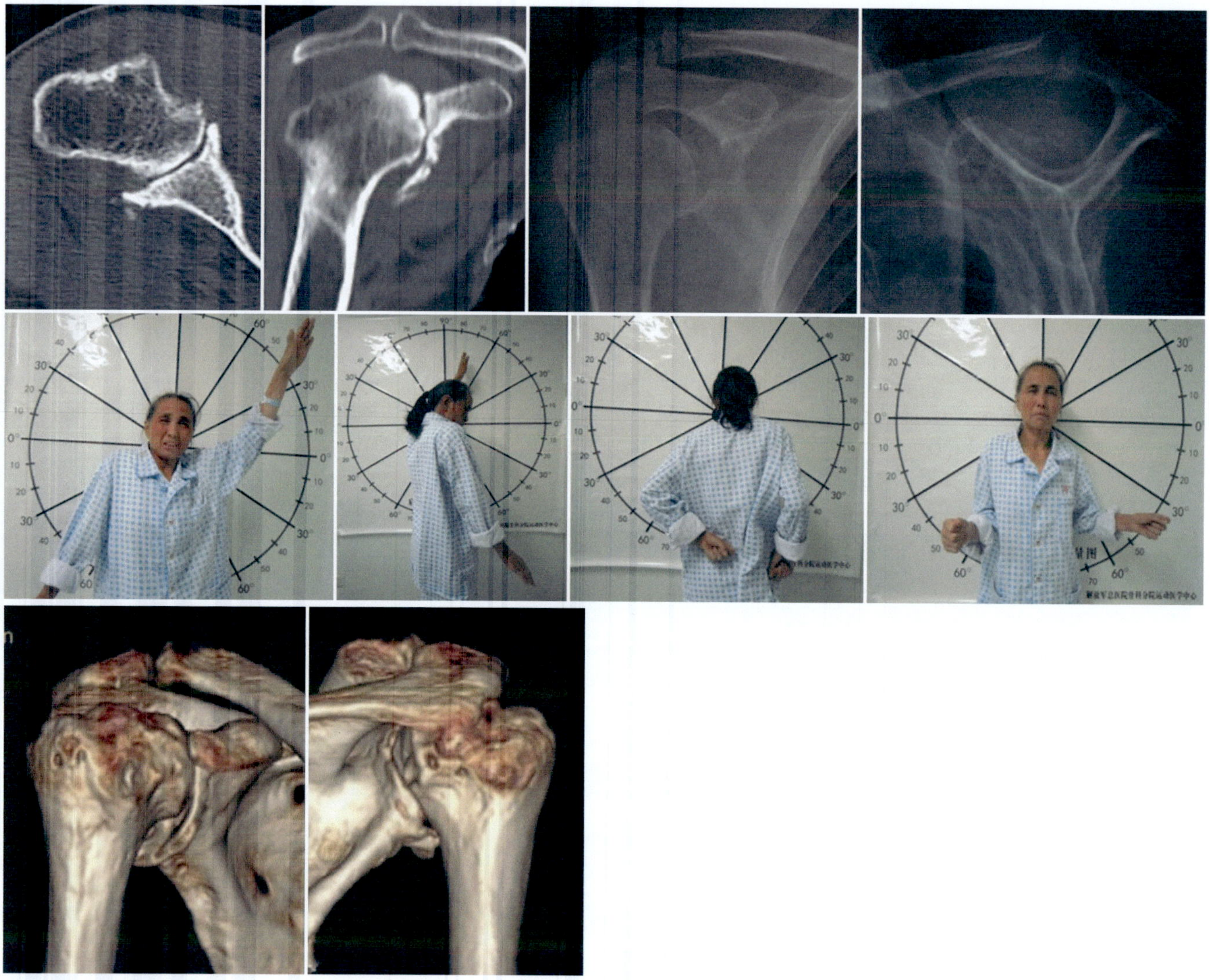

Fig. 22.3 CT scan of the shoulder joint demonstrating bone destruction and proliferation in the humeral head and glenoid

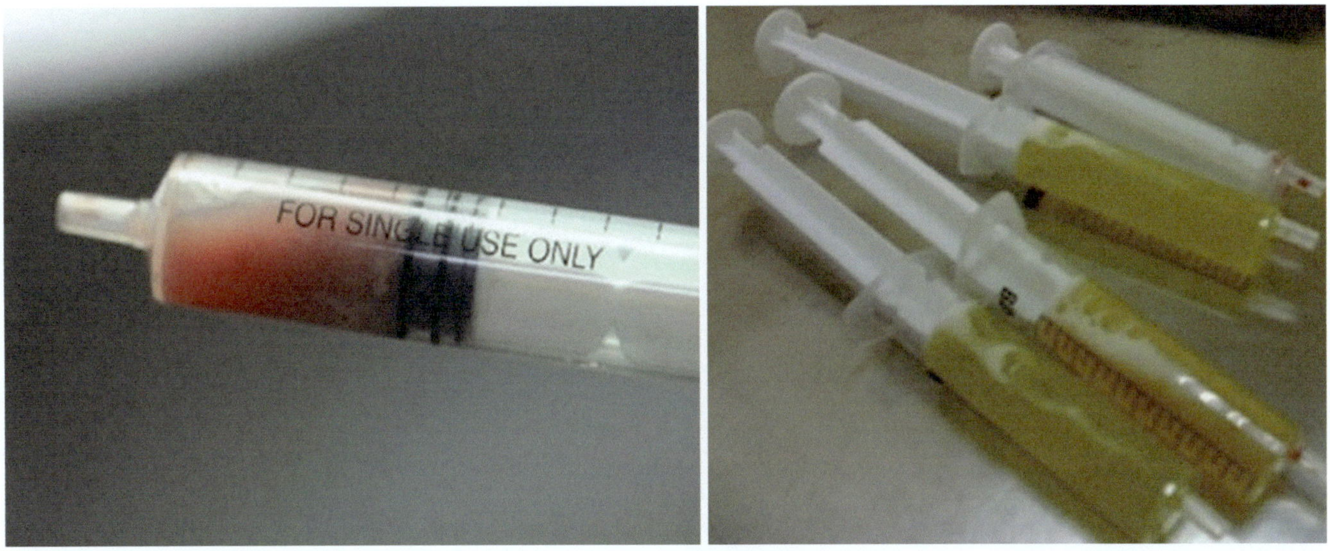

Fig. 22.4 Aspiration yielding a pale yellow, slightly turbid fluid from the shoulder joint cavity

X-ray imaging demonstrated a narrowed joint space, severe osteoporosis, and blurred articulations of the humeral head and glenoid cavity, and indicative of bone destruction (Fig. 22.2). CT scans of the shoulder joint revealed osseous destruction and proliferation at the humeral head and glenoid (Fig. 22.3). MRI showed synovial hypertrophy within the shoulder joint cavity, along with bone destruction at the humeral head and glenoid.

Complete blood count revealed normal white blood cell count, neutrophils, and lymphocytes. The rheumatoid factor was negative, the erythrocyte sedimentation rate stood at 44 mm/h, C-reactive protein levels were normal, and interleukin-6 levels remained normal. Puncture of the shoulder joint produced 50 mL of pale yellow, slightly turbid fluid (Fig. 22.4), with no acid-fast bacilli present. Cultures for aerobic and anaerobic bacteria in the synovial fluid showed no bacterial growth. Tuberculosis immunological markers were positive, with both QuantiFERON tests 1 and 2 being negative, and serological tests for syphilis antibodies were positive.

Arthroscopic examination revealed damage to the rotator cuff tissues (Fig. 22.5), destruction of the humeral head, and glenoid cavity with observable defects (Fig. 22.6). Subsequent debridement and cleaning targeted the fragmented cartilage and scar tissue of the humeral head and glenoid (Fig. 22.7). The pathology report revealed chronic inflammatory tissue, characterized by a high concentration of lymphocytes, numerous phagocytes, and significant plasma cells infiltration (Fig. 22.8).

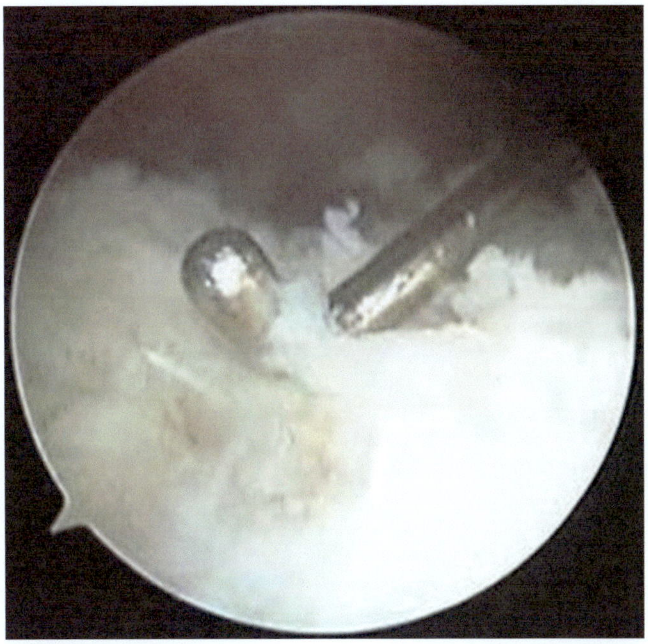

Fig. 22.5 Evidence of wear and partial tearing in the rotator cuff fibers

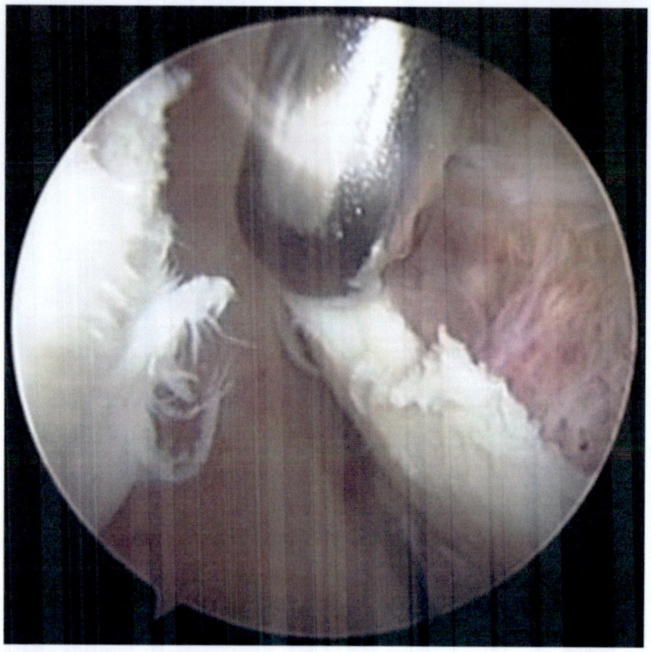

Fig. 22.6 Observations of destruction and partial loss in the humeral head cartilage

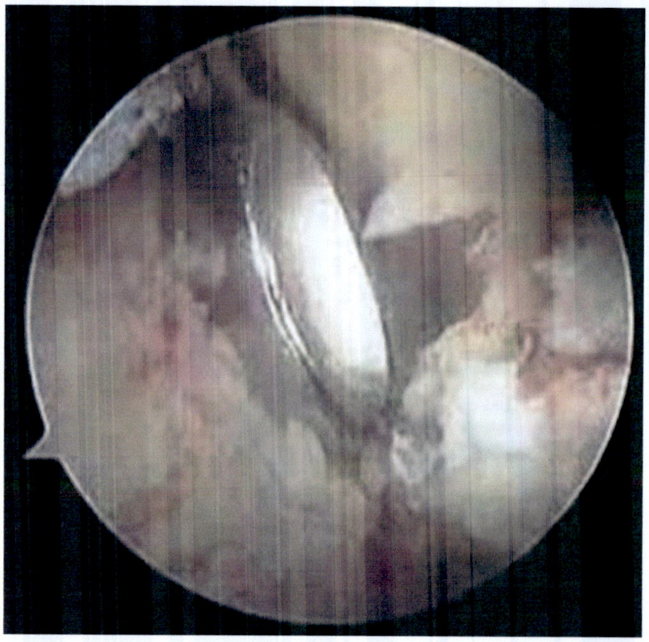

Fig. 22.7 Post-debridement of proliferative synovium and scar tissue within the joint

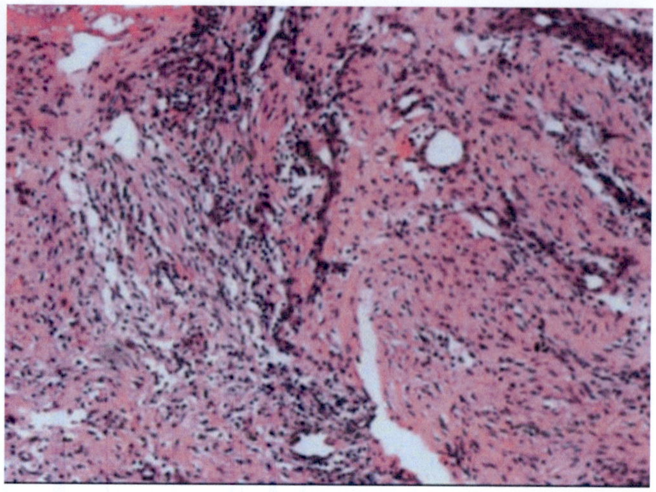

Fig. 22.8 Pathology report illustrating infiltration of inflammatory cells, comprising numerous phagocytes, lymphocytes, and plasma cells

22.2 Characteristics of the Case

The case's distinctive attributes, based on the patient's reports, include: (1) The patient had received nine intra-articular steroid injections for shoulder pain attributed to periarthritis. This was followed by the development of swelling, pain, and fever in the right shoulder joint, later identified as an infection and treated with debridement and lavage at a local hospital. (2) Imaging revealed degradation of the glenoid and humeral head cartilage in the right shoulder. (3) Puncture of the shoulder joint cavity produced 50 mL of pale yellow, slightly turbid fluid (Fig. 22.4). (4) Laboratory analyses indicated normal complete blood count, negative rheumatoid factor, and normal C-reactive protein and interleukin-6 levels. (5) Additional tests showed negative results for acid-fast bacillus and tuberculosis in the joint fluid, no growth in cultures for aerobic and anaerobic bacteria, an erythrocyte sedimentation rate of 44 mm/h, positive syphilis serology, positive tuberculosis immunological markers, but negative QuantiFERON tests 1 and 2.

22.3 Differential Diagnosis

Differential diagnosis was performed using the method of exclusion. This case required distinction from conditions such as post-traumatic arthritis, pigmented villonodular synovitis, rheumatoid arthritis, septic arthritis, hemophilic arthritis, tuberculous arthritis, syphilitic arthritis, and Charcot arthropathy. Although the patient experienced shoulder pain due to carrying loads, there is no clear history of shoulder injury, fracture, or dislocation, allowing for the exclusion of traumatic osteoarthritis of the shoulder. The joint's swelling and fluid accumulation suggest synovitis. Pigmented villonodular synovitis is more common in young to middle-aged adults and is usually found in the knee joints, characterized by villous or nodular proliferation of the synovium (Fig. 22.9), usually with bloody or yellow-brown joint fluid. Given that the extracted fluid was pale yellow and turbid, not reddish-brown, and considering the extensive damage to the humeral head and glenoid cartilage, pigmented villonodular synovitis is ruled out.

Rheumatoid arthritis, an autoimmune disorder, primarily targeting small joints like the elbows, wrists, and ankles in a symmetrical pattern, but it can also affect the hip, knee, and shoulder joints. It manifests as morning stiffness, deformities in the interphalangeal joints, elevated erythrocyte sedimentation rate, increased C-reactive protein, and positive rheumatoid factors in serum and synovial fluid.

Infections by *Staphylococcus aureus* represent 50% of cases, characterized by systemic symptoms, joint redness and swelling, increased skin temperature, pronounced tenderness, elevated white blood cell count, erythrocyte sedimentation rate, C-reactive protein, and positive bacterial cultures in blood and synovial fluid. Surgical intervention often uncovers purulent and fibrinous necrotic tissue within the joint cavity.

Shoulder joint tuberculosis: Patients with tuberculosis exhibit symptoms of tuberculous intoxication. Joint tuberculosis results from the invasion of cartilage and bone by tuberculous synovitis, leading to tuberculosis affecting the entire joint. The presence of acid-fast bacilli in blood and synovial fluid, along with tuberculous nodules and caseous changes in pathology, confirms the diagnosis.

Chronic syphilitic arthritis: This condition generally targets larger joints, leading to cartilage and subchondral bone erosion and subsequent bone destruction. Symptoms include joint swelling, pain, and restricted mobility. Specific serologic tests for syphilis antibodies and histopathological examination are essential for diagnosing and distinguishing syphilitic arthritis.

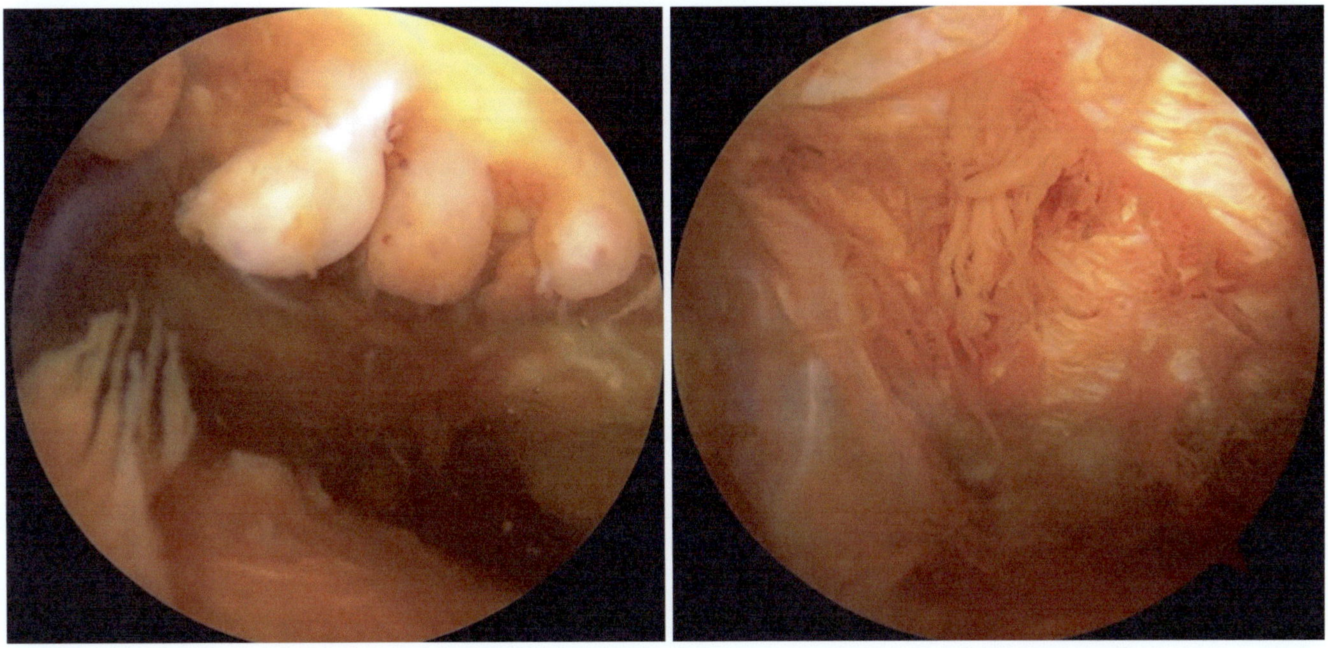

Fig. 22.9 Knee joint exhibiting pigmented villonodular synovitis, highlighted by villous and nodular synovial proliferation

Rotator Cuff Perioperative Pain Factors and Strategies

23

Ya-dong Zhang and Jun Luo

23.1 Overview of Patient Condition

The patient, a 59-year-old male, presented with a history of right shoulder joint pain and limited mobility for over six months. Physical activities exacerbate his symptoms, to the point of disrupting daily rest. While conservative treatments provided temporary relief, symptoms recurred persistently [1]. In the past month, the patient reported increased pain upon abduction and elevation of the right shoulder joint. Additionally, the patient has a medical history of diabetes.

Physical examination revealed antero-inferiorly tenderness (+) to the acromion of the right shoulder joint, along with limited external rotation (Fig. 23.1), when the right upper limb was abducted at 90°. Neer's sign, Hawkins–Kennedy sign, drop arm test, and Jobe test were all positive, while 0° abduction resistance test, Lift-off test, and Speeds sign were weakly positive. Patient's grip strength is normal for both hands. Diagnostic imaging including X-ray and MRI, X-ray showed right acromion osteophyte, type II acromion (Fig. 23.2); and MRI depicted right rota-

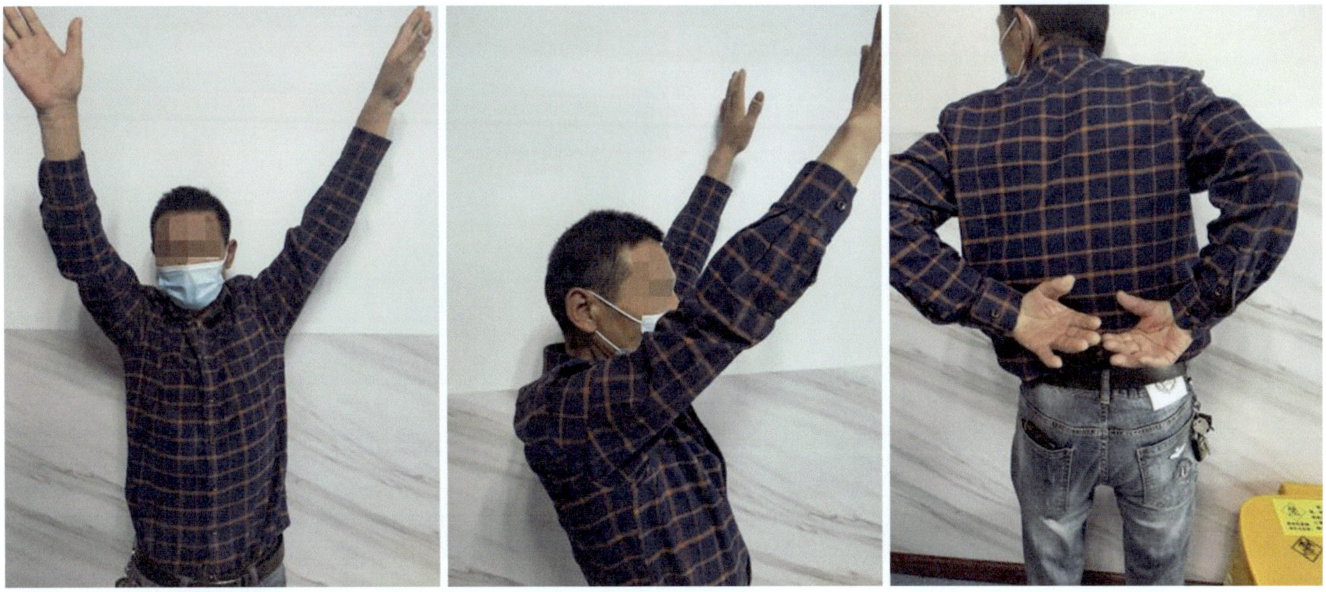

Fig. 23.1 The right shoulder joint with limited internal rotation and extension when abducted

Y.-d. Zhang (✉)
Department of Orthopedics, The Fourth Medical Center, Chinese PLA General Hospital, Beijing, China

J. Luo
Department of Orthopedics, Zhoushan Guang'an Hospital, Zhejiang, China

Y.-j. Liu et al. (eds.), *Pitfalls in Diagnosis and Treatment of Shoulder Joint Diseases*,
https://doi.org/10.1007/978-981-96-2472-0_23

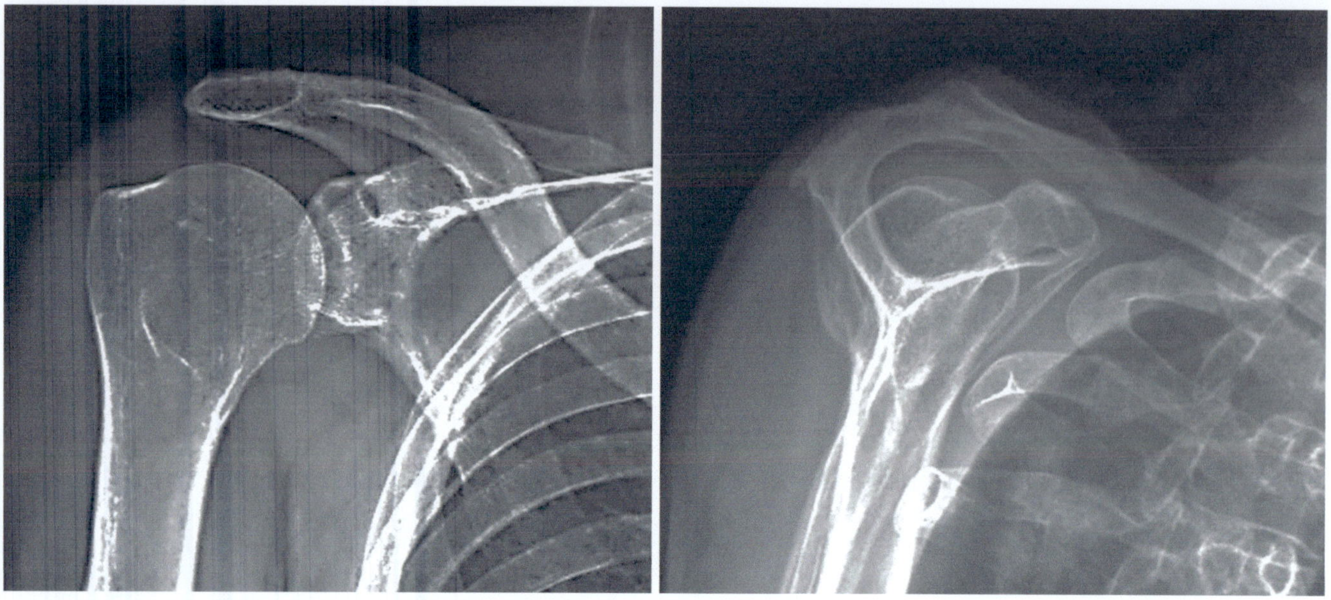

Fig. 23.2 X-ray of the right shoulder joint shows type II acromion with mild hyperplasia

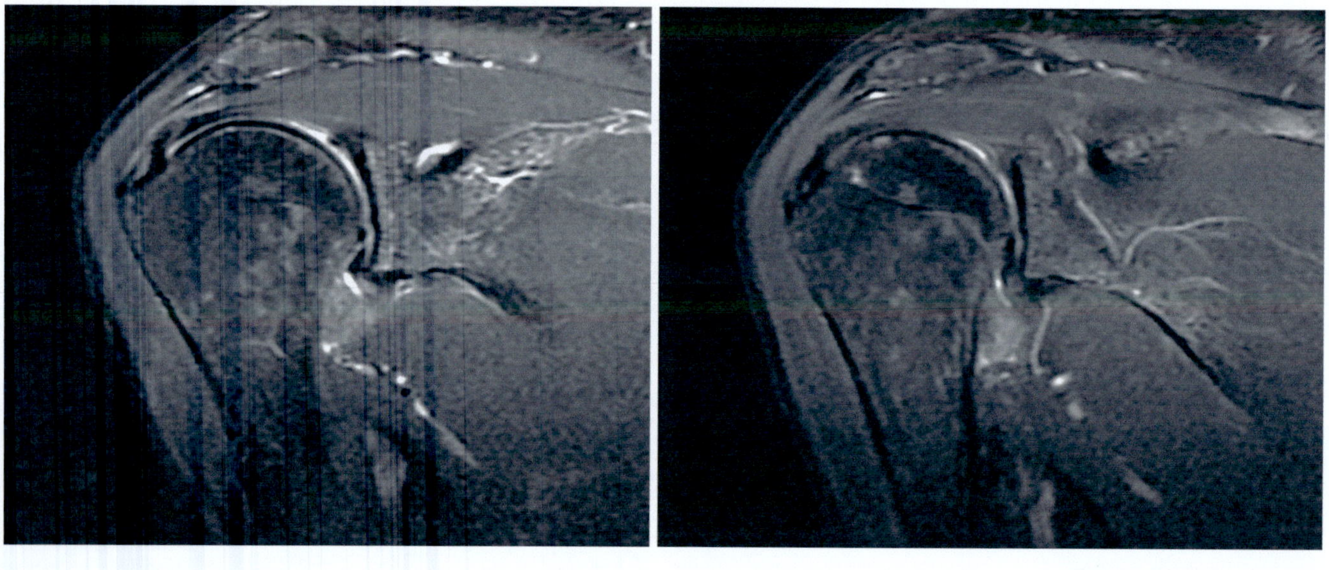

Fig. 23.3 MRI shows mild injury to the bursa layer of the right rotator cuff

tor cuff injury, mild cystic degeneration of the right humeral head, and high signal in the subacromial bursa with long head tendon of the biceps brachii (Fig. 23.3). Thus, we reached the clinical diagnosis of right rotator cuff injury, long head of biceps tendonitis, and acromion impingement syndrome.

Arthroscopic exploration and debridement under general anesthesia confirmed synovial hyperplasia (Fig. 23.4), joint space narrowing, and partial wear of the rotator cuff bursa layer (Fig. 23.5). Arthroscopic repair of the supraspinatus tendon was performed for acromial osteophyte hyperplasia (Fig. 23.6). Postoperatively, successful cuff repair was confirmed, and standard shoulder joint rehabilitation commenced. Three months postoperation, the follow-up MRI indicated satisfactory anchor position and cuff continuity (Fig. 23.7). Despite ongoing complaints of unbearable right shoulder joint pain, prompting interventions including shoulder joint cavity sealing, glycemic control, and functional training guidance resulted in gradual pain resolution over 3 months.

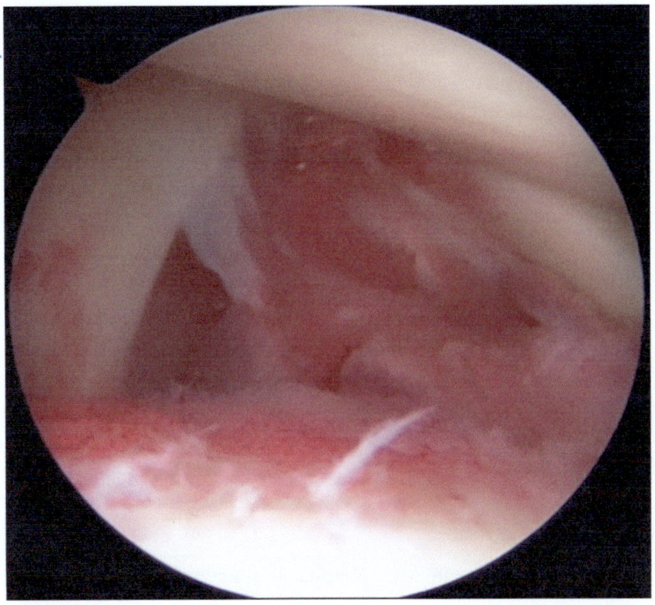

Fig. 23.4 Glenohumeral joint synovial hyperplasia, congestion, redness, and swelling

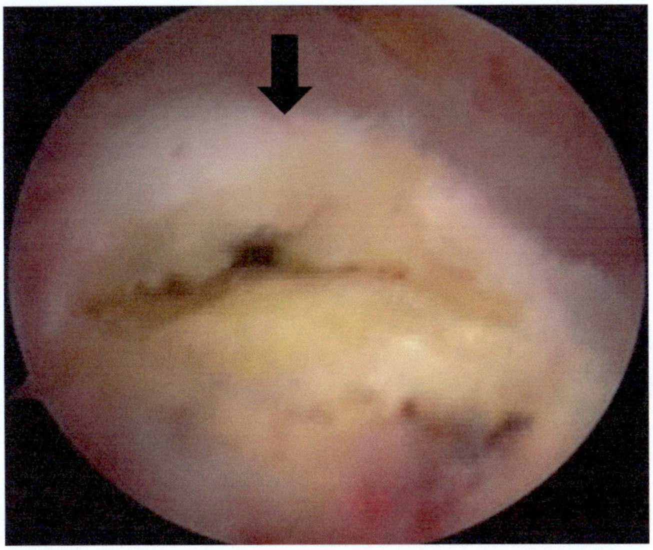

Fig. 23.5 Arthroscopic exploration shows rotator cuff tear

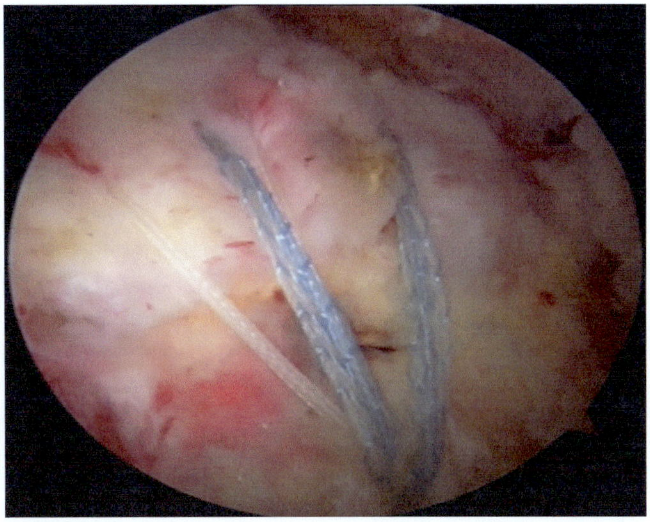

Fig. 23.6 Anchor fixation of rotator cuff suture

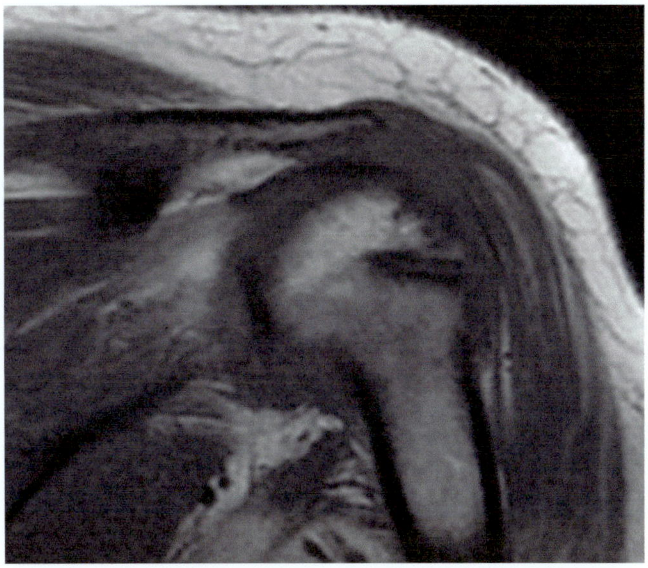

Fig. 23.7 Postoperative MRI shows good anchor position and good rotator cuff continuity

23.2 Discussion on the Causes of Pain After Rotator Cuff Surgery

The shoulder joint, characterized by extensive mobility, relies significantly on the rotator cuff for stability, with supraspinatus tendon injuries being the most common type of injuries. Postoperative pain following partial rotator cuff tears can significantly disrupt sleep and hinder functional rehabilitation, as there are various factors contributing to postoperative pain [2], and psychological anxiety being one of the prevalent causes [3]. Preoperative anxiety levels correlate with postoperative pain intensity, emphasizing the importance of preoperative assessment and intervention to mitigate postoperative pain and enhance recovery, and improve the living quality of the patient. Postoperative anxiety level evaluation and relief of the patient also needs to be closing monitored, with appropriate usage of antianxiety medicine, to help relieve the patient's pain without any heavy use of painkillers [4, 5].

Diabetic patients face three times more risk of tendon pathologies compared to those without diabetes, and rotator cuff tears being the most common one [6]. Diabetes increases the risk of rotator cuff tears, it also affects tissue healing process and heightened infection susceptibility, which all impact the recovery post-surgery. Early diabetes management and strict perioperative glycemic control are imperative to optimize surgical outcomes and minimize surgical complications. The risk of post-surgery infection needs to be clearly communicated with diabetic patients, and patients' blood sugar level needs to be closely controlled as well [7, 8].

Additionally, frozen shoulder may complicate rotator cuff tears, necessitating fully loosen shoulder joint adhesions and the removal of inflammatory synovial hyperplasia. Tenosynovitis, degeneration, and injury of the long head of the biceps brachii contribute to postoperative pain and functional impairment [9], requiring tailored interventions such as cleaning, repair, or fixation. Careful assessment of rotator cuff tension pre-suturing is crucial to prevent postoperative pain. Besides shoulder joint adhesions release, older patients might also suffer from tendonitis or injury of the long head of the biceps tendon. In these cases, the insertion point of the long head of the biceps tendon can be severed, in order to relieve shoulder joint pain and improve shoulder joint mobility. Biomechanical studies have shown that the long head tendon of the biceps brachii has the function of stabilizing the shoulder joint. Young patients should try to retain the long head tendon of the biceps brachii and fix it in situ in the intertubercular groove of the humerus without cutting. Yet, if severing is necessary, fixation on the broken end must also be performed [9].

Before suturing the rotator cuff, the tension of the rotator cuff should be carefully judged. High tension of the rotator cuff should be avoided to prevent pain.

Postoperation pain of rotator cuff surgery is mainly caused by inflammatory reaction. Multimodal analgesia such as preemptive analgesia and sequential analgesia therapy can be used for perioperative shoulder joint pain [10]. Examples of these analgesics include preoperative oral nonsteroidal anti-inflammatory analgesia, and post-surgery oral intake of oxycodone, acetaminophen, and celecoxib [11, 12]. Local ice application after surgery can reduce tissue metabolism and bleeding, reduce synovial inflammatory edema, inhibit inflammatory response, and thus perform similar analgesic effect. Caution should be exercised when injecting hormones and sodium hyaluronate into the joint cavity and subacromial area, after the rotator cuff repair surgery [13].

References

1. Itoi E. Rotator cuff tear: physical examination and conservative treatment. J Orthop Sci. 2013;18(2):197–204.
2. Kim CW, Kim JH, Kim DG. The factors affecting pain pattern after arthroscopic rotator cuff repair. Clin Orthop Surg. 2014;6(4):392–400.
3. Cho CH, Seo HJ, Bae KC, et al. The impact of depression and anxiety on self-assessed pain, disability, and quality of life in patients scheduled for rotator cuff repair. J Shoulder Elbow Surg. 2013;22:1160–6.
4. Wylie JD, Suter T, Potter MQ, et al. Mental health has a stronger association with patient-reported shoulder pain and function than tear size in patients with full-thickness rotator cuff tears. J Bone Joint Surg Am. 2016;98:251–6.
5. Menendez ME, Baker DK, Oladeji LO, et al. Psychological distress is associated with greater perceived disability and pain in patients presenting to a shoulder clinic. J Bone Joint Surg Am. 2015;97:1999–2003.
6. Abate M, Schiavone C, Salini V. Sonographic evaluation of the shoulder in asymptomatic elderly subjects with diabetes. BMC Musculoskelet Disord. 2010;11:278.
7. Bedi A, Fox AJ, Harris PE, et al. Diabetes mellitus impairs tendon-bone healing after rotator cuff repair. J Shoulder Elbow Surg. 2010;19(7):978–88.
8. Clement ND, Hallett A, MacDonald D, et al. Does diabetes affect outcome after arthroscopic repair of the rotator cuff? J Bone Joint Surg Br. 2010;92(8):1112–7.
9. Chen CH, Hsu KY, Chen WJ, et al. Incidence and severity of biceps long head tendon lesion in patients with complete rotator cuff tears. J Trauma. 2005;58(6):1189–93.
10. Fredrickson MJ, Krishnan S, Chen CY. Postoperative analgesia for shoulder surgery: a critical appraisal and review of current techniques. Anesthesia. 2010;65:608–24.
11. Singelyn FJ, Lhotel L, Fabre B. Pain relief after arthroscopic shoulder surgery: a comparison of intraarticular analgesia, suprascapular nerve block, and interscalene brachial plexus block. Anesth Analg. 2004;99:589–92.
12. Cho CH, Song KS, Min BW, et al. Efficacy of interscalene block, combined with multimodal pain control for postoperative analgesia after rotator cuff repair. Knee Surg Sports Traumatol Arthrosc. 2015;23:542–7.
13. Fredrickson MJ, Ball CM, Dalgleish AJ. Analgesic effectiveness of a continuous versus single-injection interscalene block for minor arthroscopic shoulder surgery. Reg Anesth Pain Med. 2010;35:28–33.

The Causes and Countermeasures of Perioperative Infection During Shoulder Arthroscopy

24

Chang-ming Huang, Ming-xin Wang, and Yu-jie Liu

The incidence of postoperative infection following open surgery for rotator cuff injury ranges from 0.27 to 1.9%, whereas the infection rate following arthroscopic rotator cuff reconstruction falls between 0.0016 and 0.23% [1]. Various risk factors, including but not limited to operation duration, surgical technique, use of internal fixation, obesity, diabetes, and smoking status, are associated with postoperative infection. Despite the relatively low incidence of postoperative infection in rotator cuff injuries, the potential consequences of infection are severe.

24.1 Overview

24.1.1 Case 1: Postoperative Infection of Rotator Cuff Injury

The patient was a 27-year-old male. He experienced symptoms of shoulder joint redness, swelling, and pain two weeks following anchor fixation for a rotator cuff injury. Despite undergoing shoulder joint debridement three times at a local hospital within a year, the patient did not experience improvement and required hospitalization once more.

Physical examination: A surgical scar and soft tissue bulge were observed on the lateral side of the left shoulder joint. The presence of a 5 cm × 5 cm wave sense area with slightly elevated skin temperature was noted (Fig. 24.1). There is tenderness (+ +) at the anterolateral part of acromion and intertubercular sulcus. Active shoulder movement: abduction 90° and elevation to 180°; body side: external rotation 60° and internal rotation up to lumbar 1 (L1); and in abduction 90° position: external rotation 60° and internal rotation 60°. Special examinations revealed a positive Jobe test, Hawkins sign, and lag sign, while the Neer sign and lift off test are negative. Laboratory tests showed an erythrocyte sedimentation rate of 6 mm/h, C-reactive protein level of 40 mg/dL, and a white blood cell count of $7 \times 10^3/\mu L$. The X-ray indicated a partial defect in the left humeral head bone (Fig. 24.2). Subsequent CT examination identified a bone defect in the greater tuberosity of the humerus following left rotator cuff repair (Fig. 24.3).

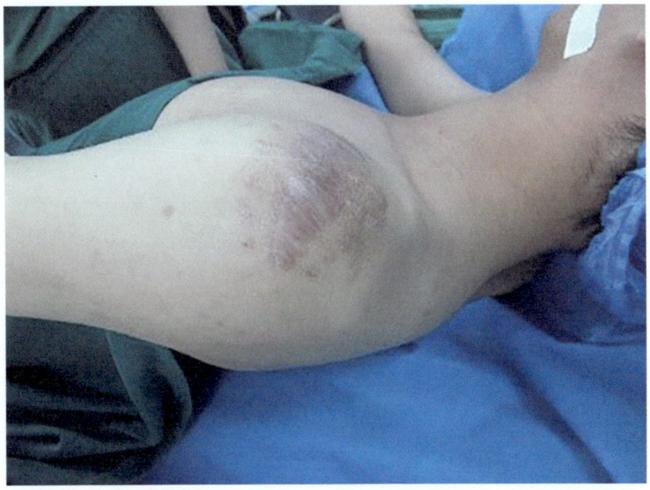

Fig. 24.1 The surgical area of the left shoulder joint is full, swollen and has a sense of fluctuation

Arthroscopic exploration revealed edematous and hyperplastic subacromial synovial tissue, with exposure of the anchor suture (Fig. 24.4), as well as dissolution and loosening of the bone surrounding the anchor. Following removal of the screws and sutures (Fig. 24.5), it was observed that the repaired rotator cuff tissue had not healed, resulting in a

C.-m. Huang
Department of Orthopedics, The 73rd Group Army Hospital, Chenggong Hospital Affiliated to Xiamen University, Xiamen, China

M.-x. Wang (✉)
Department of Orthopedics, The Fourth Medical Center, Chinese PLA General Hospital, Beijing, China

Y.-j. Liu
Orthopaedics, Chinese PLA General Hospital, Beijing, China

Y.-j. Liu et al. (eds.), *Pitfalls in Diagnosis and Treatment of Shoulder Joint Diseases*,
https://doi.org/10.1007/978-981-96-2472-0_24

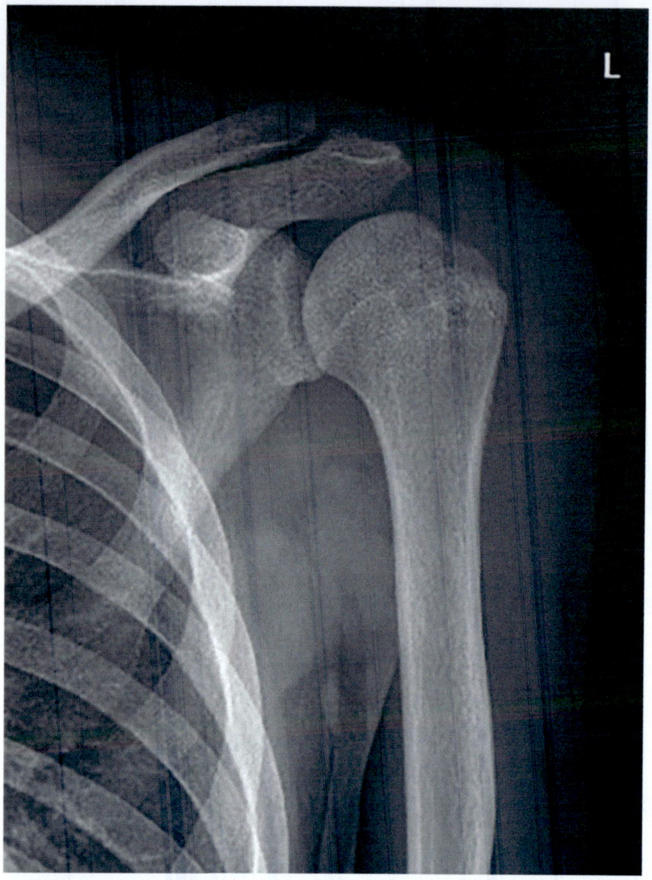

Fig. 24.2 The X-ray shows the greater tubercle of the left humerus osteoporosis with partial defects

significant local defect (Fig. 24.6). The incision successfully healed following arthroscopic debridement and administration of postoperative antibiotics to prevent infection. Pathological findings revealed chronic synovitis (Fig. 24.7), with negative bacterial culture results and resolution of postoperative pain symptoms. Six months later, the patient underwent a second-stage rotator cuff repair surgery (Figs. 24.8 and 24.9). No infection recurrence was observed during the 5-year follow-up period, and the patient experienced significant improvement in shoulder function.

24.1.2 Case 2: Inflammatory Reactive Granuloma of Suture Anchor After Rotator Cuff Surgery

The patient was a 59-year-old female, presented with symptoms 19 months postoperation for a rotator cuff injury. The lateral surgical approach exhibited redness and swelling, accompanied by mild pain and discomfort that persisted for over a month.

Physical examination revealed redness and swelling at the incision site of the lateral shoulder arthroscopic approach, measuring approximately 5 cm in diameter (Fig. 24.10). Active and passive shoulder joint movements were within normal limits.

Blood routine examination showed a white blood cell count of 5.8×10^9/L, neutrophil proportion of 64.2%, C-reactive protein level of 12.68 mg/L, and procalcitonin level of 0.08 ng/mL, ruling out tuberculosis. Color Doppler ultrasound of the rotator cuff revealed a visible subcutaneous swelling area measuring approximately 3.6×4.2 cm, displaying uneven hypoechoic characteristics with unclear boundaries. Color Doppler flow imaging (CDFI) detected a small amount of punctate blood flow signals within the area. X-ray imaging of the right shoulder joint displayed a shadow indicative of internal fixation (Fig. 24.11). CT scans showed no significant displacement of the internal fixation hardware (Fig. 24.12). MRI demonstrated focal hyperintensities surrounding the deltoid muscle and osteolytic signals adjacent to the anchors (Fig. 24.13)

Arthroscopic examination revealed a significant amount of scar tissue hyperplasia surrounding the subcutaneous tissue and suture within the deltoid bursa (Fig. 24.14). Following removal of the loose outer row anchors and scar tissue, it was evident that the supraspinatus tendon had healed effectively (Fig. 24.15).

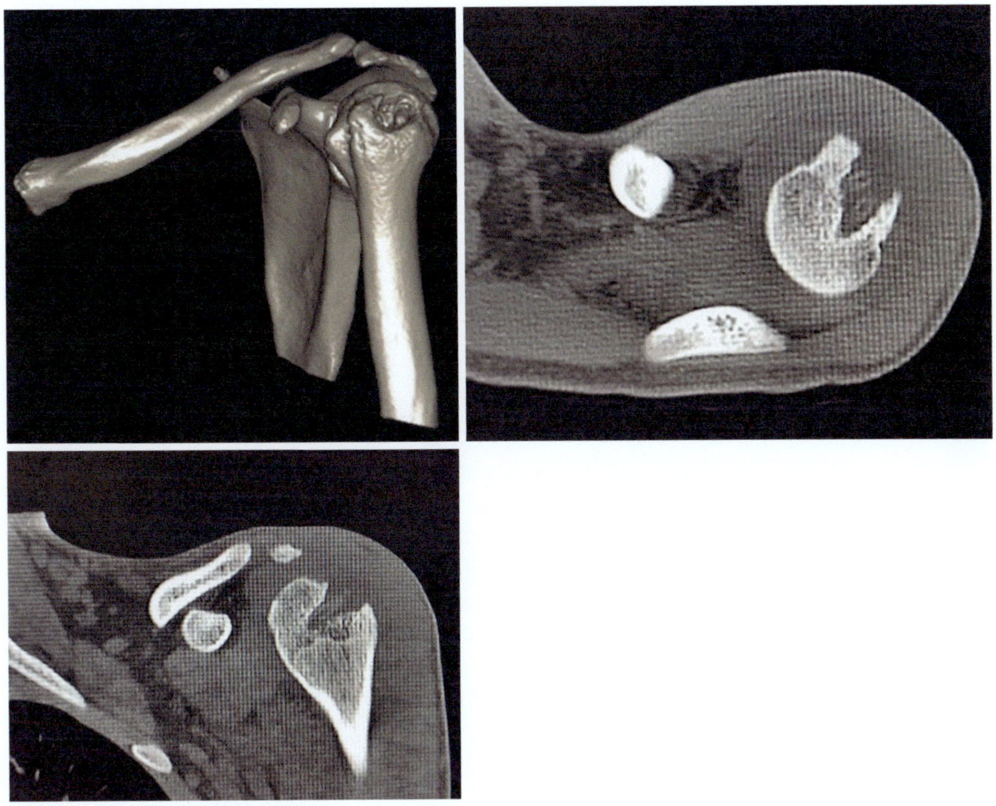

Fig. 24.3 CT shows osteolysis with bone defect around the left greater tubercle of humerus anchor

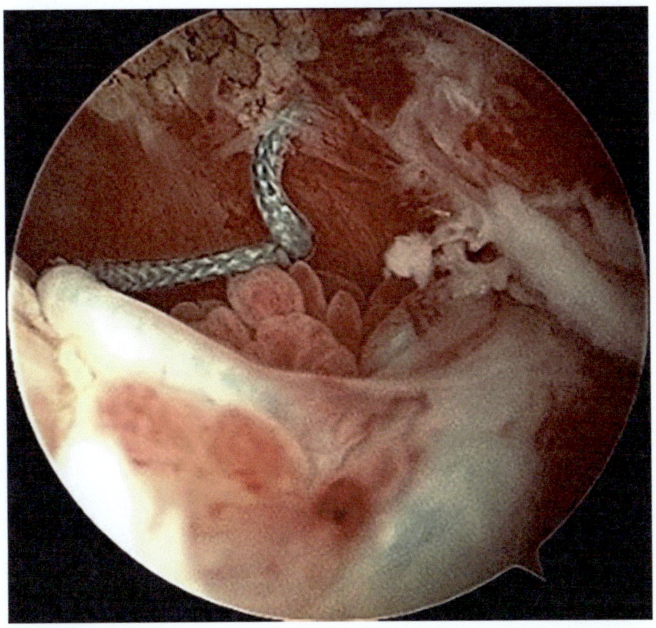

Fig. 24.4 Arthroscopy showed subacromial synovial edema with hyperplasia

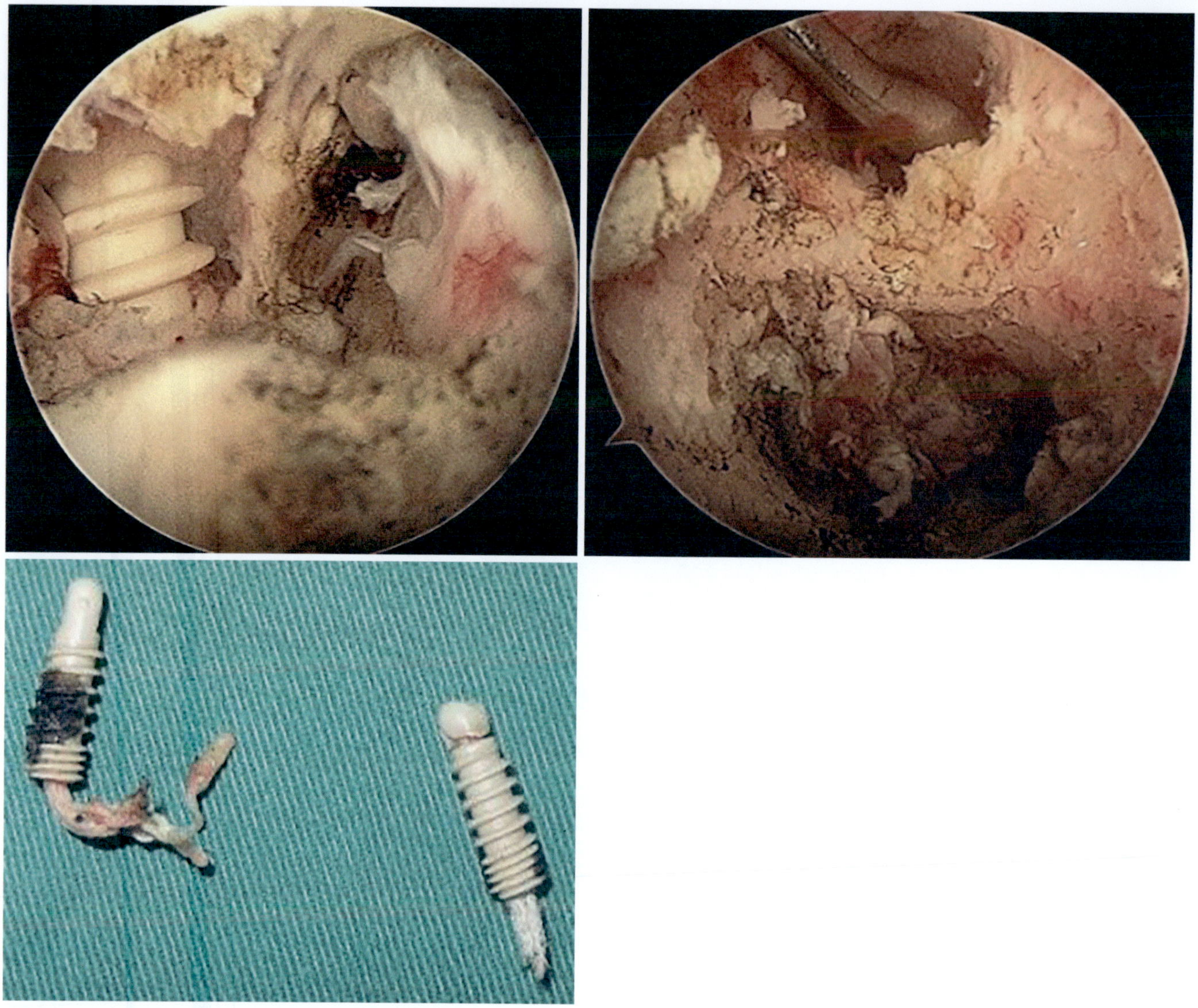

Fig. 24.5 Tack widening, anchor loose, and take out anchor

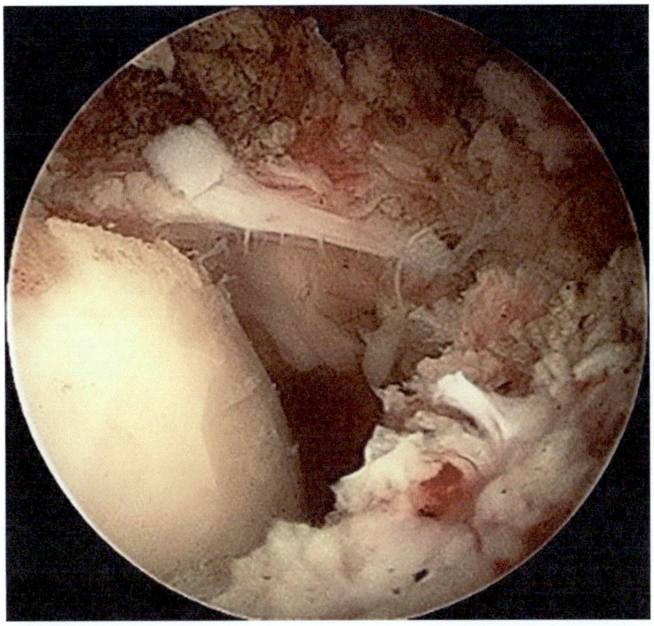

Fig. 24.6 The postoperative debridement revealed a large rotator cuff defect

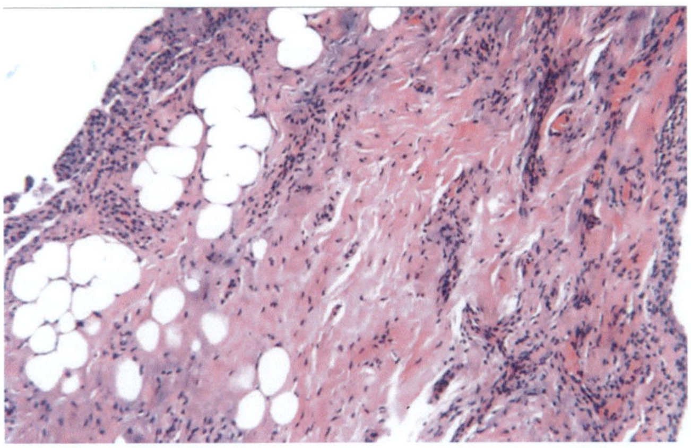

Fig. 24.7 Pathology showed chronic synovitis

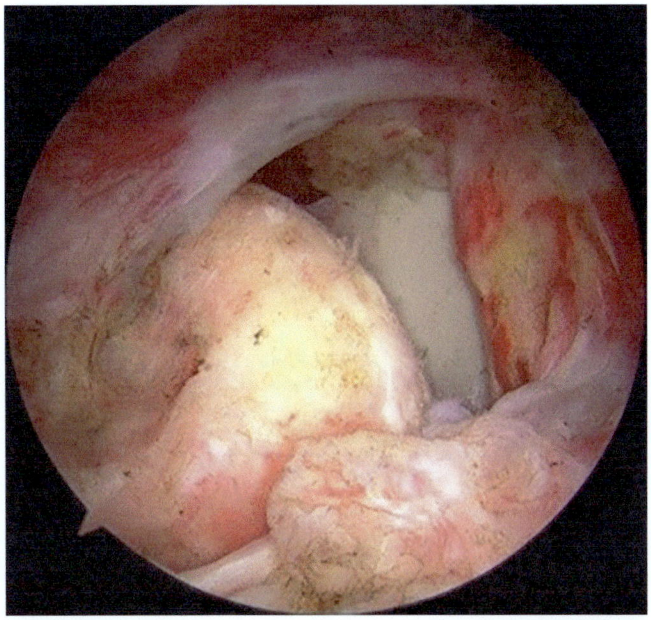

Fig. 24.8 Revision arthroscopic surgery revealed massive rotator cuff injury

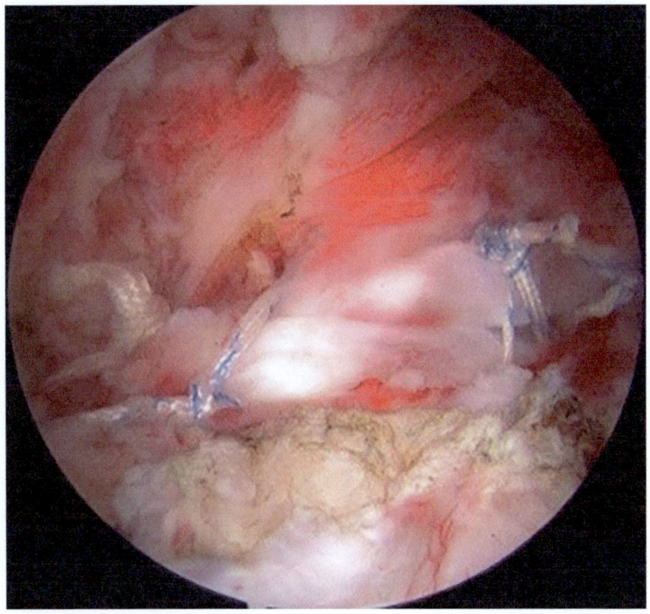

Fig. 24.9 Second surgery rotator cuff suture repair was completed

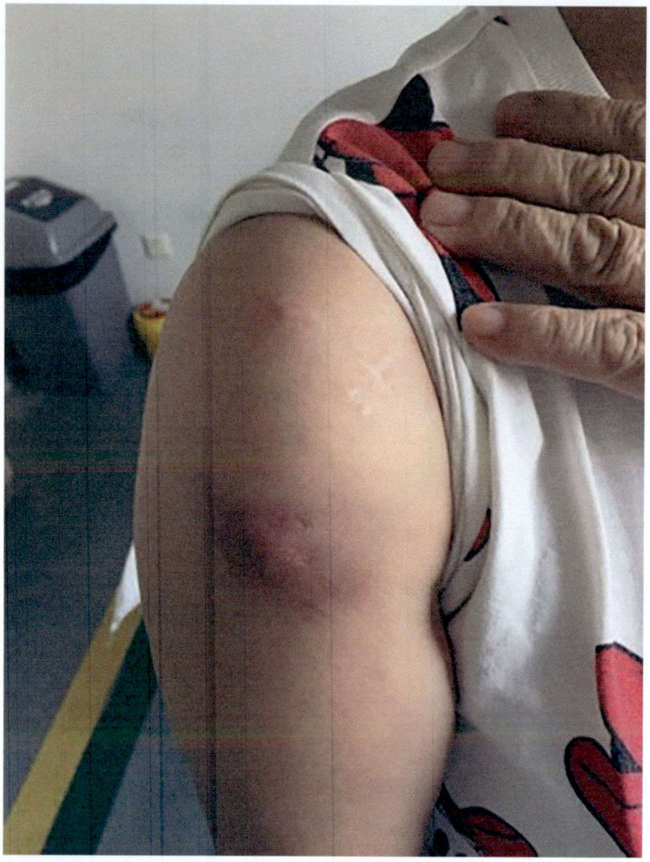

Fig. 24.10 The area around the original lateral approach incision was redness and swelling about 5 cm in diameter

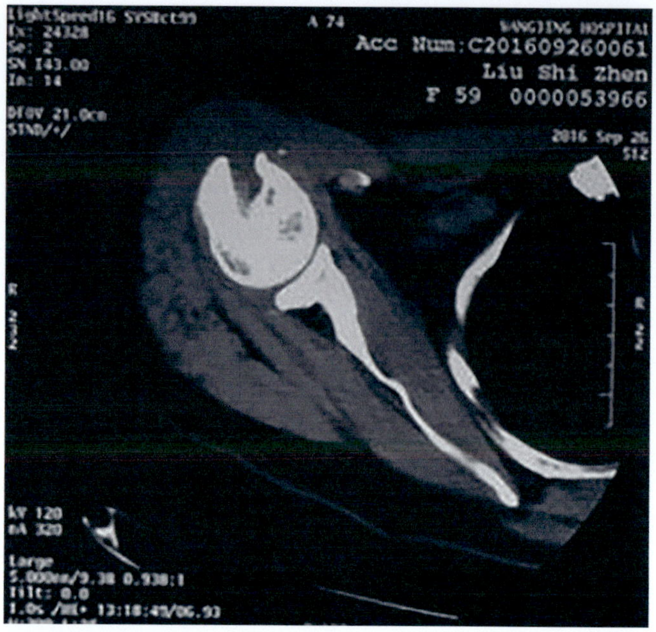

Fig. 24.12 CT showed the condition of the anchor tunnel 19 months after surgery

Fig. 24.11 Postoperative right shoulder joint X-ray showed internal fixation

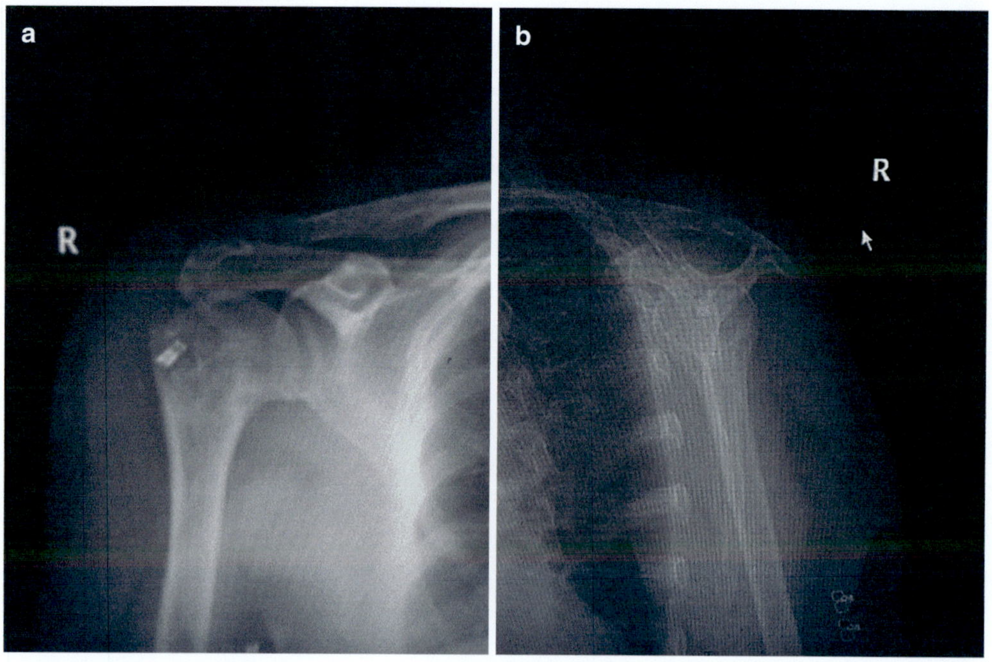

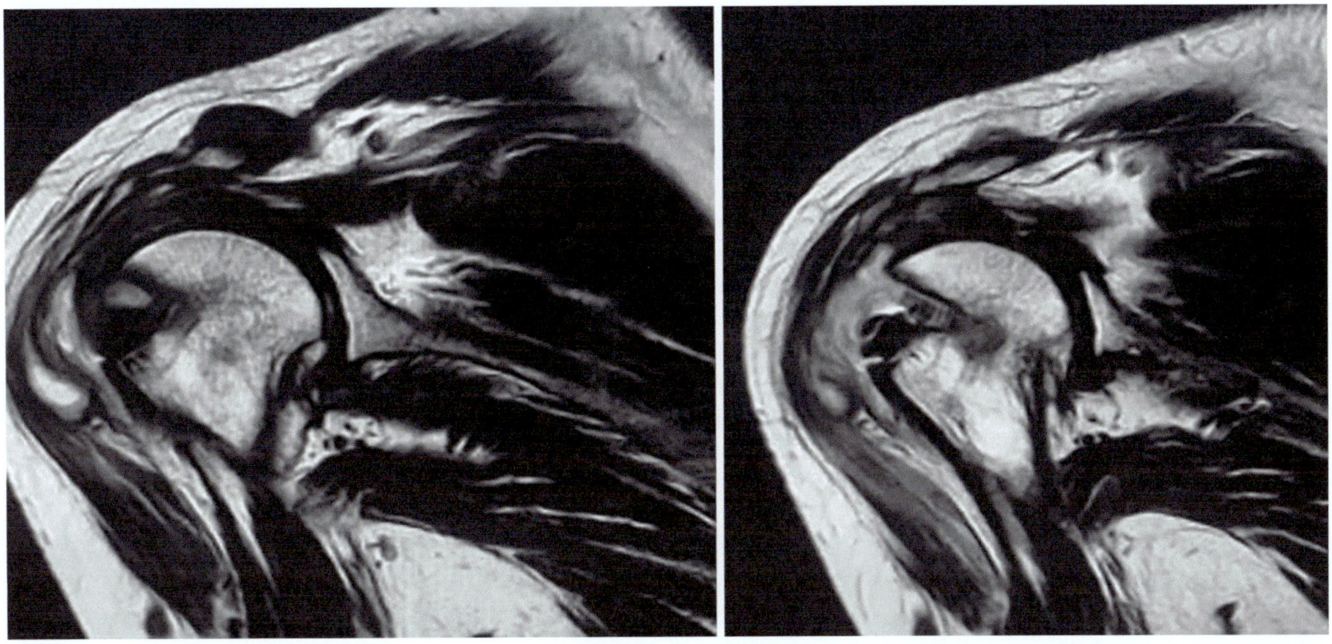

Fig. 24.13 MRI after rotator cuff surgery showed mixed signal under the acromion and high signal under the deltoid muscle

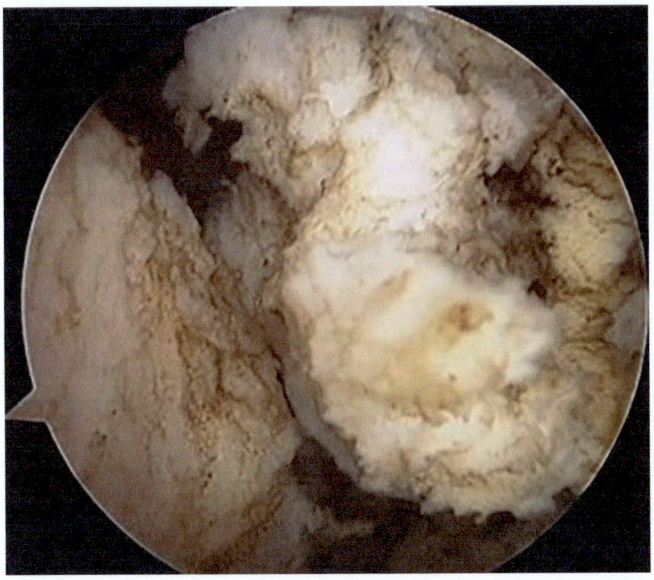

Fig. 24.14 Arthroscopic surgery was performed to clear the scar tissue of the downslide capsule of the deltoid

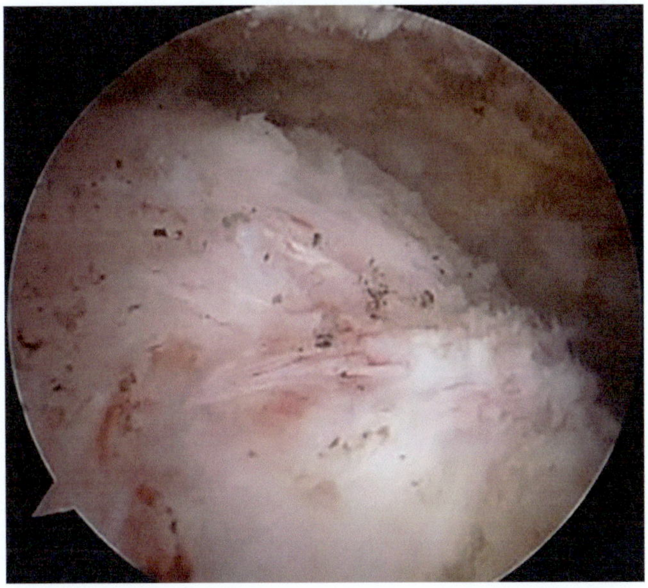

Fig. 24.15 Removal of scar tissue indicates that the supraspinatus tendon has healed

24.2 Causes of Infection After Rotator Cuff Surgery

Shoulder pain is a prevalent occurrence following rotator cuff surgery, particularly in cases where there is an elevation in white blood cell count, erythrocyte sedimentation rate, and C-reactive protein levels. X-ray imaging may reveal bone destruction in the greater tubercle of the humerus within the shoulder joint, while MRI may show abnormal signaling. Vigilance against infection is crucial in such cases.

In recent years, the utilization of small needle scalpel technology has become increasingly prevalent in the treatment of shoulder pain. However, due to a lack of anatomical knowledge among some medical practitioners, inadequate disinfection practices, and a weak understanding of aseptic principles, instances of rotator cuff injury or infection have become relatively common and warrant heightened attention. Additionally, the disintegration reaction of absorbable anchors can lead to synovial hyperplasia and localized scar formation, posing a challenge in distinguishing these effects from low toxicity infections. The prolonged duration of operation in open surgery increases the duration of tissue exposure to the open incision, providing more opportunities for bacterial contamination. As a result, open surgery is associated with a higher risk of infection compared to arthroscopic surgery [2–5]. In open shoulder surgery, the incision is typically located near the axillary front line, where bacteria can easily reside in the skin folds and hair follicle pores abundant in sebaceous glands, serving as a natural culture medium for bacterial growth. Inadequate disinfection measures can further exacerbate the risk of infection [6, 7]. Jensen et al. [4] conducted an analysis of 372,109 cases of rotator cuff repair (RCR), while Roberson et al. [8] examined 96 cases of RCR, both demonstrating an increased likelihood of infection following open surgery. Therefore, in order to mitigate the risk and incidence of postoperative infection, it is imperative to minimize operation duration and avoid open rotator cuff repair procedures.

Steroid Injection: Research indicates that preoperative intra-articular corticosteroid injections have been associated with elevated rates of postoperative infection [6, 7, 9]. Bhattachar et al. [10] reported varying infection rates following corticosteroid injections prior to surgery, with rates of 8.86% within 2 weeks, 1.56% for non-injected patients, and 0.76% for injections 3–4 weeks before surgery. Forsythe [12] similarly found differing infection rates, with 1.3% for those injected within one month and 0.8% for those not injected. No significant difference in infection rates was observed among patients who received corticosteroid injections more than 1 month before surgery.

Diabetes Mellitus: In a study conducted by Cho et al. in 2015, it was observed that patients with diabetes mellitus undergoing rotator cuff repair (RCR) may experience an elevated risk of postoperative infection [13]. This increased susceptibility to infection in diabetic patients can be attributed to compromised immune function and elevated blood glucose levels, which create a conducive environment for bacterial proliferation [13]. Furthermore, research by Chen et al. [30] indicated that diabetic patients exhibit a higher likelihood of developing postoperative infections following open RCR compared to non-diabetic individuals.

Gender, Age, and Postoperative Infection: Pauzenberger et al. [15] found that the infection rate was 3.6% in women and 96.4% in men, potentially attributed to the higher serum testosterone levels in men [6] compared to women. Additionally, the postoperative infection rate in shoulder joint patients over 60 years old is double that of patients over 40 years old [15, 16], with a postoperative complication rate of 1.13%. In a retrospective study by Padaki et al. [17] on 23,974 patients following shoulder arthroscopic RCR, 26.8% were over 65 years old, and the probability of postoperative complications was 1.13%, which was much higher than 0.46% in the group of patients <55 years old. Smoking has been identified as a potential risk factor for an increased postoperative infection rate. In a retrospective study conducted by Myles et al. [18], a total of 489 patients were included, with 173 non-smokers, 116 individuals who had quit smoking, and 200 current smokers. The postoperative infection rates for these groups were found to be 0.6%, 2.6%, and 3.7%, respectively, with statistically significant differences observed. Therefore, smoking cessation is recommended as an essential measure to mitigate the risk of postoperative incision infection.

Obesity: Cancienne conducted a regression analysis on a sample of 87,216 obese patients and 51,527 morbidly obese individuals, concluding that obesity is a significant risk factor for infection following shoulder arthroscopy [19]. Golladay et al. [20] also found that malnutrition contributed to delayed wound healing in 9–39% of cases. Factors such as malnutrition, decreased serum albumin, vitamins, adipocytes, zinc levels, and other contents were associated with an increased risk of postoperative infection.

Pathogenic Microorganisms: Identified in infected lesions following rotator cuff repair (RCR) primarily consist of *Propionibacterium acnes* (*P. acnes*), coagulase-negative staphylococcus (CNS), and *Staphylococcus aureus* (*S. aureus*) [1, 6, 7, 14]. *P. acnes* is a non-spore-forming, Gram-positive, microaerophilic bacterium. The predominant strain of postoperative shoulder joint infections following RCR is *P. acnes*, accounting for 51–86% of cases [4, 11]. This bacterium is the most common pathogen in RCR shoulder joint surgeries, with a culture time of 14–17 days or longer, and symptoms may not be immediately apparent.

24.3 Diagnosis

Rotator cuff injuries and infections typically manifest approximately 6 weeks post-surgery. Many patients may not exhibit overt early symptoms or present with specific complaints, making detection challenging. Common symptoms include shoulder pain, swelling, stiffness, and limitations in both active and passive ranges of motion. Some patients may also experience systemic symptoms such as fever, dysfunction, and localized signs of inflammation. Diagnostic evaluation for postoperative infections may involve laboratory tests such as white blood cell count, erythrocyte sedimentation rate, and C-reactive protein levels. The white blood cell count falls within the normal range and is not a reliable indicator for specific examinations. Erythrocyte sedimentation rate and C-reactive protein are commonly used markers for infection, however, they are not specific indicators for *P. acnes*. Athwal et al. [21] conducted a retrospective study on 39 patients who developed infections after RCR, finding that 60% had elevated erythrocyte sedimentation rate and 50% had abnormal C-reactive protein levels. In summary, white blood cell count, erythrocyte sedimentation rate, and C-reactive protein are not reliable diagnostic laboratory tests for infection.

Joint puncture is a standard diagnostic procedure, and when postoperative infection is suspected, obtaining synovial fluid from the glenohumeral joint for examination is highly beneficial for accurate diagnosis [22]. Normal joint fluid should have a white blood cell count of less than 0.05×10^9/L and appear light yellow, transparent, and clear. Bacterial culture, encompassing aerobic, anaerobic, acid-resistant, and fungal culture, serves as the ultimate diagnostic method for confirming infection. The initial step in this diagnostic process should involve Gram staining [23]. Subsequently, the examination of joint fluid color and transparency, along with the microscopic assessment of white blood cell count and neutrophil classification, is recommended.

In the early stages of infection, X-ray imaging may appear normal; however, as the disease progresses, X-ray findings may reveal joint space narrowing, joint surface destruction, implant dislodgement, and other pathological changes [24]. MRI and ultrasonography have the capability to identify joint effusion, abscess, and synovial changes in the initial stages, while enhanced scanning can allow for the observation of abnormal alterations in the synovial membrane.

24.4 Treatment

Following the results of bacterial culture and drug sensitivity testing, appropriate antibiotics were administered based on sensitivity. Intravenous administration led to a rapid increase in blood concentration of the antibiotics. Post-surgery, antibiotics were continued for a duration of 4–6 weeks. The predominant pathogens associated with this condition are *S. aureus* and *Propionibacterium acnes*. Timely administration of sensitive broad-spectrum antibiotics such as vancomycin, fluoroquinolones, β-lactams, clindamycin, and rifampicin is recommended for the treatment of *Staphylococcus* infections. Following surgery, a combination of broad-spectrum antibiotics and systemic nutrition support therapy can lead to a favorable therapeutic outcome.

Early arthroscopic debridement, involving the removal of inflammatory synovium, necrotic tissue, fibrous strands, and scar adhesions, is considered the optimal treatment for postoperative rotator cuff infections, facilitating early joint function rehabilitation. Intraoperative radiofrequency ablation has been shown to effectively control bleeding and reduce hemorrhage [7, 13]. Surgical debridement and local lavage have been found to alleviate symptoms of infection and impede disease progression. Existing literature suggests that an average of 2.6–3.3 debridement procedures may be necessary to eradicate the infection [21, 25]. Smith et al. [26] recommend comprehensive debridement involving the glenohumeral joint and subacromial space, particularly in cases of suppurative infection affecting bone and cartilage.

Lee et al. [27] demonstrated a significant reduction in the reinfection rate of open surgery for shoulder joint infection with bone or cartilage erosion in 57 cases. There was no notable difference in the reinfection rate among cases without bone and cartilage erosion. During the operation, infected necrotic tissue and loose anchor sutures were excised and irrigated with normal saline. Regarding the removal of sutures and anchors during debridement for infection after joint rotator cuff repair (RCR), research indicates that retaining suture anchors without looseness and fixation failure does not impact infection control. Research has indicated that maintaining secure suture anchors without experiencing loosening or fixation failure does not compromise infection control and promotes successful healing of the rotator cuff following repair. The removal of sutures and anchors is not recommended, as these materials may serve as a breeding ground for bacteria and should be extracted [25, 26]. In cases where there is insufficient coverage of the glenohumeral joint after the excision of rotator cuff tissue, the wound can be effectively covered through the transposition of either the latissimus dorsi or pectoralis major myocutaneous flap.

References

1. Hughes JD, Hughes JL, Bartley JH, et al. Infection rates in arthroscopic versus open rotator cuff repair. Orthop J Sports Med. 2017;5(7):2325967117715416.
2. Day M, Westermann R, Duchman K, et al. Comparison of short-term complications after rotator cuff repair: open versus arthroscopic. Arthroscopy. 2018;34(4):1130–6.

3. Owens BD, Williams AE, Wolf JM. Risk factors for surgical complications in rotator cuff repair in a veteran population. J Shoulder Elbow Surg. 2015;24(11):1707–12.
4. Jensen AR, Cha PS, Devana SK, et al. Evaluation of the trends, concomitant procedures, and complications with open and arthroscopic rotator cuff repairs in the medicare population. Orthop J Sports Med. 2017;5(10):2325967117731310.
5. Boddapati V, Fu MC, Schairer W, et al. Increased shoulder arthroscopy time is associated with overnight hospital stay and surgical site infection. Arthroscopy. 2018;34(2):363–8.
6. Atesok K, MacDonald P, Leiter J, et al. Postoperative deep shoulder infections following rotator cuff repair. World J Orthop. 2017;8(8):612–8.
7. Saltzman MD, Marecek GS, Edwards SL, et al. Infection after shoulder surgery. J Am Acad Orthop Surg. 2011;19(4):208–18.
8. Roberson TA, Azar FM, Miller RH III, et al. Predictors of early complications after rotator cuff repair. Tech Shoulder Elbow Surg. 2016;17(2):88–92.
9. Yeranosian MG, Arshi A, Terrell RD, et al. Incidence of acute postoperative infections requiring reoperation after arthroscopic shoulder surgery. Am J Sports Med. 2014;42(2):437–41.
10. Bhattachar JS, Lee W, Lee MJ, et al. Preoperative corticosteroid joint injections within 2 weeks of shoulder arthroscopies increase postoperative infection risk. J Shoulder Elbow Surg. 2019;28(11):2098–102.
11. Parada SA, Dilisio MF, Kennedy CD. Management of complications after rotator cuff surgery. Curr Rev Musculoskelet Med. 2015;8(1):40–52.
12. Forsythe B, Agarwalla A, Puzzitiello RN, et al. The timing of injections prior to arthroscopic rotator cuff repair impacts the risk of surgical site infection. Am J Bone Joint Surg. 2019;101(8):682–7.
13. Cho NS, Moon SC, Jeon JW, et al. The influence of diabetes mellitus on clinical and structural outcomes after arthroscopic rotator cuff repair. Am J Sports Med. 2015;43(4):991–7.
14. Zhongli A. Prevention and treatment of postoperative infection in diabetic patients. Chin J Pract Surg. 1999;3:10–1.
15. Pauzenberger L, Grieb A, Hexel M, et al. Infections following arthroscopic rotator cuff repair: incidence, risk factors, and prophylaxis. Knee Surg Sports Traumatol Arthrosc. 2017;25(2):595–601.
16. Yu M, Wang GL, Yu YQ, et al. Investigation and analysis of postoperative infection in elderly patients undergoing surgery. Chin Convalescent Med. 2014;23(2):171–3.
17. Padaki AS, Boddapati V, Mathew J, et al. The effect of age on short-term postoperative complications following arthroscopic rotator cuff repair. JSES Open Access. 2019;3(3):194–8.
18. Myles PS, Iacono GA, Hunt JO, et al. Risk of respiratory complications and wound infection in patients undergoing ambulatory surgery. Anesthesiology. 2002;97(4):842–7.
19. Cancienne JM, Brockmeier SF, Carson EW, et al. Risk factors for infection after shoulder arthroscopy in a large medicare population. Am J Sports Med. 2018;46(4):809–14.
20. Golladay GJ, Satpathy J, Jiranek WA. Patient optimization-strategies that work: malnutrition. J Arthroplasty. 2016;31(8):1631–4.
21. Athwal GS, Sperling JW, Rispoli DM, et al. Deep infection after rotator cuff repair. J Shoulder Elbow Surg. 2006;16(3):306–11.
22. Halbrecht J, Meislin RJ. Complications in knee and shoulder surgery: management and treatment options for the sports medicine orthopedist. London: Springer; 2009. p. 272.
23. Sethi PM, Sabetta JR, Stuek SJ, et al. Presence of Propionibacterium acnes in primary shoulder arthroscopy: results of aspiration and tissue cultures. J Shoulder Elbow Surg. 2015;24(5):796–803.
24. Albano D, Chianca V, Zappia M, et al. Imaging of usual and unusual complication of rotator cuff repair. J Comput Assist Tomogr. 2019;43(3):359–66.
25. Kwon YW, Kalainov DM, Rose HA, et al. Management of early deep infection after rotator cuff repair surgery. J Shoulder Elbow Surg. 2005;14(1):1–5.
26. Smith CD, Corner T, Modi CS, et al. The evidence for the management of deep infection after rotator cuff repair. Shoulder Elbow. 2011;3(3):138–42.
27. Lee DK, Rhee SM, Jeong HY, et al. Treatment of acute shoulder infection: can osseous lesion be a rudder in guideline for determining the method of debridement? J Shoulder Elbow Surg. 2019;28(12):2317–25.

Part IX

Fracture of the Greater Tuberosity and Chronic Tear of the Pectoralis Major Muscle: An Introduction and Summary

Jing Xue

Introduction

This part introduces the underlying factors contributing to misdiagnosis of greater tuberosity fracture in the management of shoulder dislocation while proposing effective strategies for mitigating diagnostic errors. At the same time, it focuses on the key points, difficulties, and causes of error in the treatment of greater tuberosity fracture, especially introduces the anchor fixation technique and the plate fixation technique, and puts forward a feasible method for better reduction of greater tuberosity fracture during operation. Through the implementation of these methods, postoperative re-displacement of fractures can be prevented, thereby ensuring the efficacy of the surgical procedure.

It is difficult to diagnose pectoralis major laceration in the early stage, which is prone to missed diagnosis and misdiagnosis. This part focuses on the diagnosis of pectoralis major injury and introduces the technics and precautions of arthroscopic minimally invasive treatment of old pectoralis major injury in detail.

Summary

1. Shoulder dislocation is easy to cause greater tuberosity fracture. Physicians must be more vigilant and aware of greater tuberosity fracture in patients with shoulder dislocation. The physician must thoroughly inquire about the patient's complete medical history and conduct a meticulous physical examination. The imaging examination should be conducted both prior to and following the treatment, with comprehensive documentation of the diagnosis and treatment records. The blind manual reduction of shoulder joint dislocation should not be performed solely based on personal experience without the use of imaging examination, in order to prevent any potential treatment errors. The selection of appropriate internal fixation is crucial for managing comminuted fractures of the greater tuberosity of the humerus, as improper fixation can easily result in failure to stabilize the fracture.
2. The advantages of arthroscopic surgery for humeral greater tuberosity fractures include reduced soft tissue trauma, decreased risk of postoperative infection and adhesion, minimal blood loss, and early initiation of functional exercise. For different types of humeral greater tuberosity fractures, such as avulsion, compression, and splitting, careful preoperative evaluation should be performed to optimize the treatment plan in order to obtain the best results.

J. Xue (✉)
Orthopaedics, Air Force Medical Center of Chinese PLA, Beijing, China

3. Lacerations of the pectoralis major muscle are often neglected. Once they are delayed and become chronic injuries, it will increase the difficulty of treatment. Arthroscopic-assisted minimally invasive surgical repair and reconstruction for chronic laceration of pectoralis major muscle further expand the application field of arthroscopic technique beyond the joint, and the clinical results are satisfactory.

Errors in Diagnosis and Treatment of Humerus Macrotuberous Fracture and Countermeasures

25

Yu-jie Liu and Jun-liang Wang

25.1 Overview of the Diagnosis and Treatment Process

The patient, a 62-year-old female, was accidentally knocked down while riding a bicycle and suffered anterior dislocation of the shoulder joint. The emergency department was treated in the local county hospital without imaging examination. The doctor on duty performed pedal pull manipulation. No postoperative imaging review was conducted, and a triangular bandage sling was applied. Three weeks after the injury, the patient still had shoulder pain, swelling and limited outreach activities, and went to the hospital outpatient clinic again.

Physical examination: right shoulder deltoid atrophy, greater tubercle of humerus tenderness (++), subcutaneous soft tissue with ecchymosis. The muscles of supraspinatus, deltoid, biceps, triceps were significantly atrophy, and the shoulder joint active and passive abduction, external rotation, forward flexion, backward extension and lift were significantly limited.

Radiographic examinations: Shoulder joint radiographs (Fig. 25.1) and three-dimensional CT reconstruction revealed comminuted fractures of the greater tubercle of the humerus (Fig. 25.2). MRI revealed compression fracture of the greater tubercle of humerus (Fig. 25.3) and injury of supraspinatus tendon.

Arthroscopic investigation under general anesthesia revealed that there was old hemorrhage in the right shoulder joint cavity, intraarticular tissue adhesion (Fig. 25.4), and displacement of the greater tubercle fracture of humerus (Fig. 25.5). After the scar tissue was debrided, the fracture was reduced. The humerus greater tubercle was fixed with a hollow screw, and the supraspinatus tendon was fixed and repaired with two suture anchors. Postoperative radiographs showed that the protrusion of the screw impinged on the acromion (Fig. 25.6). The shoulder joint abduction and upward lifting activities were limited, and there were friction and pain with internal and external rotation.

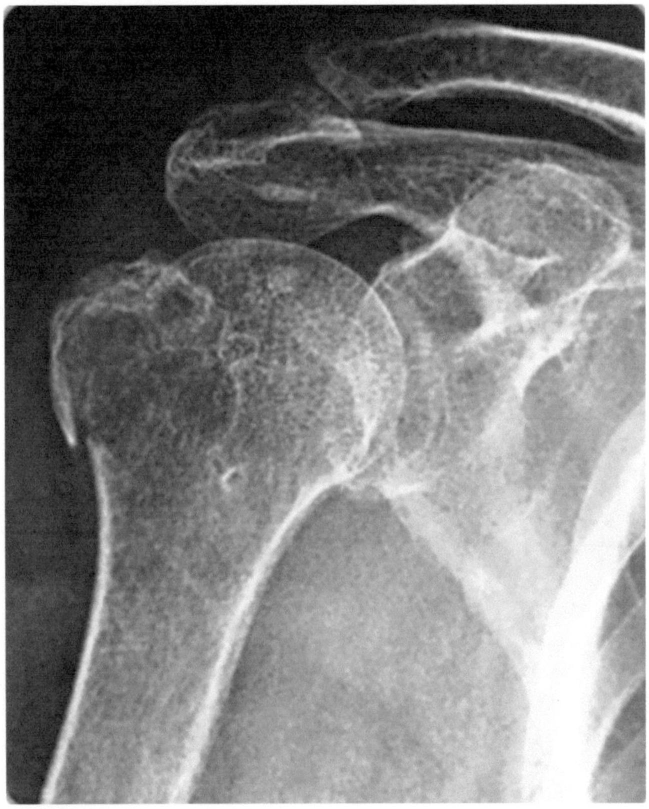

Fig. 25.1 Radiographs of the right shoulder joint showed a displaced fracture of the greater tubercle of the humerus

Y.-j. Liu
Orthopaedics, Chinese PLA General Hospital, Beijing, China

J.-l. Wang (✉)
Department of Orthopedics, Hainan Hospital of Chinese PLA General Hospital, Sanya, China

Y.-j. Liu et al. (eds.), *Pitfalls in Diagnosis and Treatment of Shoulder Joint Diseases*,
https://doi.org/10.1007/978-981-96-2472-0_25

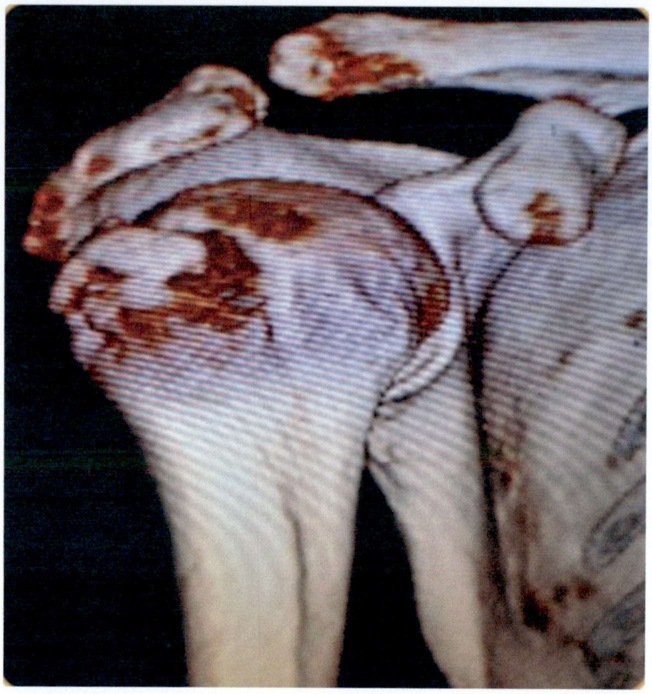

Fig. 25.2 3D-CT reconstruction of the right shoulder joint shows a fracture of the greater tubercle of humerus

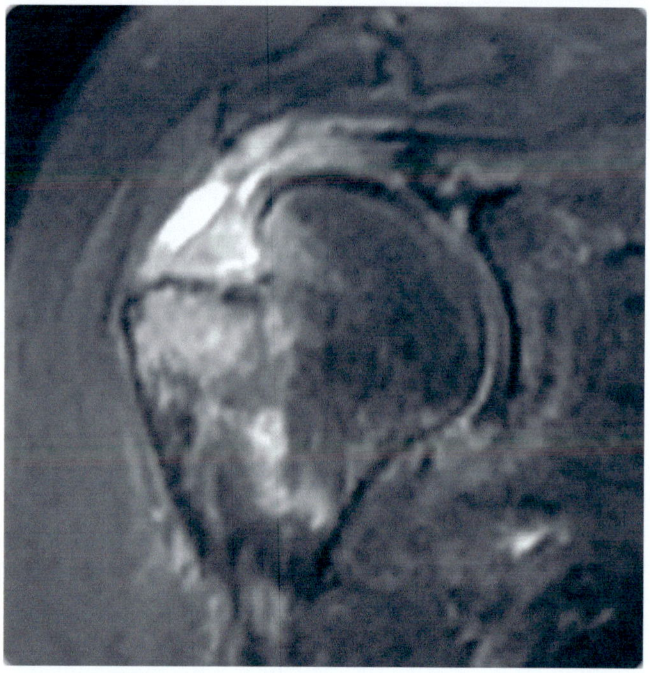

Fig. 25.3 MRI of the right shoulder joint showed fracture of the greater tubercle of the humerus and compression fracture of the humerus head

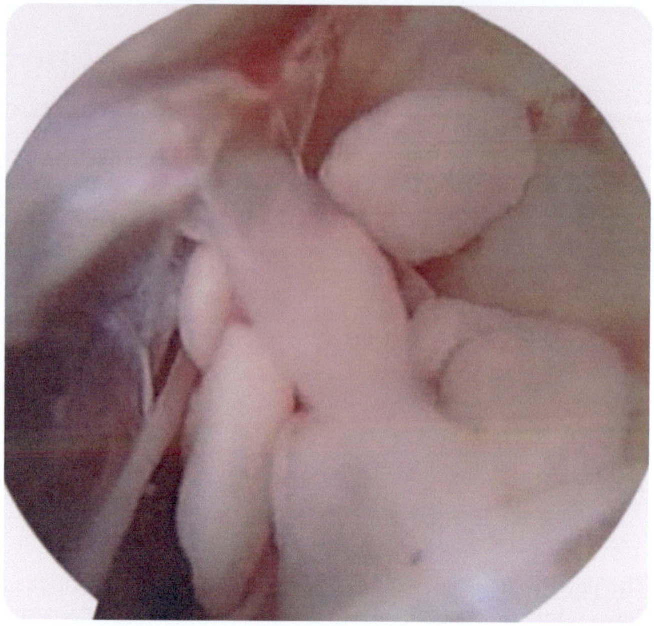

Fig. 25.4 Arthroscopy revealed intracavitary adhesions of the shoulder joint

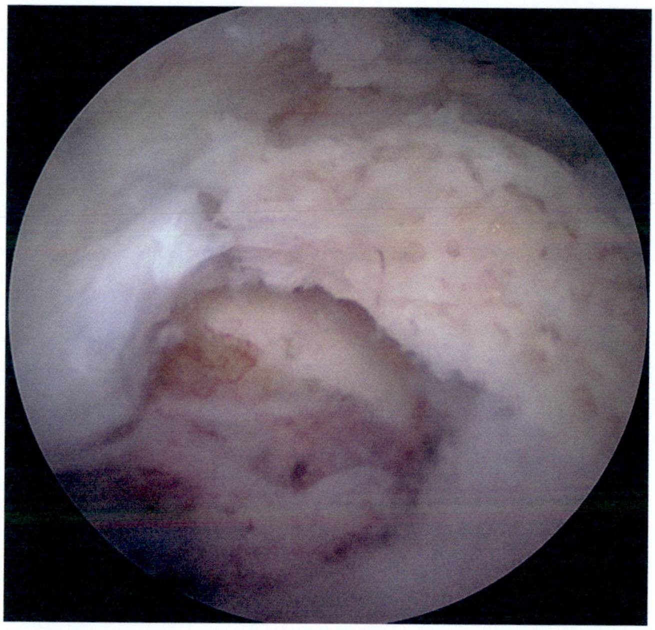

Fig. 25.5 Surgical exploration revealed that the greater tubercle fracture of the humerus was displaced in the subacromial space

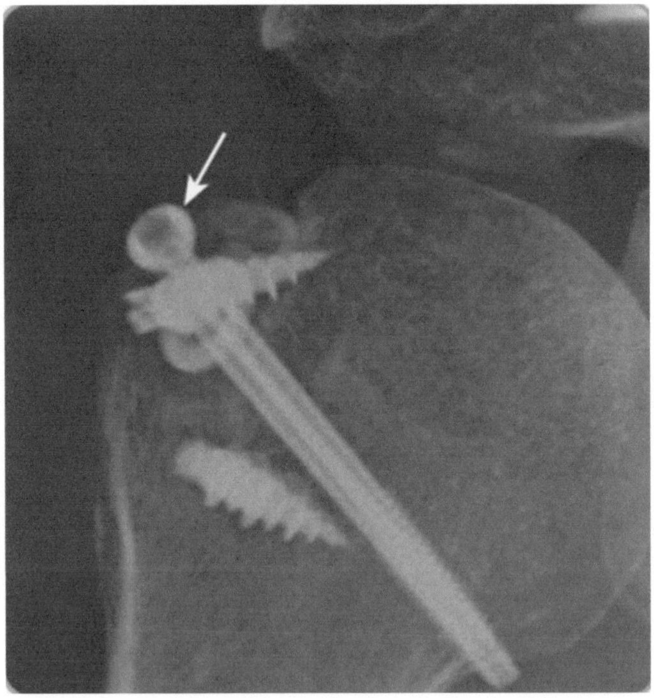

Fig. 25.6 Postoperative radiographs of the right shoulder joint showed a hollow screw protrusion (arrow) higher than the bone fragment

25.2 Missed Diagnosis, Misdiagnosis, and Reflection

Elderly people with osteoporosis suffered shoulder joint trauma or dislocation, easy to cause humeral tubercle fracture. Awareness of humerus greater tubercle fracture due to shoulder dislocation must be enhanced. When receiving medical treatment, the doctor must ask for a detailed medical history, carefully carry out a physical examination, and imaging examination. Then doctor evaluated according to clinical manifestations and examination results and formulated diagnosis and treatment plan. Imaging examination should be obtained before and after treatments, and diagnosis and treatment records should be made. Without imaging examination, the shoulder joint manual reduction should not be carried out blindly based on personal experience. After treatment, it is necessary to explain the precautions, functional exercises, and follow-up time to the patient in detail to avoid misdiagnosis and missed diagnosis.

The choice of hollow screw fixation for comminuted fractures of the greater tubercle of humerus is not an appropriate indication, because the diameter of the bone fragment fixed by screw must be more than three times the diameter of the screw, otherwise the bone fragment is prone to fragmentation. The tip of the screw must bite the opposite bone cortex, otherwise the anti-withdrawal force is weak, and it is easy to pull out. The X-ray film of the patient showed that there was a distance of 3 mm between the screw and the gasket, and the screw did not really exert pressure, and the screw impinged with the acromion, affecting lift, abduction, and rotation of the shoulder joint. Therefore, the selection of surgical methods and fixation materials must be considered comprehensively.

26 Surgical Errors and Strategies of Humerus Greater Tubercle Fracture

Yu-jie Liu and Jun-liang Wang

26.1 Overview of the Diagnosis and Treatment Process

A 72-year-old male accidentally slipped down with left hand supporting the ground. He suffered left shoulder joint pain, swelling, and limited movement after injury. Emergency radiographs showed a fracture of the left humerus greater tubercle with an upward displacement of the fracture fragments (Fig. 26.1).

The physical examination revealed swelling in the left shoulder joint, restricted abduction, extensive bruising on the upper arm (Fig. 26.2), and marked tenderness (++) over the greater tubercle of the humerus beneath the acromion. Further history-taking indicated that the patient had been on a regimen of enteric-coated aspirin for management of hyperlipidemia.

Open reduction and plate and screw fixation were performed under general anesthesia. After surgery, the patient reported left shoulder pain with abduction, rotation, and shoulder lifting. The radiographs showed that the tip of the plate was elevated above the greater tubercle of the humerus and that the plate had impinged with the acromion, and the fracture fragment of the greater tubercle was located within the glenohumeral joint (Fig. 26.3). CT examination showed that the tip of the plate was elevated above the greater tubercle of the humerus and the fracture fragment was located in the glenohumeral joint (Fig. 26.4).

Three months after surgery, the patient had shoulder joint pain and severely limited movement, and strongly requested the removal of the plate and screw. Under brachial plexus anesthesia, the shoulder joint was investigated with arthroscopy. Narrowing of the subacromial space and adhesion of intra-articular scar tissue were found (Fig. 26.5). Scar tissue was cleaned under arthroscopy (Fig. 26.6), and the subacromial adhesive band was cleaned with radiofrequency ablation (Fig. 26.7). A subacromial investigation revealed that the greater tubercle of the humerus was displaced and protruded into the subacromial space (Fig. 26.8), impinging on the acromial at 60° of passive joint abduction.

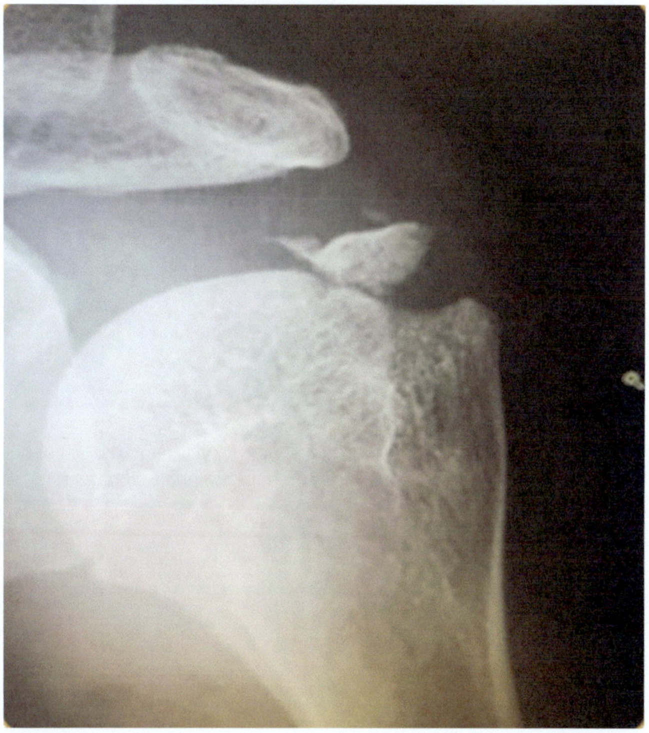

Fig. 26.1 X-rays of the left shoulder joint showed a displaced fracture of the greater tubercle of the humerus

Y.-j. Liu
Orthopaedics, Chinese PLA General Hospital, Beijing, China

J.-l. Wang (✉)
Department of Orthopedics, Hainan Hospital of Chinese PLA General Hospital, Sanya, China

Y.-j. Liu et al. (eds.), *Pitfalls in Diagnosis and Treatment of Shoulder Joint Diseases*,
https://doi.org/10.1007/978-981-96-2472-0_26

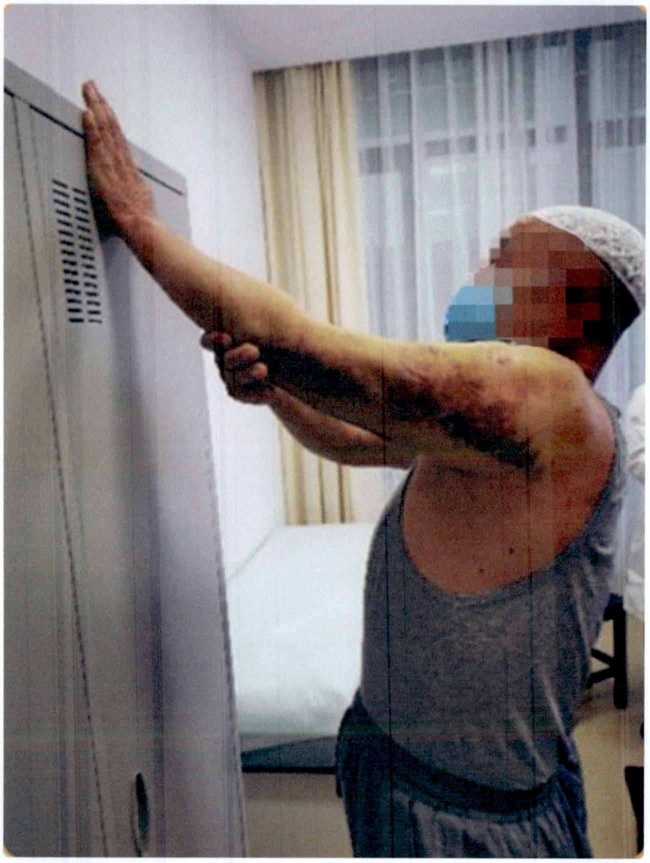

Fig. 26.2 Large area of subcutaneous congestion around the left upper arm and shoulder joint, and limited shoulder abduction and uplift movement

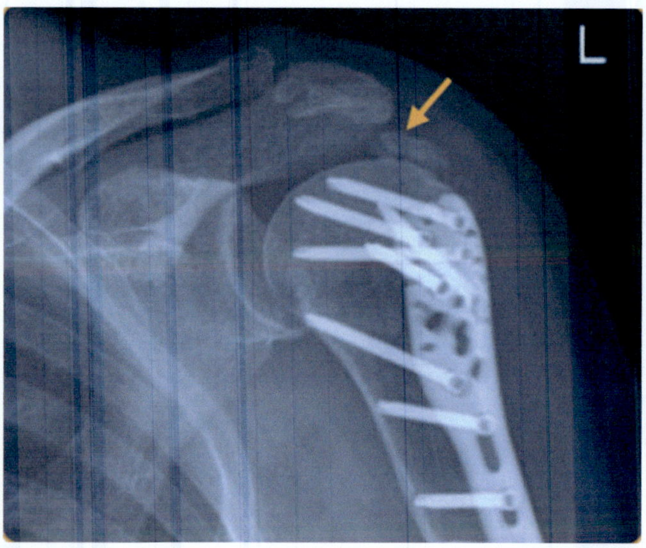

Fig. 26.3 Postoperative radiographs of the left shoulder joint showed displacement of the fracture to the glenohumeral joint (arrow)

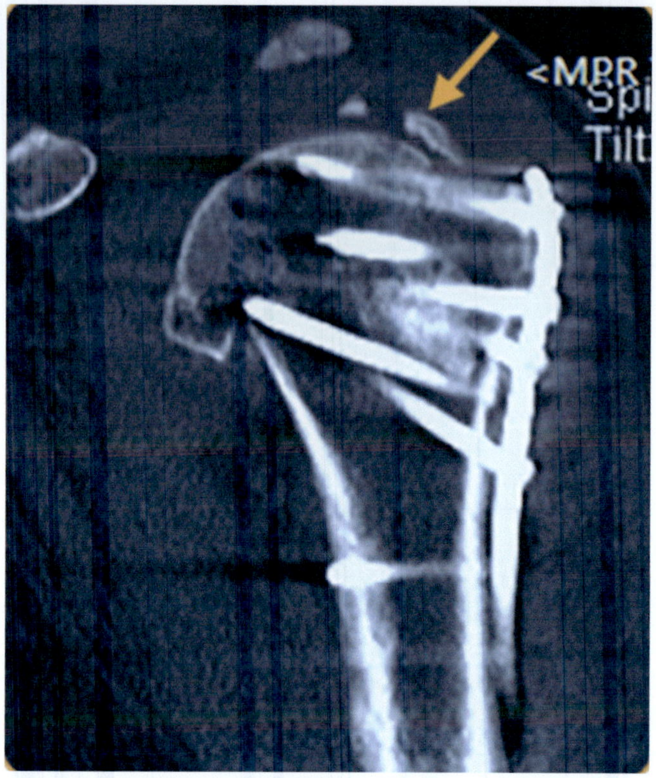

Fig. 26.4 Postoperative coronal 3D-CT reconstruction showed that the tip of the plate was above the greater tubercle of the humerus and the fracture fragment was located in the glenohumeral joint (arrow)

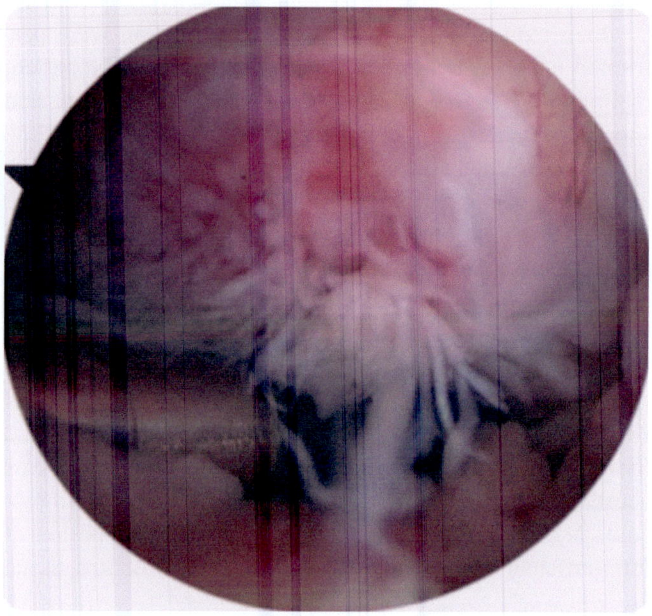

Fig. 26.5 Arthroscopy showed narrowing of the subacromial space and hyperplasia of synovium and scar

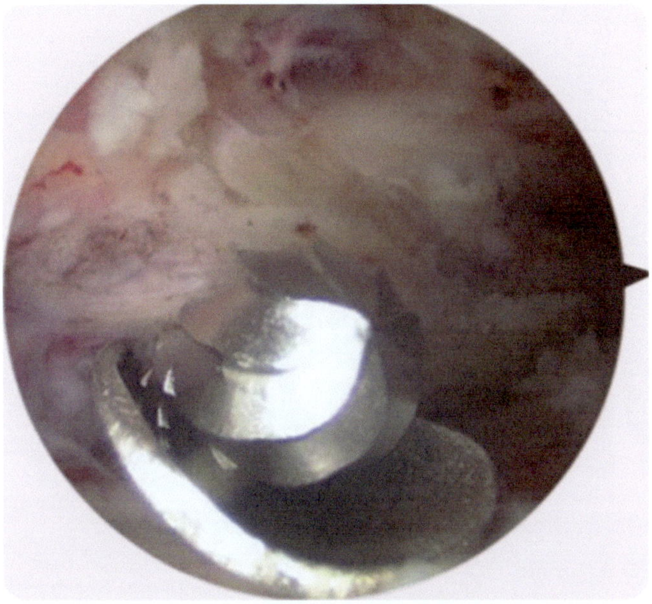

Fig. 26.6 The adhesive tissue was cleaned under arthroscopy

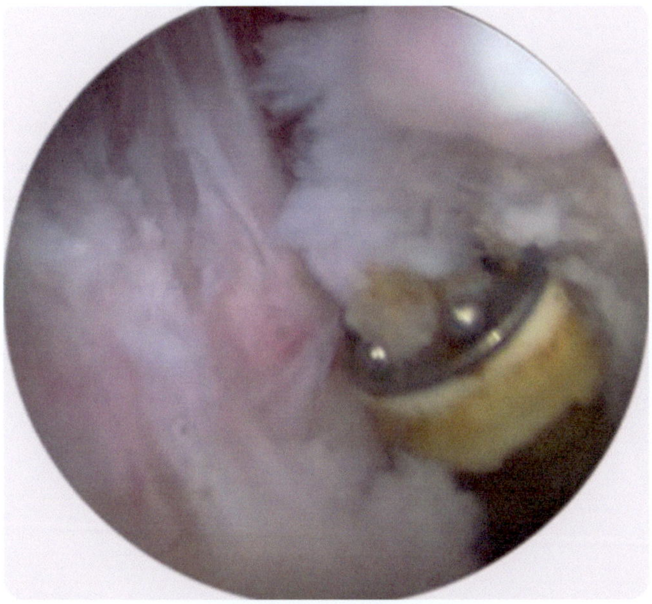

Fig. 26.7 Radiofrequency ablation cleared the subacromial adhesive band

Removing plate and screw under arthroscopy: A periosteal stripper was used to push away scar tissue along the surface of the plate to reveal the plate and screw caps (Fig. 26.9). The screw caps were inserted with a rotary screwdriver, and the screws were removed one by one, then the plate were extracted (Fig. 26.10).

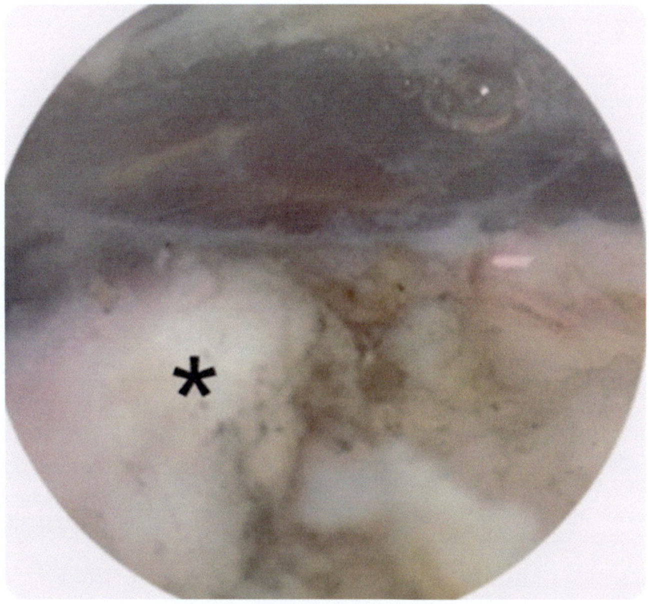

Fig. 26.8 Subacromial exploration revealed displacement of fracture fragment (*) of the greater tubercle of humerus

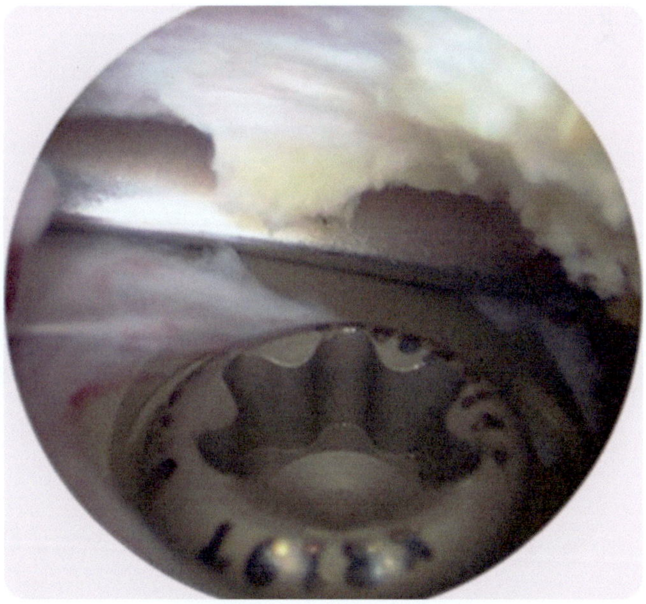

Fig. 26.9 The screw cap was exposed arthroscopically by removing the scar

The fracture fragment of the greater tubercle of humerus was reduced under arthroscopy and fixed with anchor and suture bridge technique to repair the rotator cuff injury (Fig. 26.11).

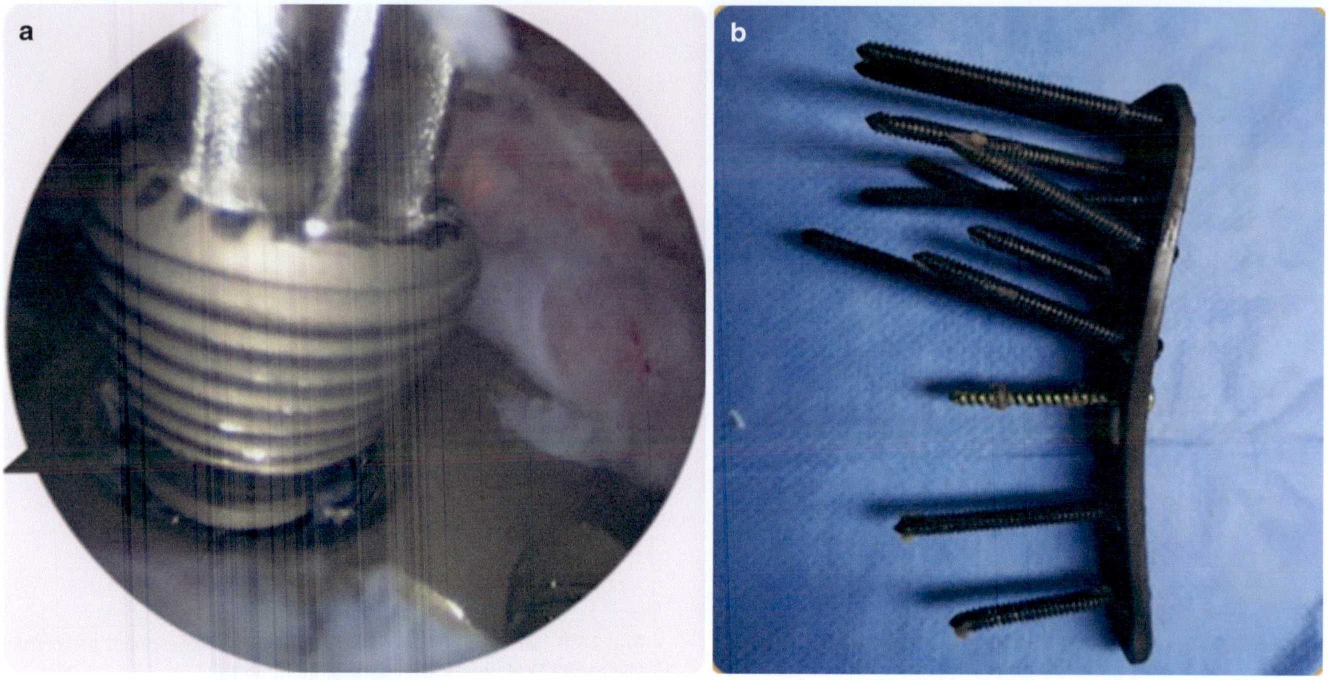

Fig. 26.10 Removing plate and screw under arthroscopy. (**a**) Inserting the screwdriver into the screw caps; (**b**) the removed plate and screws

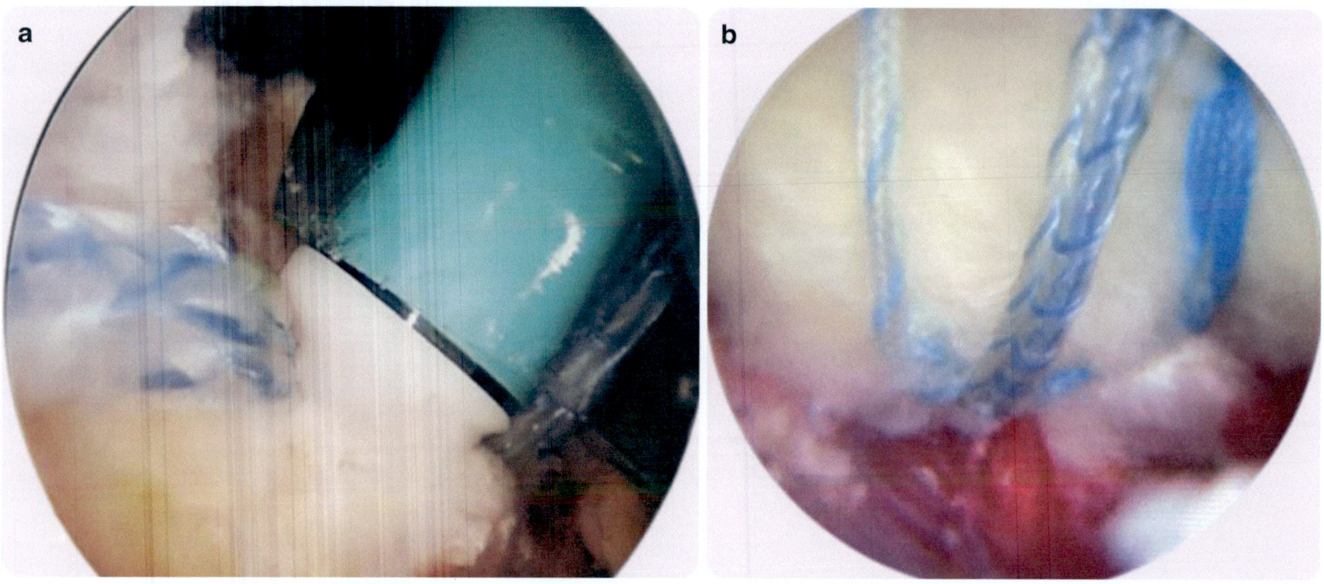

Fig. 26.11 Anchor and suture bridge techniques were used to fix fracture fragment and repair rotator cuff injuries. (**a**) Inserted lateral row suture anchor; (**b**) completed fixation

26.2 Selection of Treatment Methods for Fracture of Greater Tubercle of Humerus

The majority of minor or non-displaced humeral tubercula fractures do not require surgery. There is still debate as to how much of the displacement requires surgical treatment [1]. Some scholars [2] believed that there were complications of ectopic ossification in surgical treatment, and if the fracture is mildly displaced (≤5 mm) and moderately displaced (6–10 mm), non-surgical treatment can be adopted. Clinical studies have found that shoulder dislocation combined with humerus greater tubercle fracture has the risk of displacement, and some scholars believe that displacement >3 mm affects over-the-top activity, especially in young people, and surgical treatment should be chosen [3, 4].

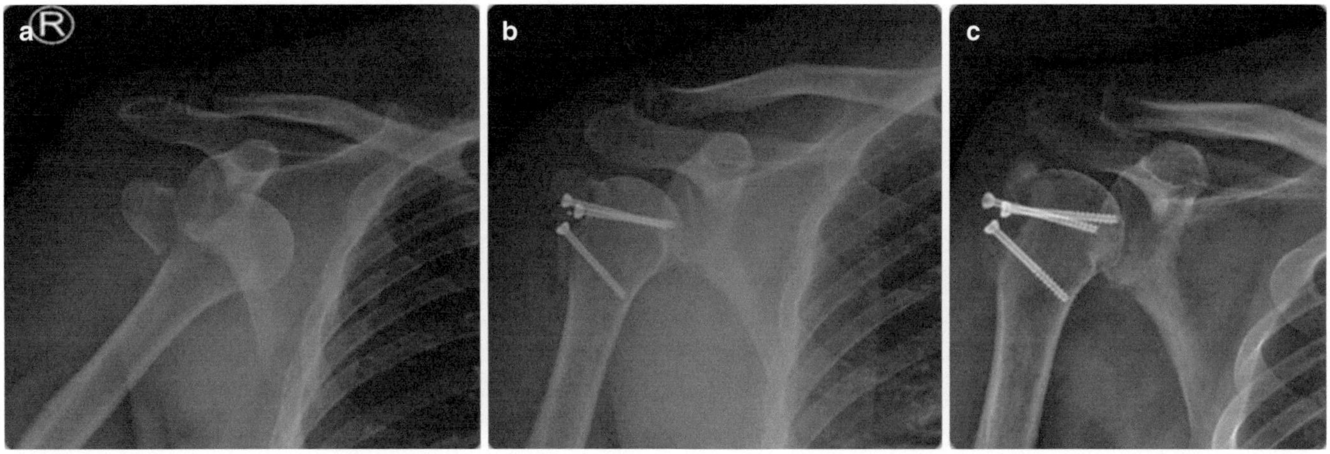

Fig. 26.12 X-ray of right shoulder joint. (**a**) Preoperative findings showed dislocation of the right shoulder joint and displacement of the greater tubercle of the humerus. (**b**) The fracture was well reduced and fixed after operation. (**c**) Bone resorption and fracture displacement were observed 4 months after operation

Displacement of greater humeral tubercle fractures over 5 mm may result in malunion, which may affect the motor function of the shoulder joint [5].

In the past, open reduction and internal fixation of proximal humerus fractures were commonly used. The fixation techniques, such as hollow screw, Kirschner needle and steel plate, were performed through the deltopectoral approach or Deltoid-split approach. However, if the fracture fragment is small or comminuted, the above materials and methods are difficult to achieve accurate reduction and firm fixation, and many complications may occur, such as bone absorption and fracture displacement after hollow screw fixation (Fig. 26.12).

Some surgeons use plate screws to fix humerus greater tubercle fractures and do not pay much attention to the repair and reconstruction of rotator cuff injuries. They attempt to achieve the purpose of fixation by pressing the fracture fragment of the humerus greater tubercle attached to the rotator cuff with the plate. However, because the tip of the plate is too high and too long, impingement with the acromion was occurred (Fig. 26.13). Following plate and screw fixation, displacement of the greater tubercle fracture may occur due to the traction forces exerted by the rotator cuff (Fig. 26.14). Therefore, if the fracture fragment is fixed with plate screws, the rotator cuff tissue must be repaired. Otherwise, the fracture fragment will be displaced after surgery leading to surgical failure (Fig. 26.15).

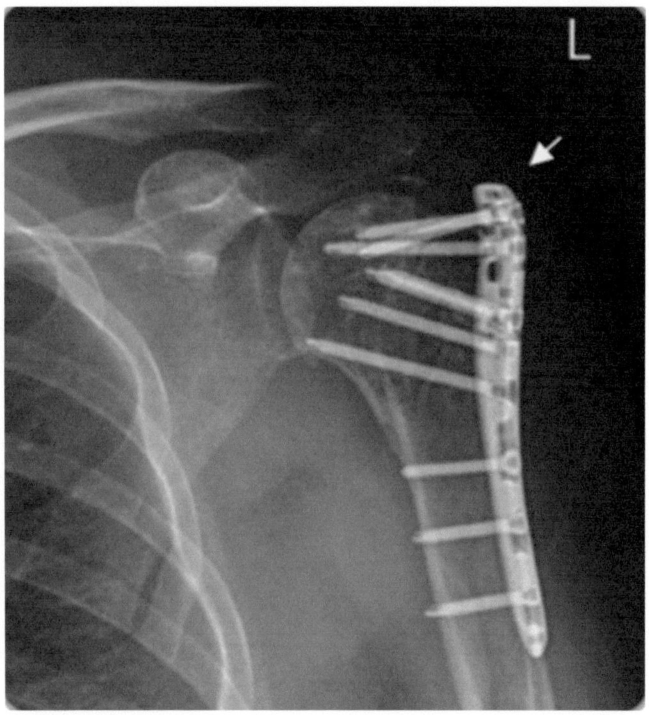

Fig. 26.13 Postoperative X-ray of left shoulder showing excessively high plate (arrow)

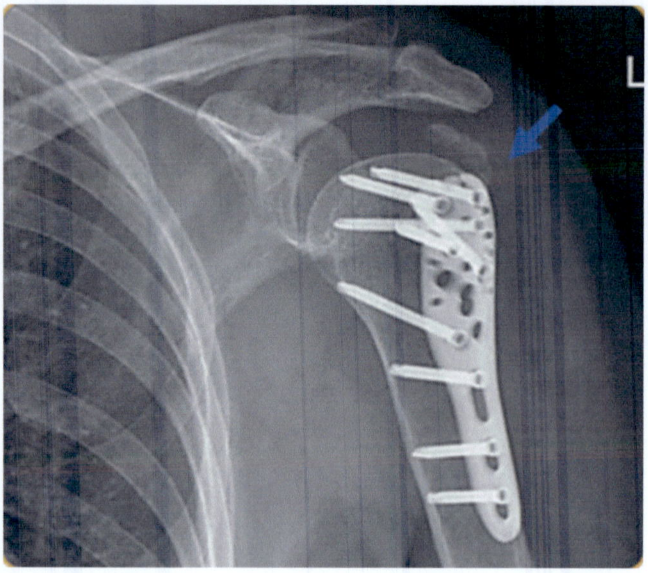

Fig. 26.14 One-month post-surgery, X-ray of left shoulder showing displacement of the greater tubercle of humerus pulled by supraspinatus tendon (arrow)

Suture anchors provide a new option for the treatment of greater tubercle fractures of humerus. Arthroscopic surgery can repair fractures of the greater tubercle of the humerus and rotator cuff injuries with less displacement [6–8]. Compared with open surgery, arthroscopic surgery reduces the incidence of shoulder adhesion and minimizes the impact on shoulder function [9]. For split fractures of the greater tubercle of the humerus, open surgery with plate screw fixation is recommended.

Arthroscopic surgery is not suitable for cases with large bone fragment, because the fracture fragment of the greater tubercle is large, and the operation space will be small, which increases the difficulty of surgical operation and risks damage to the axillary nerve [10, 11]. The average distance between the acromial edge and the axillary nerve was 6 cm [12].

Huntleya et al. [13] reported that shoulder stiffness, pain, and ectopic ossification were the most common complications of humeral greater tuberosity fracture surgery, with a complication rate of 15.1%. The overall complication rate

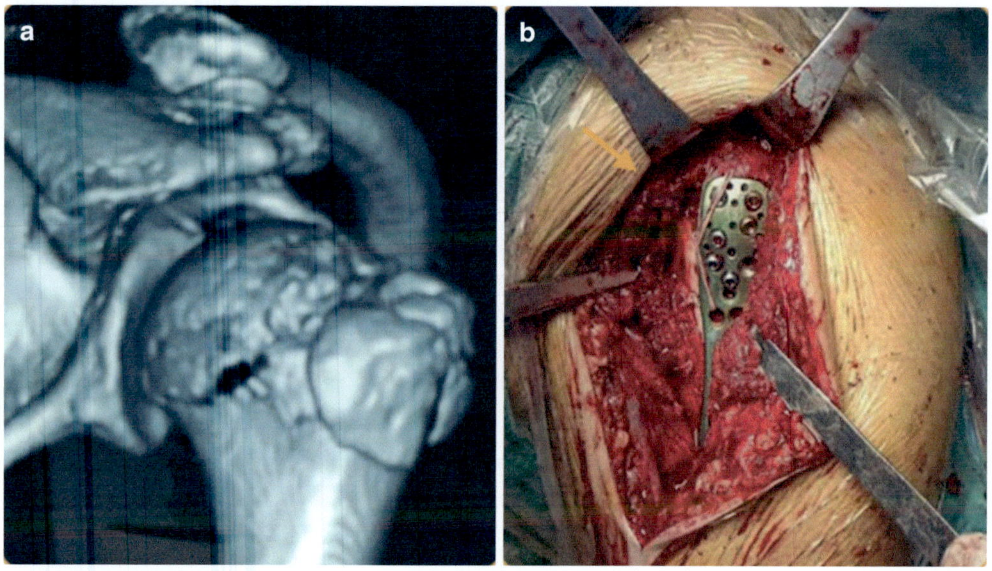

Fig. 26.15 The rotator cuff was fixed by suture and the fracture of the greater tubercle of humerus was fixed by plate. (**a**) Preoperative 3D-CT reconstruction showed surgical neck fracture of humerus combined with greater tubercle fracture. (**b**) Intraoperative lock-plate fixation of proximal humerus and rotator cuff sutured to plate (arrow)

was 22.6% (43/190) for open surgery and 7.3% (9/124) for arthroscopic surgery.

In conclusion, arthroscopic surgery has the advantages of less soft tissue trauma, lower risk of postoperative infection and adhesion, less blood loss, and is conducive to early functional exercise. Therefore, for different types of fractures with avulsion, compression and split of the greater tubercle of humerus, the preoperative evaluation should be carefully optimized to obtain the best effect.

References

1. Neer CS. Displaced proximal humeral fractures: part I. Classification and evaluation. Clin Orthop. 2006;442:77–82.
2. Mattyasovszky SG, Burkhart KJ, Ahlers C, et al. Isolated fractures of the greater tuberosity of the proximal humerus, a long-term retrospective study of 30 patients. Acta Orthop. 2011;82(6):714–20.
3. George MS. Fractures of the greater tuberosity of the humerus. J Am Acad Orthop Surg. 2007;15(10):607–13.
4. Park TS, Choi IY, Kim YH, et al. A new suggestion for the treatment of minimally displaced fractures of the greater tuberosity of the proximal humerus. Bull Hosp Jt Dis. 1997;56(3):171–6.
5. Bono CM, Renard R, Levine RG, et al. Effect of displacement of fractures of the greater tuberosity on the mechanics of the shoulder. J Bone Joint Surg Br. 2001;83(7):1056–62.
6. Ji JH, Kim WY, Ra KH. Arthroscopic double-row suture anchor fixation of minimally displaced greater tuberosity fractures. Arthroscopy. 2007;23(10):1133–4.
7. Ji JH, Shafi M, Song IS, et al. Arthroscopic fixation technique for comminuted displaced greater tuberosity fracture. Arthroscopy. 2011;26(5):600–9.
8. Song HS, Williams GR. Arthroscopic reduction and fixation with suture-bridge technique for displaced or comminuted greater tuberosity fractures. Arthroscopy. 2008;24(8):956–60.
9. Park SE, Jeong JJ, Panchal K, et al. Arthroscopic-assisted plate fixation for displaced large-sized comminuted greater tuberosity fractures of proximal humerus: a novel surgical technique. Knee Surg Sports Traumatol Arthrosc. 2016;24(12):3892–8.
10. Bono CM, Grossman MG, Hochwald N, et al. Radial and axillary nerves.anatomic considerations for humeral fixation. Clin Orthop Relat Res 2000;(373):259.
11. Gardner MJ, Boraiah S, Helfet DL, et al. The anterolateral acromial approach for fractures of the proximal humerus. J Orthop Trauma. 2008;22(2):132–7.
12. Samart S, Apivatgaroon A, Lakchayapakorn K, et al. The correlation between acromion-axillary nerve distance and upper arm length; a cadaveric study. J Med Assoc Thai. 2014;97(Suppl 8):S27–33.
13. Huntleya SR, Lehtonena EJ, Robina JX, et al. Outcomes of surgical fixation of greater tuberosity fractures:a systematic review. Orthop Traumatol Surg Res. 2020;106:1119–26.

27 Arthroscopic-Assisted Minimally Invasive Surgery for Chronic Tear of the Pectoralis Major

Jun-liang Wang and Yu-jie Liu

Tear of pectoralis major muscle is a rare sports injury. Patisser [1] first reported tear of pectoralis major in 1822. With the increase of sports population and fitness enthusiasts, reports of tear of pectoralis major muscle have gradually increased [2, 3]. Pectoralis major muscle tears predominantly occur in young males during weightlifting activities, particularly bench press, or horizontal bar exercises. These injuries are typically managed conservatively as soft tissue injuries, although select cases may require open surgical intervention [4–6]. Tear of pectoralis major muscle is often neglected, and once becomes an old injury, it will increase the difficulty of diagnosis and treatment and affect the curative effect. In our department, three patients with chronic tear of pectoralis major were treated by ultrasonography and magnetic resonance imaging, and minimally invasive surgery with the assistance of arthroscope.

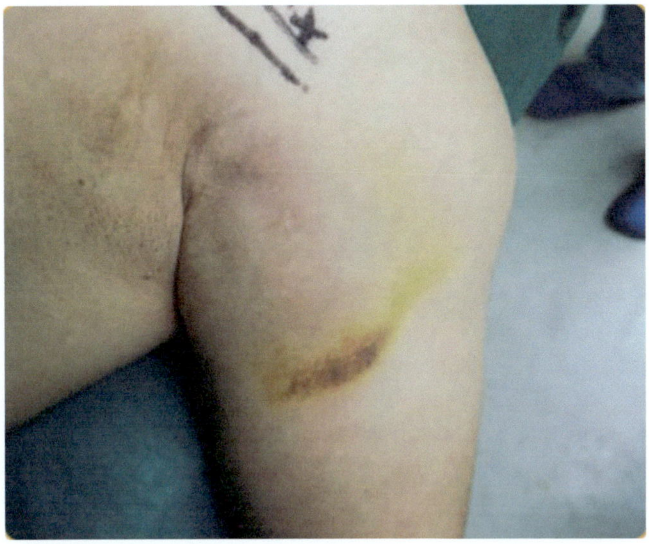

Fig. 27.1 There were old ecchymosis on the upper arm and anterior chest wall of the affected side 5 weeks after injury

27.1 Overview of the Diagnosis and Treatment Process

A 40-year-old male patient suddenly experienced severe pain in the left thorax and shoulder with a tearing sound during bench press barbell (90 kg) training. Subsequently, the patient developed swelling of the subcutaneous tissue of the left anterior axillary fold, and a large area of ecchymosis appeared in the subcutaneous tissue of the anterior chest wall and the medial upper arm. The upper limb was suspended and fixed in the emergency department, and the pain symptoms gradually eased, and the ecchymosis of the anterior axillary fold gradually subsided 5 weeks after the injury (Fig. 27.1). An outpatient review 8 weeks after the injury revealed an egg-like mass bulge in the chest during contraction of the pectoral major muscle (Fig. 27.2). The mass is more apparent, when the pectoralis major muscles contract.

Physical examination: Bilateral pectoralis major muscles were asymmetrical, there was a deep groove at the junction of pectoralis major and deltoid muscle on the affected side, and the papillary sag sign on the affected side was positive (Fig. 27.3). Local touch has a feeling of emptiness with tenderness. The ultrasound showed a retraction of the torn end of the pectoralis major. MR Gradient echo sequences showed focal effusion in the pectoral major muscle with high intra-

J.-l. Wang (✉)
Department of Orthopedics, Hainan Hospital of Chinese PLA General Hospital, Sanya, China

Y.-j. Liu
Orthopaedics, Chinese PLA General Hospital, Beijing, China

Y.-j. Liu et al. (eds.), *Pitfalls in Diagnosis and Treatment of Shoulder Joint Diseases*,
https://doi.org/10.1007/978-981-96-2472-0_27

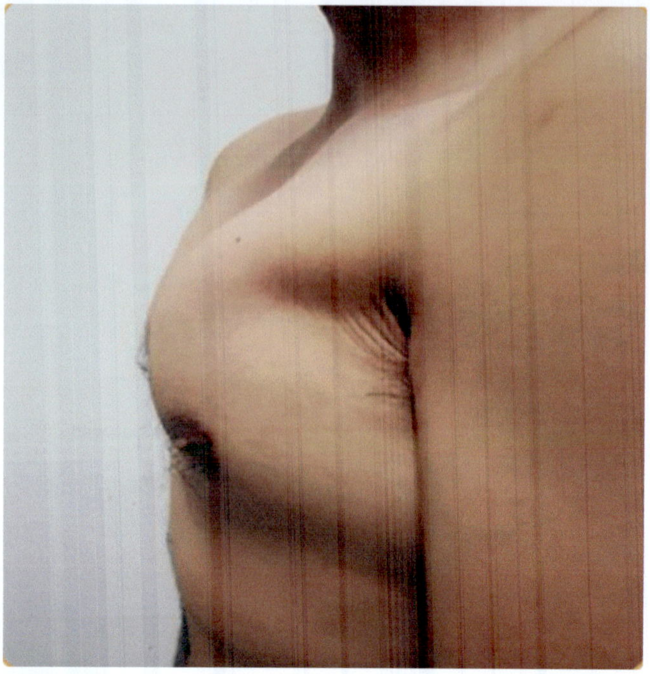

Fig. 27.2 Left breast bulge

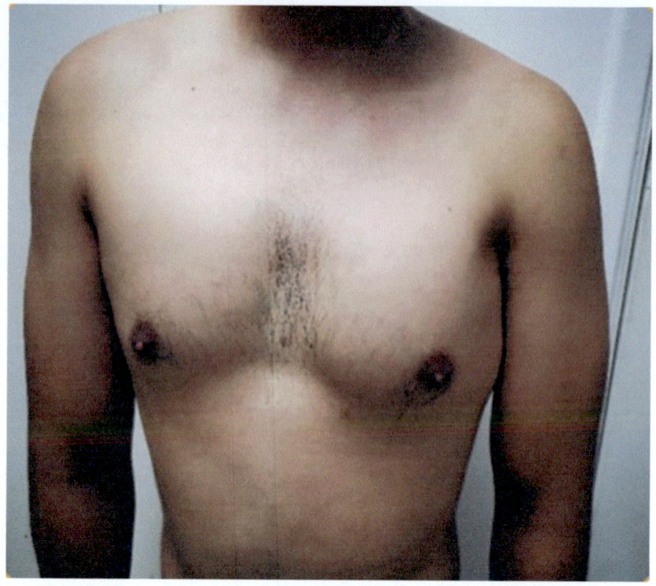

Fig. 27.3 The left nipple sagged, and the two nipples were asymmetrical

muscular signal, indicating complete tear of the pectoral major muscle, retraction of the tear end of the tendon (Fig. 27.4), and local soft tissue edema. A complete routine examination was performed to determine the location of pectoralis major muscle tear and humeral shaft insertion, and to measure the distance and position of muscle and tendon break end stop point. After routine examination, the location of pectoralis major muscle tear and humeral shaft insertion were marked, and the distance between tear point and insertion was measured.

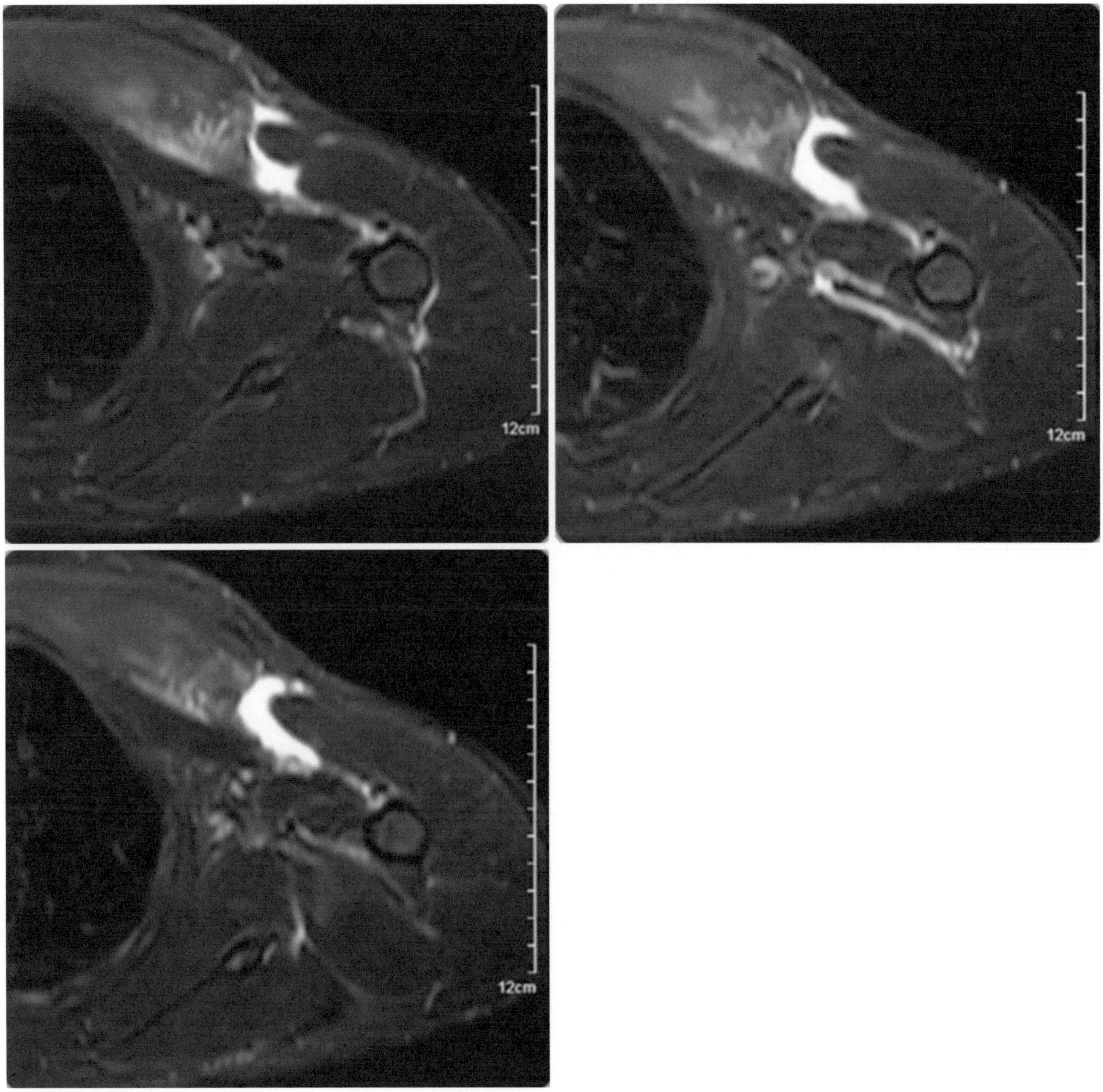

Fig. 27.4 Preoperative MRI showed rupture and retraction of pectoralis major tendon

27.2 Arthroscopic-Assisted Minimally Invasive Repair of Thoracic Major Muscle Tear

General anesthesia was used, and the patient was placed on a beach chair. Before the operation, the anatomical markers of shoulder joint surface and surgical approach were marked (Fig. 27.5). After routine skin sterilization, 60 mL saline containing epinephrine was injected into the surgical area of the anterior axillary wall for clear visual field. A stripper was inserted between the subcutaneous tissue at the anterior axillary fold and the pectoralis major muscle to separate the working space of the surgical procedure. The scar tissue was cleared with shaver blade and radiofrequency under the surveillance of arthroscope. The injured stump of the pectoralis major was explored with the assistance of arthroscopy, and the torn stump of the pectoralis major was sutured using a rotator cuff suture passer (Fig. 27.6). The contracture band of the pectoralis major was further explored with suture traction, and the stump of the pectoralis major was sutured with No. 2 high-strength suture. Then the stump of the pectoralis major was close to the attachment of the proximal humerus (Fig. 27.7).

Through deltopectoral approach, the cephalic vein and deltoid muscles were separated and retracted. The insertion of the pectoral major muscle was debrided near the tendon groove of the long head tendon of the biceps humerus. The traction suture at the residual tendon of the pectoralis major was pulled to the insertion of the proximal humerus (Figs. 27.8 and 27.9). A bone hole was drilled at the insertion of the pectoral major muscle, then the high-strength sutures were passed through the footprint anchor hole. The stump was sutured and reinforced with the surrounding tissue (Fig. 27.10).

The patients had no nerve, vascular injury, infection, and other complications. The elbow joint, wrist joint, and shoulder joint function exercise were carried out according to the rehabilitation plan after the operation to avoid the adhesion of the shoulder and elbow joint after the operation. Upper limb abduction, forward flexion, and backward extension exercises were performed passively at the sixth week after surgery. Breaststroke training began at the eighth week after surgery. The shoulder joint function fully recovered to the pre-injury level 3 months after surgery. Postoperative MRI showed good fixation position and anatomical morphology of pectoralis major tendon (Fig. 27.11).

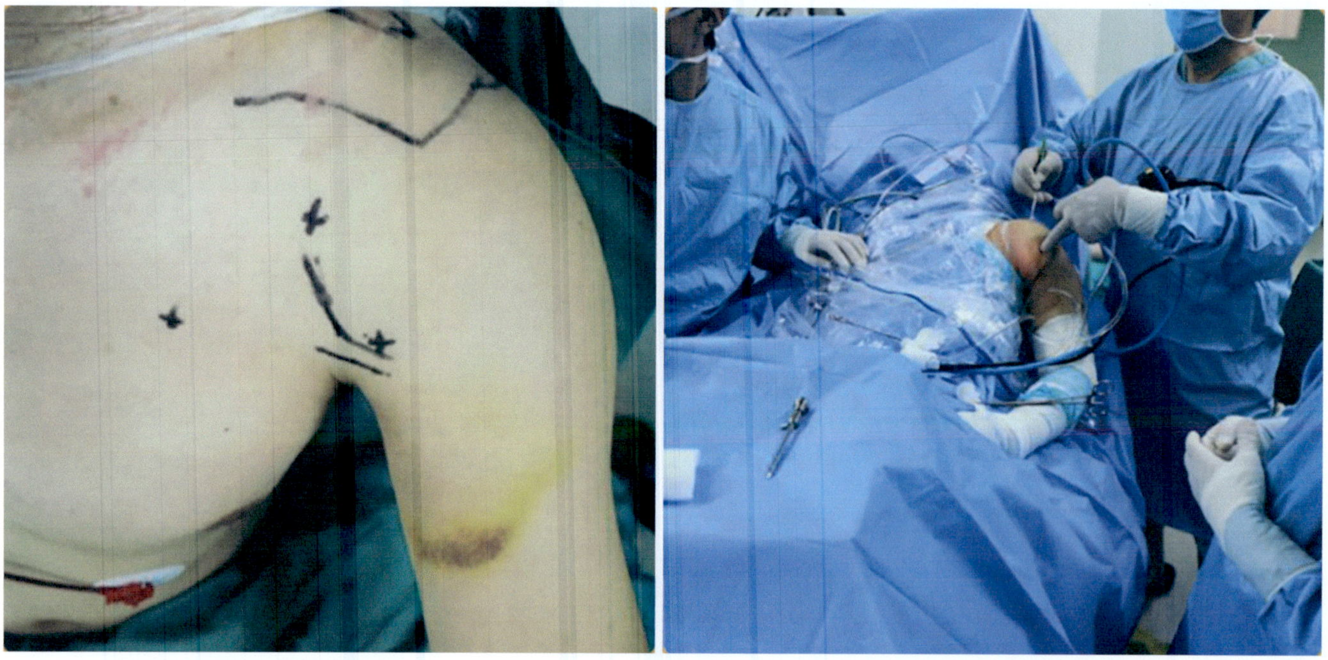

Fig. 27.5 Surgical position and approach marker

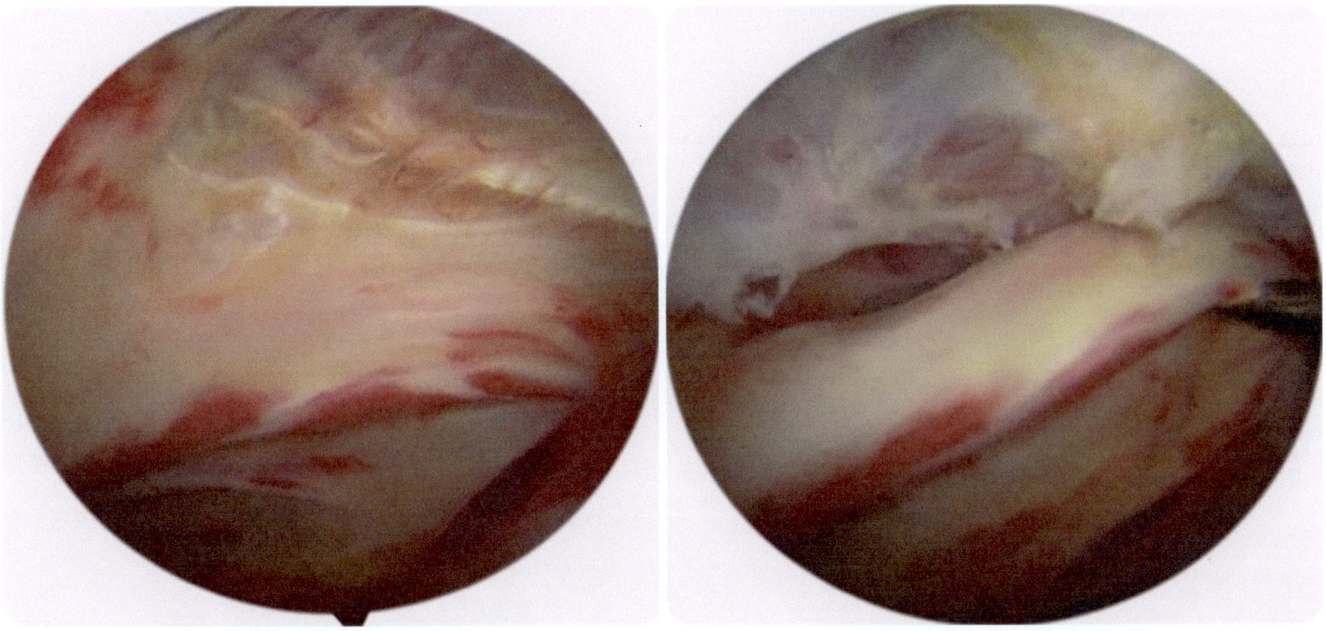

Fig. 27.6 Release the pectoral major muscles

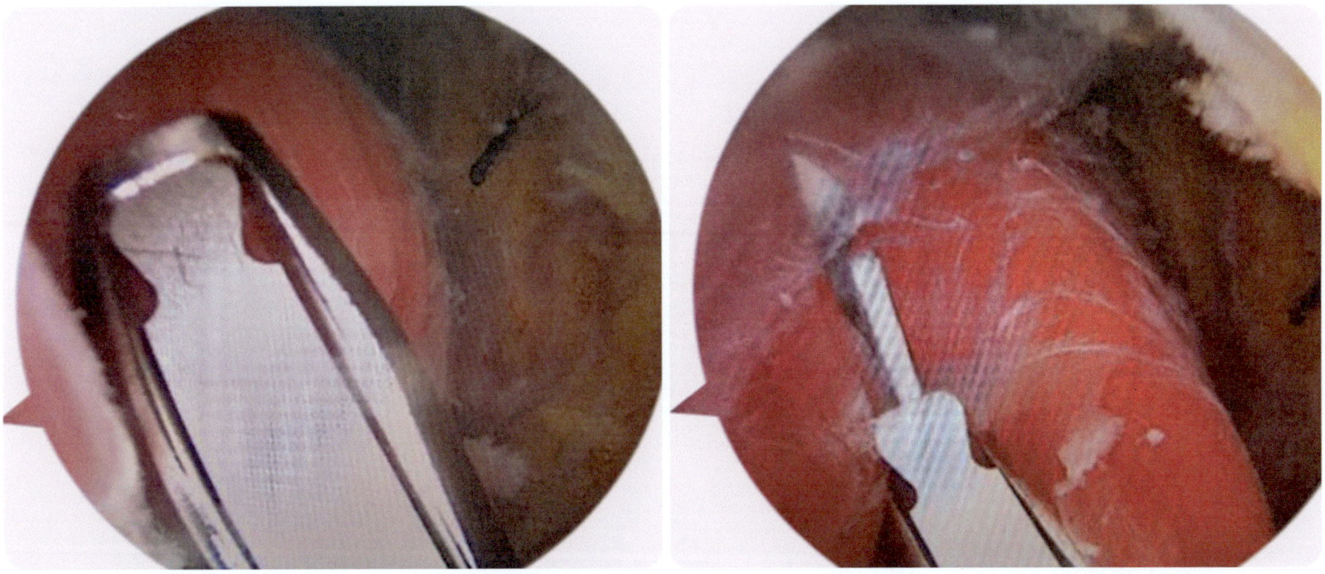

Fig. 27.7 Suture the pectoralis major stump with rotator cuff suture passer

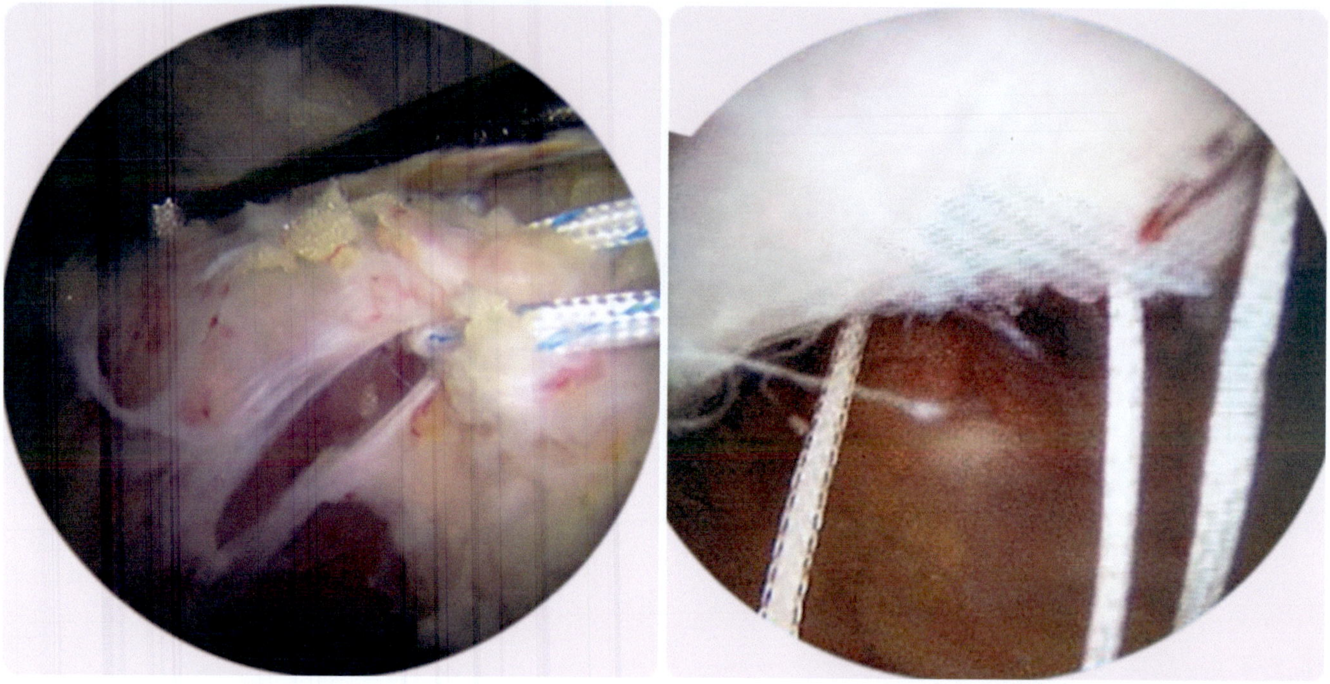

Fig. 27.8 Release the stump of the pectoralis major

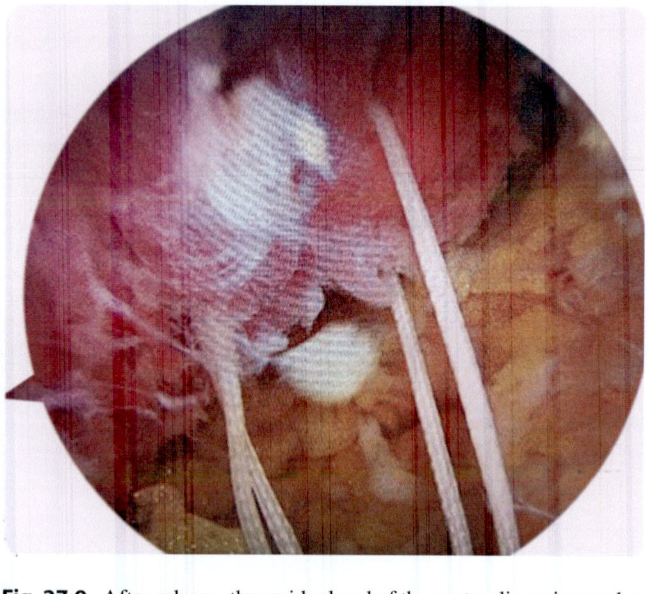

Fig. 27.9 After release, the residual end of the pectoralis major tendon was close to the attachment of the proximal humerus

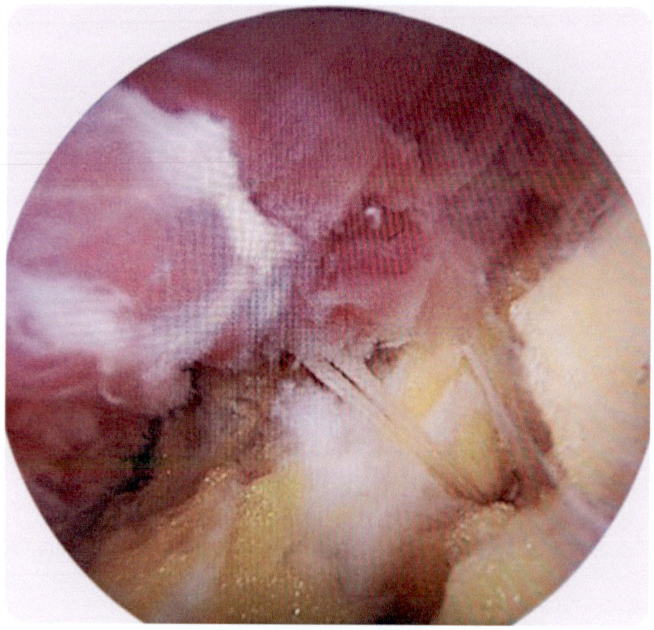

Fig. 27.10 The pectoralis major was anchored to the proximal humerus

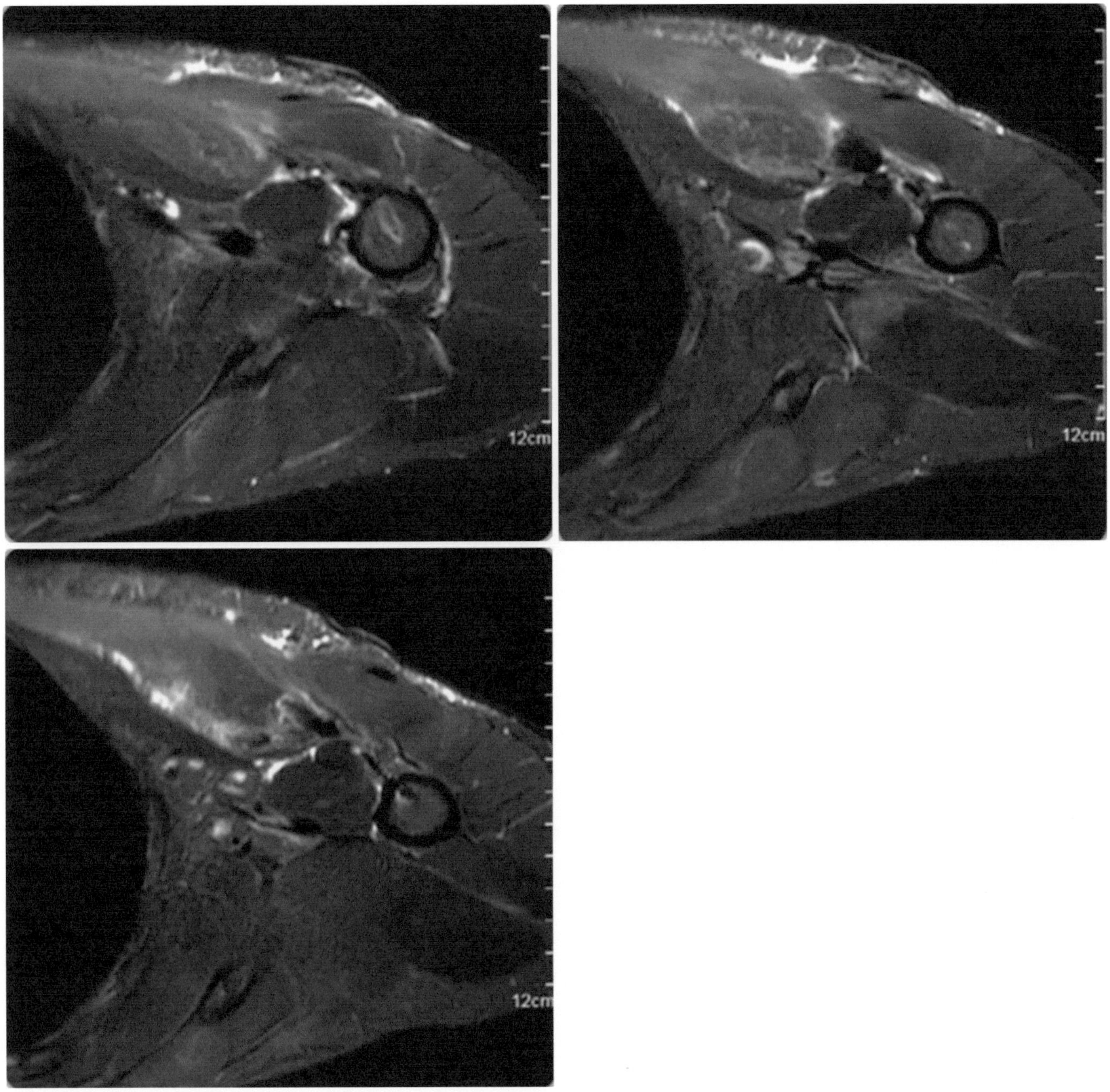

Fig. 27.11 Postoperative MRI showed that the pectoralis major tendon was well fixed to the proximal humerus

27.3 Discussion

The pectoralis major is divided into the head of the clavicle and the pectoral head, and the two heads end together at the lateral margin of the biceps tendon groove. The main functions of the pectoralis major muscle are the adduction and rotation of the upper arm. The injury of pectoralis major muscle can be divided into direct injury and indirect injury, which can occur in any part from the starting point to the ending point. Direct injuries usually lead to lacerations in the muscular abdomen, while indirect injuries lead to injuries at the humerus attachment or muscle–tendon junction. In clinical practice, the most common injuries caused by indirect injuries were tendon and attachment tears, while the injuries of the attachment points of the clavicle and sternum of the pectoralis major and the muscular abdomen were relatively rare [7]. The location of the tear is age-related. Young people tend to tear at the tendon junction, while older people usually tear at the attachment of the tendon to the bone [8].

According to the injury location, pectoralis major muscle tears can be divided into muscle origin or abdominal tear, muscle–tendon junction tear, intramuscular tear, humeral insertion, and bone avulsion of humeral insertion [9]. It is divided into partial tear and complete tear according to the degree of tear. The typical early manifestations of a laceration of the pectoralis major muscle are pain, local swelling, weakened muscle strength, and large subcutaneous hematoma.

Conservative treatment is suitable for elderly patients with medical disease and incomplete tear. Conservative treatment can restore the range of motion of the limbs despite muscle weakness. Bodendorfer et al. [4] showed that the curative effect of acute repair was significantly better than that of chronic repair. Thompson et al. [10] suggest that repair surgery was best performed within 6 weeks of injury. Studies have shown that the efficacy satisfaction and treatment results of delayed surgical repair are still better than those of nonsurgical treatment [10–12], so it is recommended to take surgical treatment as far as possible even if early misdiagnosis or the optimal time of surgical treatment is delayed. Early correct diagnosis and timely surgical treatment are very important. It is important to evaluate the location and degree of contracture of pectoralis major muscle injury to select the surgical method. Autologous or allogeneic tendons such as fascia lata and semi-tendinous tendons can be used for repair, reconstruction, or reinforcement fixation for severe muscle and tendon contracture [10, 13].

Due to the limited length of tendon available for repair of a torn pectoralis major muscle [13], if the disease course exceeds 8 weeks, muscle and tendon contracture, scar adhesion, surgical exploration is difficult to distinguish from the tear end. Ultrasonography is cheap and convenient, and it is of great value in the diagnosis. However, because this injury is relatively rare, even experienced musculoskeletal ultrasound experts sometimes have difficulty in making an accurate diagnosis and evaluation of chronic injuries. Therefore, ultrasound is mainly used for the preliminary examination of injuries, while the preoperative evaluation of surgical patients must rely on MRI [9]. MRI examination is of great significance in the diagnosis and evaluation of chronic tear injury of pectoralis major muscle, in determining the specific location of the tear of pectoralis major muscle, the situation of the broken end of the tendon and the degree of retraction, and in formulating the surgical treatment plan. Lee et al. have shown that MRI helps to better assess pectoral major muscle injury and rule out other pathological changes compared to ultrasound.

In three patients with chronic contracture of pectoralis major muscle injury, axial MRI imaging technology was used before surgery to further identify the location, severity, and length of contracture of pectoralis major muscle tear. The measurement showed that the distance between the tear end of pectoralis major and the end of proximal humerus was 55~65 mm. Arthroscopic surgical exploration was performed on patients with chronic contracture of pectoralis major injury to accurately identify the tear site and clearly display the tear location of pectoralis major muscle and the degree of retraction of the tear end of tendon under arthroscopy. The tendon was fixed with the aid of arthroscopy to avoid open surgery with large incisions. After the operation, the patient underwent functional rehabilitation training according to the established rehabilitation program, and the patient returned to exercise 3 months after the operation and achieved a good effect. Follow-up was performed according to Bak evaluation criteria. The clinical results of these three cases were considered to be excellent.

In conclusion, arthroscopy-assisted minimally invasive surgery for the treatment of chronic pectoralis major lacerations has further expanded the field of application of arthroscopic technology in the extra-articular field and achieved satisfactory clinical efficacy.

References

1. Patissier P. Traite des maladies des artisans. Paris. 1822. pp. 162–164.
2. Sahota S, Gibbs DB, Lawton CD, et al. Pectoralis major injuries in the National Football League. Sports Health. 2020;12(2):116–23.
3. Pedrazzini A, Banchi M, Bertoni N, et al. Pectoralis major tendon rupture in a weight lifter: a rare case. Acta Biomed. 2017;88(1):86–90.
4. Bodendorfer BM, Wang DX, McCormick BP, et al. Treatment of pectoralis major tendon tears: a systematic review and meta-analysis of repair timing and fixation methods. Am J Sports Med. 2020;48(13):3376–85.
5. Sephien A, Orr J, Remaley DT. Pectoralis major tear in a 23-year-old woman while performing high-intensity interval training: a rare presentation. BMJ Case Rep. 2020;13(3):e232649.
6. Cordasco FA, Mahony GT, Tsouris N, et al. Pectoralis major tendon tears: functional outcomes and return to sport in a consecutive series of 40 athletes. J Shoulder Elbow Surg. 2017;26(3):458–63.
7. Orvets ND, Bhale R, Budge MD. Surgical management of pectoralis major tears of the sternal origin because of seat belt trauma: a report of 2 cases. JBJS Case Connect. 2021;11(3)
8. Berson BL. Surgical repair of pectoralis major rupture in an athlete. Case report of an unusual injury in a wrestler. Am J Sports Med. 1979;7(6):348–51.
9. Lee YK, Skalski MR, White EA, et al. US and MR imaging of pectoralis major injuries. Radiographics. 2017;37(1):176–89.
10. Thompson K, Kwon Y, Flatow E, et al. Everything pectoralis major: from repair to transfer. Phys Sports Med. 2020;48(1):33–45.
11. Abbas MJ, Buckley P, Shah S, et al. Simultaneous repair of bilateral pectoralis major tendons: a case report. World J Orthop. 2021;12(10):802–10.
12. Choudhary M, Shah N, Arshad MS, et al. The outcome of surgical management of chronic pectoralis major ruptures in weightlifters. Acta Orthop Belg. 2017;83(3):433–7.
13. Long M, Enders T, Trasolini R, et al. Pectoralis major tendon reconstruction using semitendinosus allograft following rupture at the musculotendinous junction. JSES Open Access. 2019;3(4):328–32.

Part X

Shoulder Joint Free Body, Rice Grain Body, and Calcified Tendonitis: An Introduction and Summary

Jing Xue

1.1 Introduction

This part focuses on the reasons why it is difficult to find the lesion in the operation of calcifying tendinitis of the shoulder joint. At the same time, the relationship between the pathological stage of calcifying tendinitis and shoulder pain, clinical characteristics, and diagnostic points are introduced in detail. The methods of conservative treatment and surgical treatment are described in detail. The arthroscopic manifestations, advantages, challenges, and corresponding strategies of treating calcifying tendinitis in the shoulder joint are presented.

This part also introduces the diagnostic ideas and causes of misdiagnosis of shoulder loose bodies and rice bodies. The causes of rice body formation and the differences between rice bodies and loose bodies in shoulder joint are analyzed. Arthroscopic shoulder surgery is helpful for the diagnosis. Synovial debridement and removal of loose bodies are the key points of treatment.

1.2 Summary

1. Many patients with calcifying tendinitis of the shoulder joint can be treated with conservative treatment measures, such as oral non-steroidal anti-inflammatory drugs, local block, and physiotherapy, and the symptoms can be completely relieved. If the interval between diagnosis and surgery exceeds 2 to 4 weeks, it is recommended to routinely repeat X-ray and CT examinations the day before the operation. This ensures accurate assessment of the calcification lesion's presence, size, and location, thereby preventing potential intraoperative complications due to the inability to locate the lesion. When conservative treatment is ineffective in acute stage, subacromial injection of local anesthetics under X-ray fluoroscopy and epidural needle puncture decompression of calcified lesions can be used for treatment, and most of the pain symptoms can be significantly relieved after treatment. Arthroscopic surgery can accurately treat the lesion, and the necessary acromioplasty and rotator cuff repair can be performed, and the curative effect is more exact.
2. Rice bodies of shoulder joint are easily misdiagnosed as lipoma. Joint puncture, ultrasound, and magnetic resonance imaging have important reference value for diagnosis and differential diagnosis. Arthroscopic rice bodies removal and synovectomy are the key to reduce recurrence.

J. Xue (✉)
Orthopaedics, Air Force Medical Center of Chinese PLA, Beijing, China

28 Pitfalls and Strategies in the Diagnosis and Treatment of Calcified Supraspinatus Tenosynovitis

Hai-peng Li, Jing-bing Zhou, and Yu-jie Liu

Calcific tendinitis of the rotator cuff (CTR) is common in women aged 30–60 years, accounting for 5–40% of the causes of shoulder pain. The supraspinatus tendon accounts for about 80%, the infraspinatus tendon accounts for 15%, and the subscapularis tendon accounts for 5% [1]. About 20% of patients may have no clinical symptoms, and about 50% of patients have no obvious cause. The etiology is still unclear and may be related to degeneration, trauma, hypoxia, endocrine, metabolic disorders, etc. [2, 3]. Due to the deposition of hydroxyapatite [$Ca_{10}(PO_4)_6(OH)_2$] and inflammatory stimulation, the onset is sudden, knife-like severe pain and limited shoulder joint activity [4]. There are many theories about the pathological changes of CTR, and the theory of reactive calcification proposed by Uhthoff et al. [4] has been widely recognized.

Calcifying tendonitis of rotator cuff is divided into three stages: precalcification, calcification, and postcalcification. The calcification stage is divided into formation stage, dormancy stage, and absorption stage (i.e., attack stage). During this period, the calcified lesions are absorbed, macrophages and multinucleated giant cells are active, leading to severe inflammatory reactions and the most severe pain. Some patients need surgical treatment to relieve pain. However, calcifying tendonitis of rotator cuff is a self-limited disease, and the calcified lesions can be absorbed and healed by themselves. Therefore, preoperative clinical and imaging examinations are very important for judging and confirming the lesion situation and surgical treatment location, otherwise blind surgery will cause the situation that the lesions are difficult to find.

28.1 Overview of Diagnosis and Treatment

A 57-year-old female patient had unexplained paroxysmal severe pain in the right shoulder joint at night for 3 days. During the attack, the pain was like needle pricking and knife cutting, which was unbearable and seriously affected sleep and quality of life.

Physical examination: painful expression, right shoulder joint in passive position, left hand holding elbow joint (Fig. 28.1). The right subacromial area was tender to touch and pressure examination, and the shoulder joint movement was limited. The shoulder joint X-ray film showed a lamellar high-density shadow under the right subacromial (Fig. 28.2), diagnosed as calcified supraspinatus tendonitis. The patient strongly requested hospitalization for surgery, because the bed was tight, so anti-inflammatory analgesics and physiotherapy were given first, waiting for hospitalization. The patient had no history of diabetes, drinking, excessive exercise, and trauma. Five weeks later, the patient was admitted to hospital. After completing routine preoperative examinations, arthroscopic exploration was performed under general anesthesia. The subacromial and glenohumeral joint space were repeatedly explored during the operation, and no calcification was found. X-ray fluoroscopy was also used during the operation to find no calcification. The radiofrequency was used to clean the hypertrophic inflammatory synovial membrane and flush the joint cavity, and the operation was completed. The shoulder joint X-ray film was taken on the day after the operation (Fig. 28.3), and no calcification lesions of the shoulder joint were found at the time of visit.

H.-p. Li (✉)
Department of Orthopedics, The Fourth Medical Center, Chinese PLA General Hospital, Beijing, China

J.-b. Zhou
Sports Medicine and Rehabilitation Department, Beijing Chaoyang Hospital, Capital Medical University, Beijing, China

Y.-j. Liu
Orthopaedics, Chinese PLA General Hospital, Beijing, China

Y.-j. Liu et al. (eds.), *Pitfalls in Diagnosis and Treatment of Shoulder Joint Diseases*,
https://doi.org/10.1007/978-981-96-2472-0_28

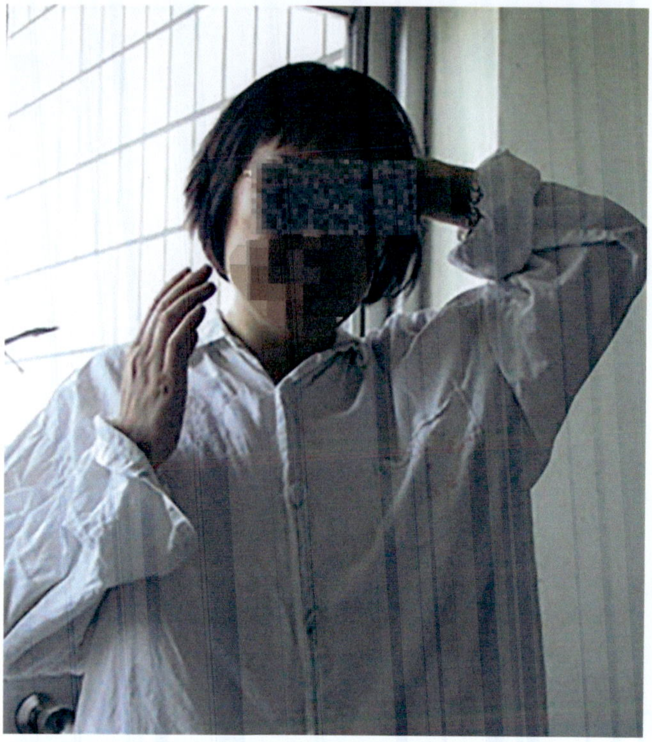

Fig. 28.1 Right shoulder pain with limited shoulder lifting

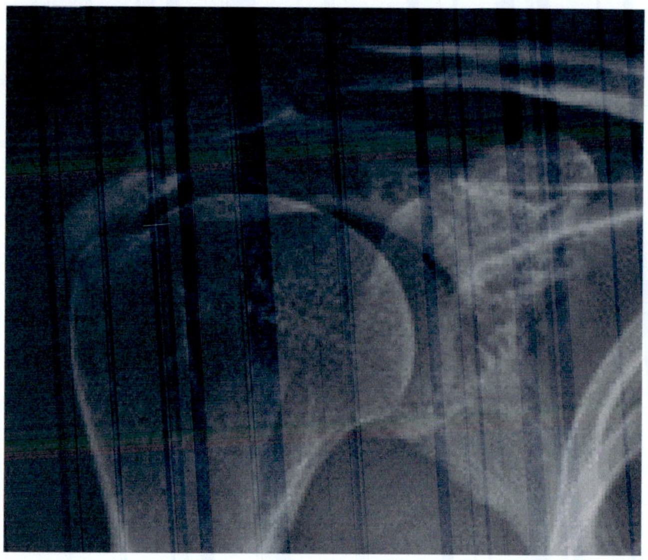

Fig. 28.2 X-ray of right shoulder showing subacromial high density

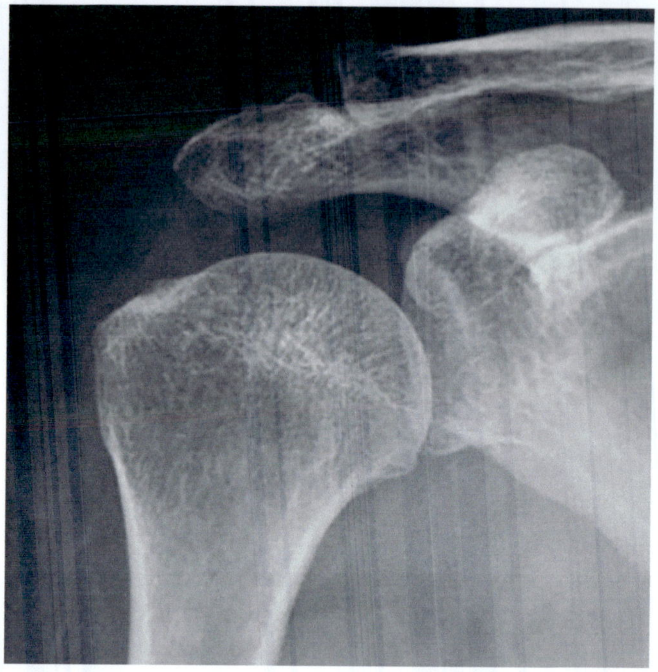

Fig. 28.3 X-ray of right shoulder showing complete disappearance of calcified supraspinatus tendon shadow

28.2 Experience

In this case of calcified supraspinatus tendonitis of the shoulder joint, why was no lesion found during the operation? What should we learn? It is worth further discussion. From the onset of the disease to the interval of 1 month, the patient underwent a series of conservative treatments, and the complete absorption of calcified spots is possible. The author once treated a patient with calcified tendonitis (Fig. 28.4) with conservative treatment for 5 weeks, and the absorption of calcified spots disappeared (Fig. 28.5). It has been reported in literature that 50.4~70% of patients can completely relieve their symptoms with conservative treatments such as oral nonsteroidal anti-inflammatory drugs, local block, and physiotherapy [1], indicating that calcified supraspinatus tendonitis is self-limited. Although the diagnosis is confirmed by X-ray examination at the time of visit, it is necessary to have a further imaging review before surgery. Imaging examina-

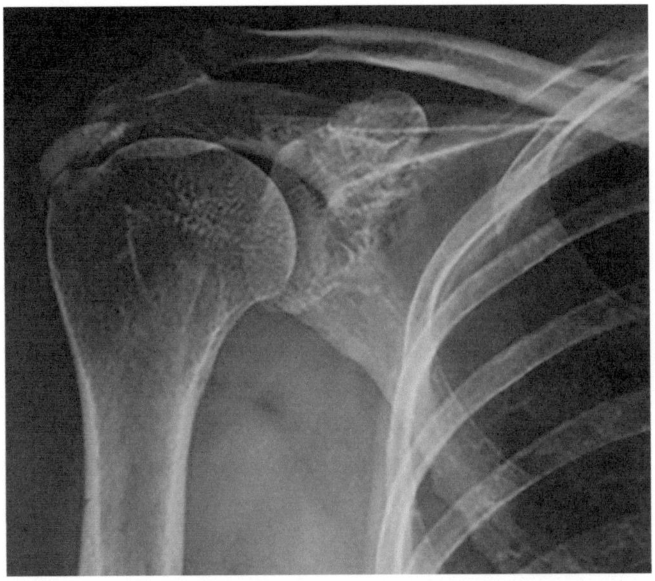

Fig. 28.4 Calcified supraspinatus tendon under right acromion

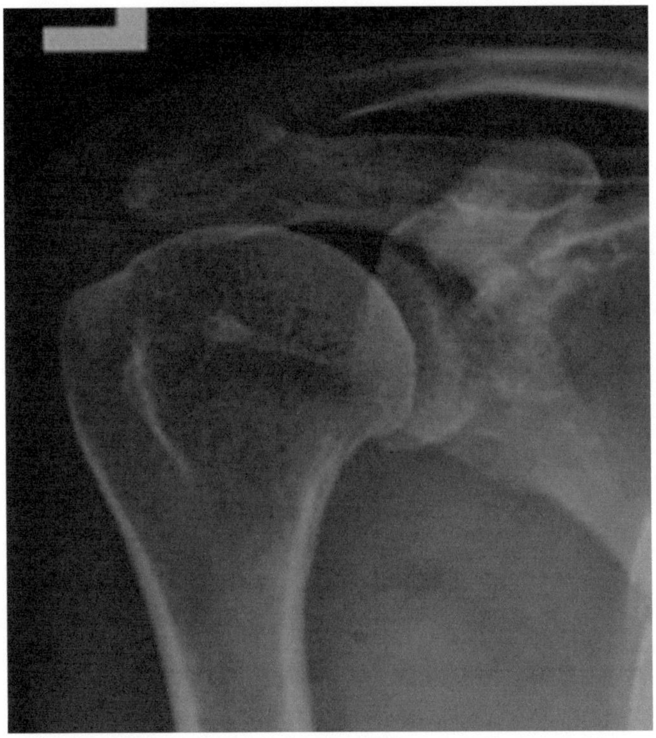

Fig. 28.5 Disappearance of calcified lesion after needle puncture decompression under local anesthesia

tion has important value in the diagnosis and differential diagnosis. X-ray examination has the advantages of being quick, convenient, and inexpensive and is the first choice of imaging examination method for calcified rotator cuff tendonitis. In typical cases, high-density calcified spots 1.5~2 cm away from the humeral attachment of the rotator cuff tendon can be seen. Gartner and Heyer [5] proposed to classify calcified spots according to X-ray imaging. Type I: calcified spots with high-density and obvious boundaries; Type II: calcified spots with high-density but unclear boundaries, or obvious boundaries but low density; Type III: calcified spots with low-density and unclear boundaries, which are cloudy. CT can show calcification more clearly and locate calcification accurately, especially can clearly find the calcification of the subscapular tendon that is easy to miss. CT should be used as a further examination method before surgical treatment or nonsurgical treatment of rotator cuff calcifying tendonitis. Ultrasonography can effectively detect calcification lesions, clarify the location of calcification lesions, observe the volume and shape of calcification lesions without radiation, and can be used in pregnant women and other populations, but it is highly dependent on the experience and technology of the examiner [6]. MRI is helpful in the differential diagnosis and discovery of rotator cuff accompanied by injury, but the examination time is long and the cost is high. Only when the clinician has a profound understanding of the epidemiology, pathological process, auxiliary examination, and other basic knowledge of rotator cuff calcifying tendonitis, he can correctly choose the treatment method and the timing of surgical treatment. Rotator cuff calcifying tendonitis needs to be differentiated from rotator cuff injury, subacromial impingement syndrome, cervical spondylosis, biceps tendonitis, gouty arthritis, and other diseases, especially from degenerative or malnutrition calcification. The latter two are prone to occur in older people, and the lesion is at the tendon–bone junction, which is not a self-limited disease. Absorption phase calcification involves the subacromial sac, the long head of the biceps tendon or the greater tuberosity of the humerus bone tissue, and may also involve the short head of the biceps tendon. There is controversy about whether there is a correlation between rotator cuff calcification and rotator cuff injury. Some scholars found that there is a significant correlation between cloudy calcification and rotator cuff injury, but it is impossible to predict whether there is rotator cuff injury by the location or volume of calcification. Retrospective studies found that there was no statistically significant difference in the prevalence of rotator cuff injury between the calcified rotator cuff tendonitis group and the shoulder pain control group, suggesting that the calcified rotator cuff tendonitis and rotator cuff injury are two different pathological processes.

28.3 Nonsurgical Treatment of Calcified Rotator Cuff Tendinitis

Conservative treatment is preferred for calcified rotator cuff tendinitis, including immobilization, ice therapy, physical therapy, and the use of nonsteroidal anti-inflammatory drugs. Many patients can be cured by conservative treatments such as the use of nonsteroidal anti-inflammatory drugs or closure. The application of nonsteroidal anti-inflammatory drugs as the preferred treatment can effectively relieve the shoulder pain symptoms of most patients. Invasive nonsurgical treatment is suitable for patients with severe or protracted calcified rotator cuff tendinitis, among which subacromial corticosteroid injection (SAI) is the most commonly used treatment in clinic due to its low cost and fewer complications [7]. De Witte et al. [8] found that 73% of patients with calcified rotator cuff tendinitis had complete absorption of calcified lesions after SAI treatment, and the symptoms were relieved. Extracorporeal shock wave therapy (ESWT) is a physical therapy method that can effectively promote the fragmentation and absorption of calcified lesions in calcified rotator cuff tendinitis and achieve good clinical efficacy [9]. The energy flux density (EFD) of low-intensity shock wave is <0.08~0.12 mJ/mm^2, while the EFD of high-intensity shock wave is >0.12~0.28 mJ/mm^2 [10]. Verstraelen et al. [11] found that high-intensity shock wave can more effectively promote the absorption of calcified lesions in patients with calcified rotator cuff tendinitis and relieve shoulder pain. The latest randomized controlled trials show that the short-term clinical efficacy of ESWT for rotator cuff calcification tendonitis is worse than that of ultrasound-guided percutaneous irrigation of calcific tendinopathy (US-PICT). The probability of persistent shoulder pain after ESWT treatment is 41%, and residual symptoms require SAI, US-PICT, and other interventions [11]. However, as a noninvasive treatment, ESWT has advantages of short treatment time, low cost, and easy operation, which is the first treatment method that patients with rotator cuff calcification tendonitis are willing to try.

US-PICT is currently considered to be the first-line treatment for rotator cuff calcification tendonitis, which can effectively relieve pain and has almost no obvious complications [12].This technique uses a syringe to inject 4 mL of 0.9% NaCl solution into the calcification lesion under ultrasound guidance, and then the solution of dissolved calcium salts is sucked out of the body, repeated several times, until the salt solution sucked out of the body does not contain calcified substances. Studies have shown that the saline solution heated to 42 °C is more effective than the saline solution at room temperature in dissolving calcified lesions [13]. Some scholars have proposed that the double-needle technique is suitable for hard calcified lesions in order to completely crush calcified substances, while the single-needle technique is more suitable for liquid calcified lesions [14]. Lanza et al. [15] conducted a systematic review of 15 articles on US-PICT for rotator cuff calcification tendonitis and found that US-PICT is a safe and effective treatment, relieving 55% of shoulder pain on average, and only 10% of mild complications. Studies have shown that US-PICT combined with SAI can improve the short-term clinical efficacy of rotator cuff calcifying tenosynovitis.

In the case of failure of conservative treatment in acute attack, the calcified lesions can be punctured and sucked repeatedly with epidural needles to decompress and release calcified substances, which can significantly relieve the pain symptoms of patients. Oudelaar et al. [15] used this method to treat 431 patients with rotator cuff calcifying tenosynovitis, conducted a 6-week follow-up, and found that 74% of patients with shoulder pain were completely relieved of pain, achieving good curative effect. The author used subacromial injection of local anesthetics and decompression of calcified lesions under X-ray fluoroscopy for patients with unbearable pain at onset and poor effect of conservative treatment in acute attack (Fig. 28.4), and the patient's symptoms were relieved, and good curative effect was achieved. Postoperative X-ray examination showed that the calcified spots disappeared (Fig. 28.5). After puncture and suction of calcified lesions, subacromial sac injection of glucocorticoids or platelet-rich plasma (PRP) can effectively inhibit the inflammatory reaction of calcified lesions and promote tendon healing. Studies have shown that nonsteroidal anti-inflammatory drugs (NSAIDs) combined with SAI can early relieve the pain symptoms of patients with rotator cuff calcifying tenosynovitis, restore shoulder joint function, and reduce the probability of complications such as bursitis and periarthritis of shoulder.

28.4 Arthroscopic Debridement for the Treatment of Calcifying Tenosynovitis

With the development of arthroscopy technology, arthroscopic surgery can precisely treat the lesions, and at the same time, it can explore and treat rotator cuff injuries, clean up synovitis, and perform acromionoplasty. For patients whose symptoms do not obviously improve after conservative treatment, surgical treatment can be performed. Shoulder arthroscopy for the treatment of calcified rotator cuff tendonitis is a treatment method with small trauma, quick recovery, and good effect, mainly including calcification removal, subacromial decompression, and the treatment of accompanying injuries. Preoperative X-ray examination is used to confirm the location and type of calcified lesions. X-ray type III, that is, the calcified shadow is cloudy and low in density, indicating that this is the absorption period, and surgical treatment should be considered carefully [16]. CT, ultrasound, and MRI examinations should be selected according to the specific situation, which can help develop a precise surgical plan. Arthroscopic calcification removal: the glenohumeral joint is explored from the posterior approach, and the strawberry spot of inflammatory stimulation and hyperemia and edema on the supraspinatus tendon joint cavity can be seen (Fig. 28.6). The needle is inserted into the strawberry spot, and a nylon thread is inserted along the needle core to explore the subacromial space. The location of the calcified lesion is determined by finding the suture. The calcified lesion cyst wall is punctured with an epidural needle, and the white calcified spot is shown in the subacromial space (Fig. 28.7). The tip of the needle can bring out lime slag-like calcification (Fig. 28.8). Due to high pressure, the calcified lesion erupts like a volcanic eruption. The lesion and adhesion band were cleaned with a radiofrequency plasma knife (Fig. 28.9). In most cases, repair of the rotator cuff is not necessary, but if the full-thickness rotator cuff tear is large, the damaged rotator cuff can be sutured side to side. The morphology of the acromion and the wear of the coracoclavicular arch were used to determine whether acromionoplasty was performed. Functional exercises were performed after 3–4 weeks of immobilization.

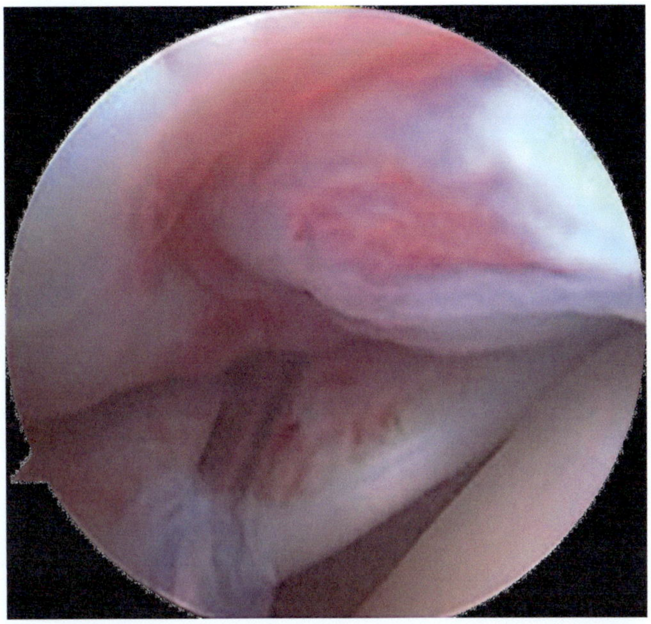

Fig. 28.6 Arthroscopic display of hyperemic, edematous strawberry patches of supraspinatus tendon in the glenohumeral joint space

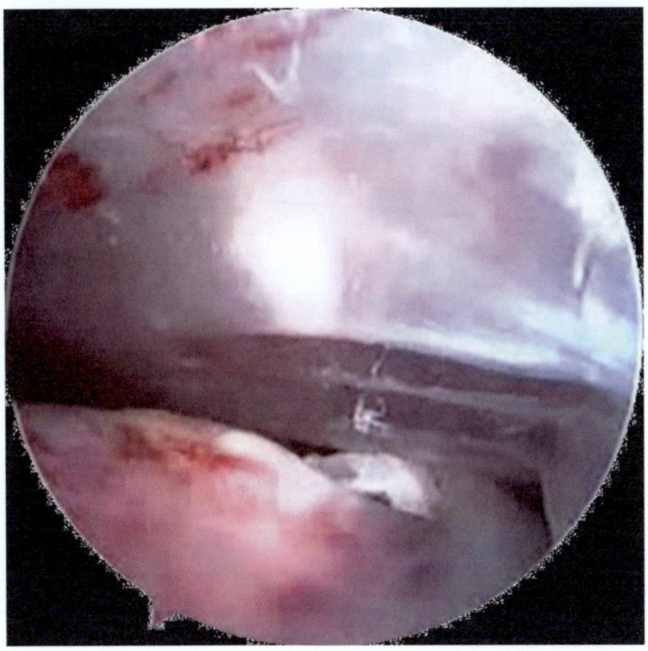

Fig. 28.7 White calcified lesion found in the subacromial space

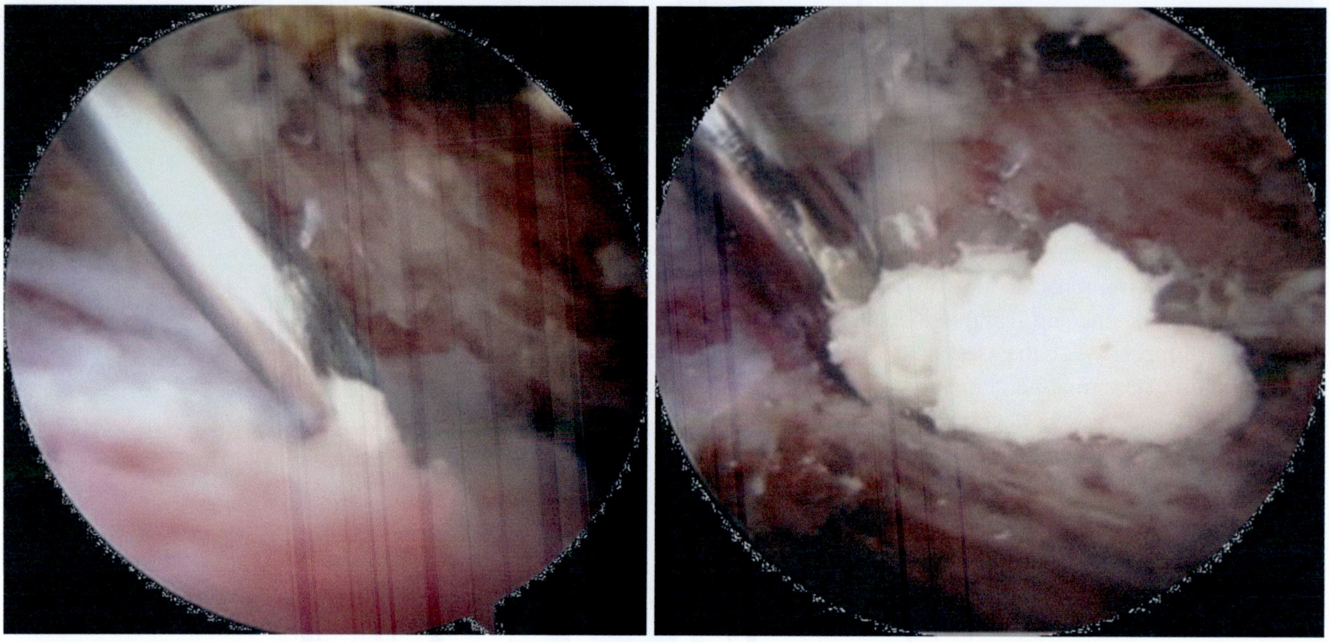

Fig. 28.8 Puncture needle penetrates calcified lesion, lime slag-like calcified material erupts

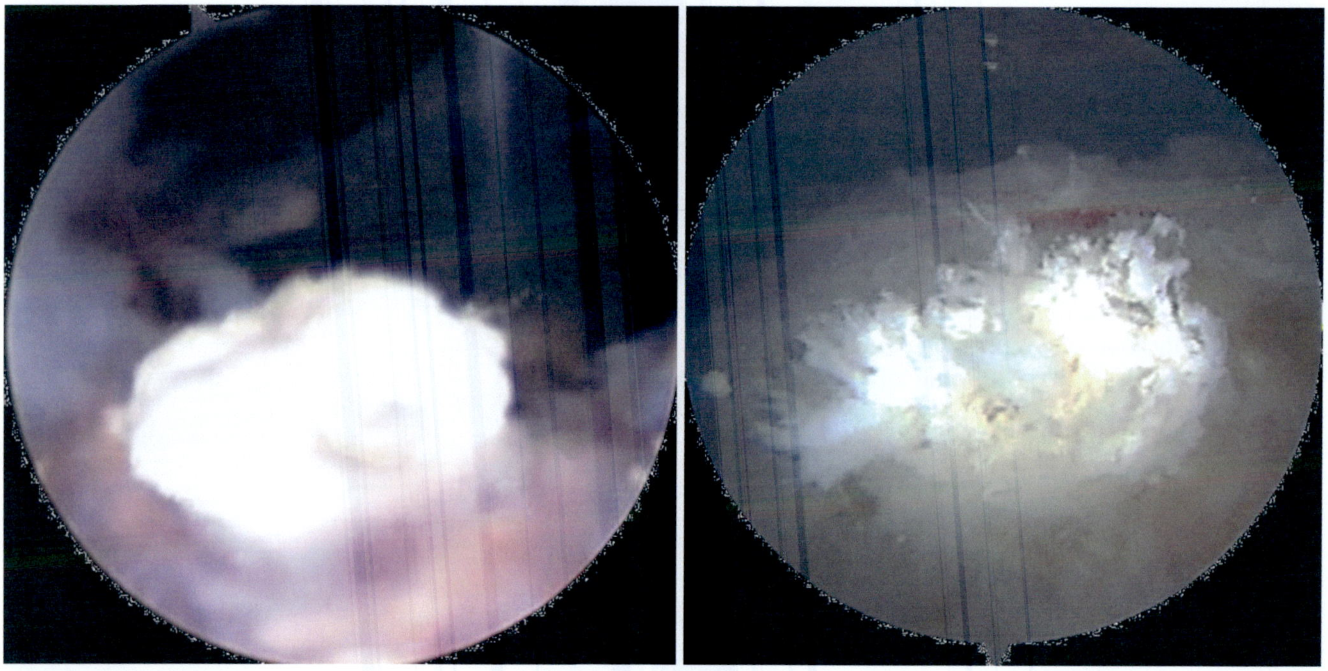

Fig. 28.9 Cleaning calcified supraspinatus tendon

28.5 Calcifying Tendonitis Does Not Always Occur in the Supraspinatus Tendon

Calcifying tendonitis does not always occur in the supraspinatus tendon. The supraspinatus tendon accounts for about 80%, the infraspinatus tendon accounts for 15%, and the subscapularis tendon accounts for 5% [1]. Sometimes, simple anterior–posterior X-ray films (Fig. 28.10) are difficult to accurately locate the location of calcified lesions, and unclear localization will affect the accurate treatment of the lesions. Therefore, CT examination (Fig. 28.11) or CT three-dimensional reconstruction (Fig. 28.12) are of important reference value for accurate localization. Calcifying tendonitis

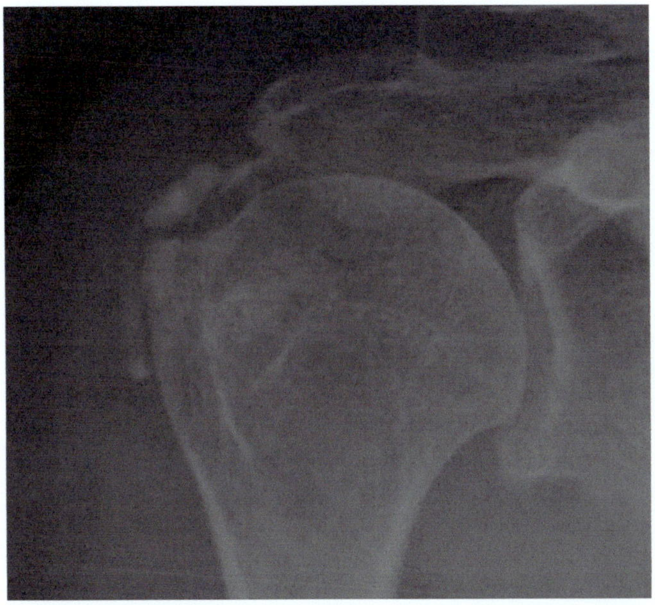

Fig. 28.10 Anterior and posterior x-ray of shoulder showing calcified lesion of shoulder

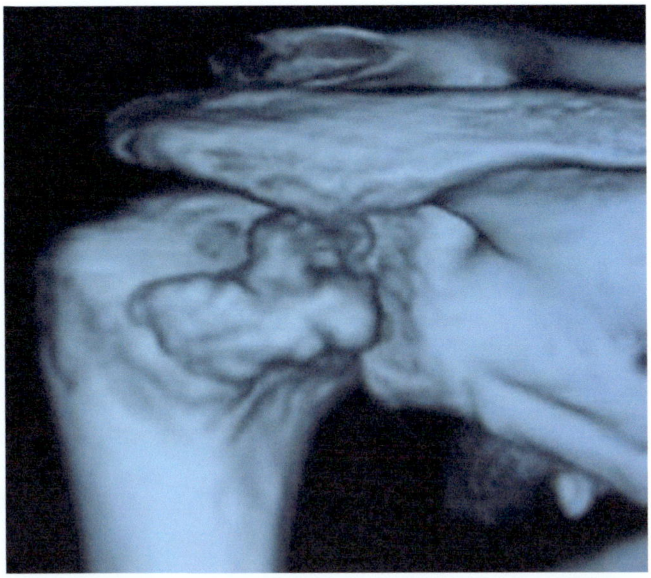

Fig. 28.12 CT three-dimensional reconstruction showing large high-density calcified lesion in the infraspinatus

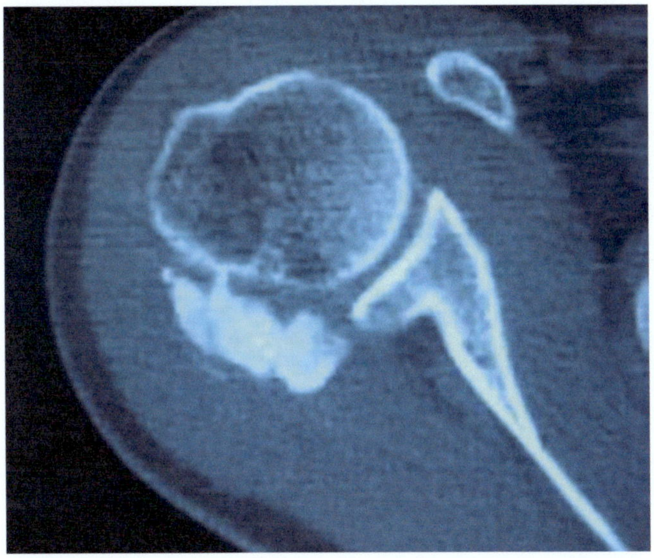

Fig. 28.11 CT examination showing calcified lesion in the infraspinatus

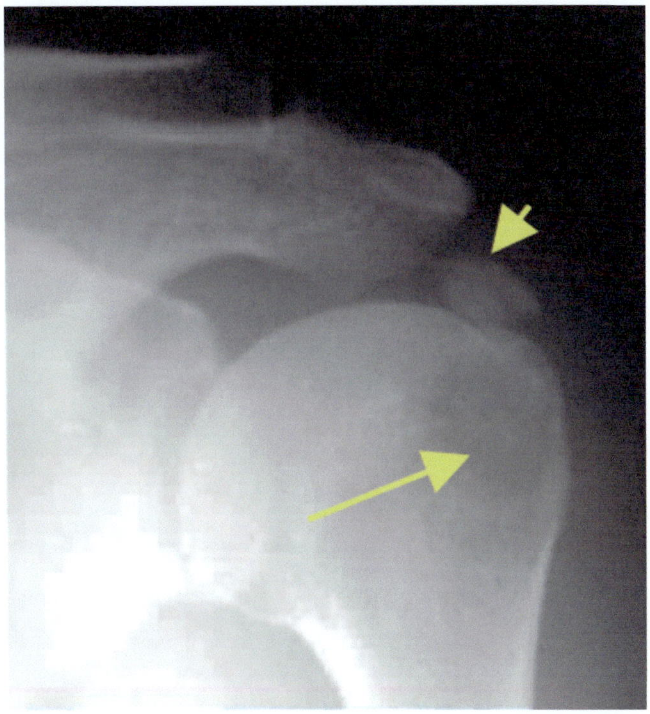

Fig. 28.13 X-ray showing calcified lesion under the acromion (short arrow) and reduced bone density in the greater tuberosity (long arrow)

involving the humeral greater tuberosity bone accounts for 9–34%, showing an oval area of reduced bone density (Fig. 28.13). MRI shows that calcification involves the humeral head bone (Fig. 28.14). After cleaning and curettage of the lesions under arthroscopy, the lesions in the humeral head are shown (Fig. 28.15). Bone grafting or hydroxyapatite filling of the bone defect can be used in the cavity (Fig. 28.16). Before operation, attention should be paid to the identification with avulsion fracture. The high-density area of avulsion fracture is small, with clear and sharp edges, discontinuous humeral bone edges, and the absence of fracture fragments can be found. In the short term, edema signals appear at the fracture site (Fig. 28.17). With the development

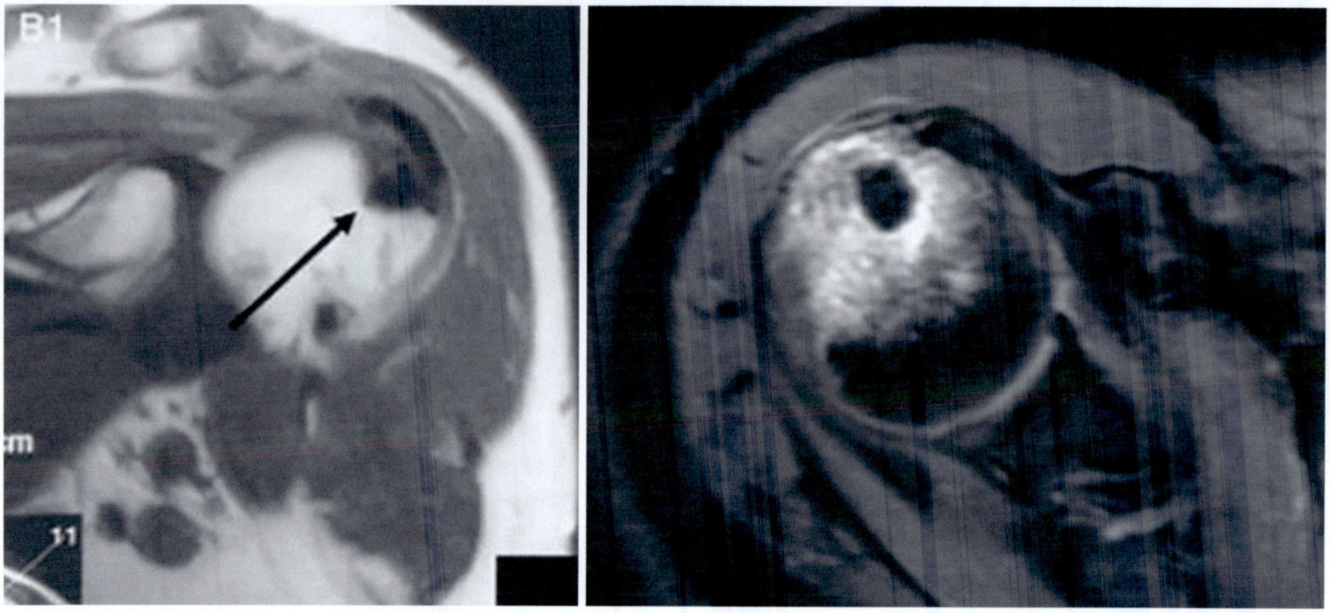

Fig. 28.14 MRI showing calcification involving the supraspinatus tendon attachment point of the greater tuberosity

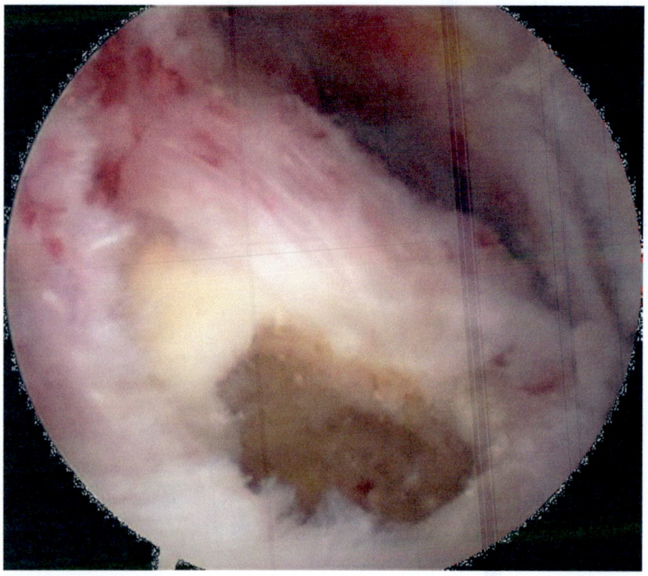

Fig. 28.15 Arthroscopic curettage of lesion, showing a cavity in the greater tuberosity

of arthroscopy technology, shoulder arthroscopy can precisely treat the lesions, and at the same time it can explore and treat rotator cuff injuries, clean synovitis, and perform acromioplasty. Studies have shown that calcified rotator cuff tendonitis may cause bursitis, rotator cuff injury, myositis ossificans, acromion impingement, and other complications. Arthroscopic surgery is used to treat calcified rotator cuff tendonitis only when other treatments fail.

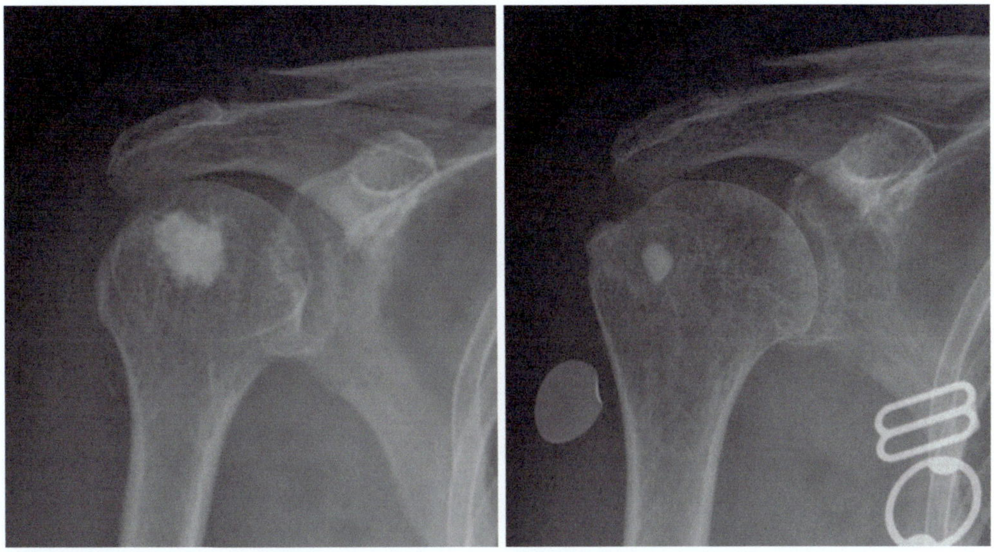

Fig. 28.16 Hydroxyapatite implanted into the greater tuberosity cavity to fill bone defect

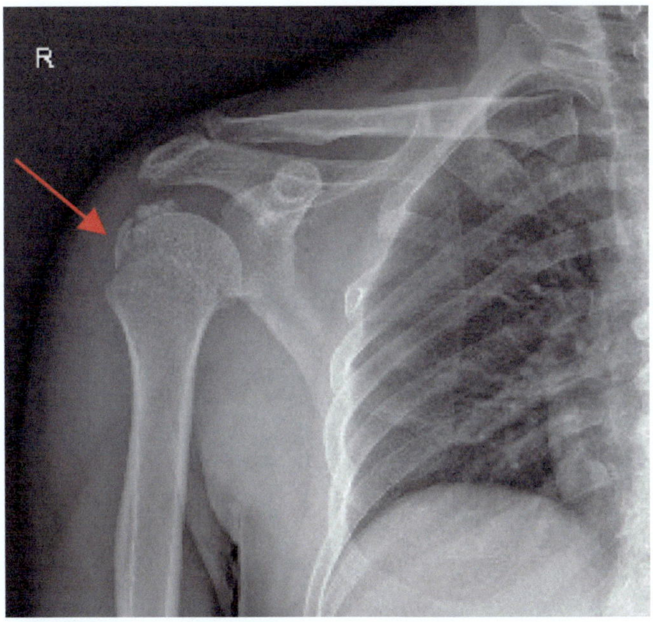

Fig. 28.17 Avulsion fracture of the greater tuberosity

References

1. Cocco G, Ricci V, Boccatonda A, et al. Migration of calcium deposit over the biceps brachii muscle, a rare complication of calcific tendinopathy: ultrasound image and treatment. J Ultrasound. 2018;21(4):351–4.
2. Messina C, Banfi G, Orlandi D, et al. Ultrasound-guided interventional procedures around the shoulder. Br J Radiol. 2016;89(1057):20150372.
3. Orlandi D, Mauri G, Lacelli F, et al. Rotator cuff calcific tendinopathy: randomized comparison of US-guided percutaneous treatments by using one or two needles. Radiology. 2017;285(2):518–27.
4. Uhthoff HK, Sarkar K. Calcifying tendinitis. Baillieres Clin Rheumatol. 1989;3(3):567–81.
5. Becciolini M, Bonacchi G, Galletti S. Intramuscular migration of calcific tendinopathy in the rotator cuff: ultrasound appearance and a review of the literature. J Ultrasound. 2016;19(3):175–81.
6. Kamawal Y, Steinert AF, Holzapfel BM, et al. Case report—calcification of the medial collateral ligament of the knee with simultaneous calcifying tendinitis of the rotator cuff. BMC Musculoskelet Disord. 2016;17(1):283.
7. Nörenberg D, Ebersberger HU, Walter T, et al. Diagnosis of calcific tendonitis of the rotator cuff by using susceptibility-weighted MR imaging. Radiology. 2016;278(2):475–84.
8. De Witte PB, Kolk A, Overes F, et al. Rotator cuff calcific tendinitis: ultrasound-guided needling and lavage versus subacromial corticosteroids: five-year outcomes of a randomized controlled trial. Am J Sports Med. 2017;45(14):3305–14.
9. Arirachakaran A, Boonard M, Yamaphai S, et al. Extracorporeal shock wave therapy, ultrasound-guided percutaneous lavage, corticosteroid injection and combined treatment for the treatment of rotator cuff calcific tendinopathy: a network meta-analysis of RCTs. Eur J Orthop Surg Traumatol. 2017;27(3):381–90.
10. Malliaropoulos N, Thompson D, Meke M, et al. Individualised radial extracorporeal shock wave therapy (rESWT) for symptomatic calcific shoulder tendinopathy: a retrospective clinical study. BMC Musculoskelet Disord. 2017;18(1):513.
11. Verstraelen F, Verhagen S, Giesberts A, et al. Needle aspiration of calcific deposits versus shock wave therapy for conservative therapy resistant calcifying tendinitis of the shoulder: protocol of a randomized, controlled trial. BMC Musculoskelet Disord. 2022;23(1):308.
12. Louwerens JKG, Sierevelt IN, Kramer ET, et al. Comparing ultrasound-guided needling combined with a subacromial corticosteroid injection versus high-energy extracorporeal shockwave therapy for calcific tendinitis of the rotator cuff: a randomized controlled trial. Arthroscopy. 2020;36(7):1823–1833.e1.
13. Sconfienza LM, Vigano S, Martini C, et al. Double-needle ultrasound-guided percutaneous treatment of rotator cuff calcific tendinitis: tips & tricks. Skeletal Radiol. 2013;42(1):19–24.
14. Spinnato P, Ponti F, D'Agostino V, et al. Ultrasound-guided percutaneous irrigation of calcific tendinopathy outside the rotator cuff: short-term evaluation. Skeletal Radiol. 2022;51(10):2039–44.
15. Lanza E, Banfi G, Serafini G, et al. Ultrasound-guided percutaneous irrigation in rotator cuff calcific tendinopathy: what is the evidence? A systematic review with proposals for future reporting. Eur Radiol. 2015;25(7):2176–83.
16. Wei J, Cai X, Liuyu J, et al. Extra-articular arthroscopic treatment of rotator cuff calcifying tendonitis. Orthop J China. 2008;2008(7):501–3.

Misconceptions and Countermeasures in the Diagnosis and Treatment of Shoulder Loose Body and Rice Body

29

Yu-jie Liu, Chun-bao Li, and Ming-xin Wang

29.1 Case

A 62-year-old male retiree presented with a longstanding mass in his right shoulder joint, which had progressively enlarged over the course of four months. The pain associated with the mass worsened following physical exertion and improved with rest. There was no examination report for joint dysfunction or locking. The patient denied any history of trauma, fever, night sweats, or weight loss. Previous medical evaluations had identified the mass as a lipoma, with further investigation warranted for possible tumor involvement.

Physical examination: A lump was identified anterior to the right shoulder joint, measuring approximately the size of a duck egg (Fig. 29.1). The local temperature of the skin is normal, with no erythema or edema. Dilated capillaries and obvious tenderness points were not observed either. Palpation revealed a soft lump with a fluctuant quality, which did not demonstrate mobility with shoulder joint movements or positional changes. The abduction, supine, and supine rotation movements of the shoulder joint are mildly restricted, but no significant abnormalities in upper limb muscle strength were observed.

The X-ray and CT examination of the right shoulder joint revealed no evident abnormalities. Ultrasonography indicated dilation of the subacromial and subdeltoid bursa with reduced intracapsular translucency, as well as hyperplasia of synovial tissue with flocculent and cornified echoes (Fig. 29.2). Additionally, partial damage to the right rotator cuff was observed (Fig. 29.3). MRI imaging displayed pomegranate seed–like low signal images in the anterior joint capsule of the shoulder joint, subdeltoid muscle, and subacromial bursa (Fig. 29.4)

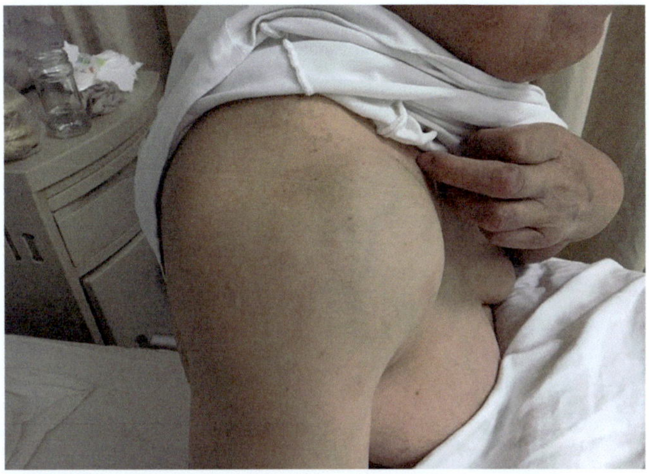

Fig. 29.1 The lump located in front of the right shoulder joint

The patient underwent shoulder arthroscopy under general anesthesia. The results showed mild degeneration on the surface of shoulder joint cartilage, as well as wear of the rotator cuff tissue below the acromion. Synovial hyperplasia (Fig. 29.5) was observed in both the subacromial and the subdeltoid bursa, with the presence of rice-like particles (Fig. 29.6) in the latter. Additionally, the axillary bursa also contained rice bodies resembled pomegranate seeds (Fig. 29.7). Subsequently, a large amount of rice bodies were successfully filtered out through arthroscopic surgery (Fig. 29.8), smaller ones were removed using negative pressure suction, while larger ones were extracted using nucleus pulposus forceps.

Y.-j. Liu
Orthopaedics, Chinese PLA General Hospital, Beijing, China

C.-b. Li (✉) · M.-x. Wang
Department of Orthopedics, The Fourth Medical Center, Chinese PLA General Hospital, Beijing, China

Y.-j. Liu et al. (eds.), *Pitfalls in Diagnosis and Treatment of Shoulder Joint Diseases*,
https://doi.org/10.1007/978-981-96-2472-0_29

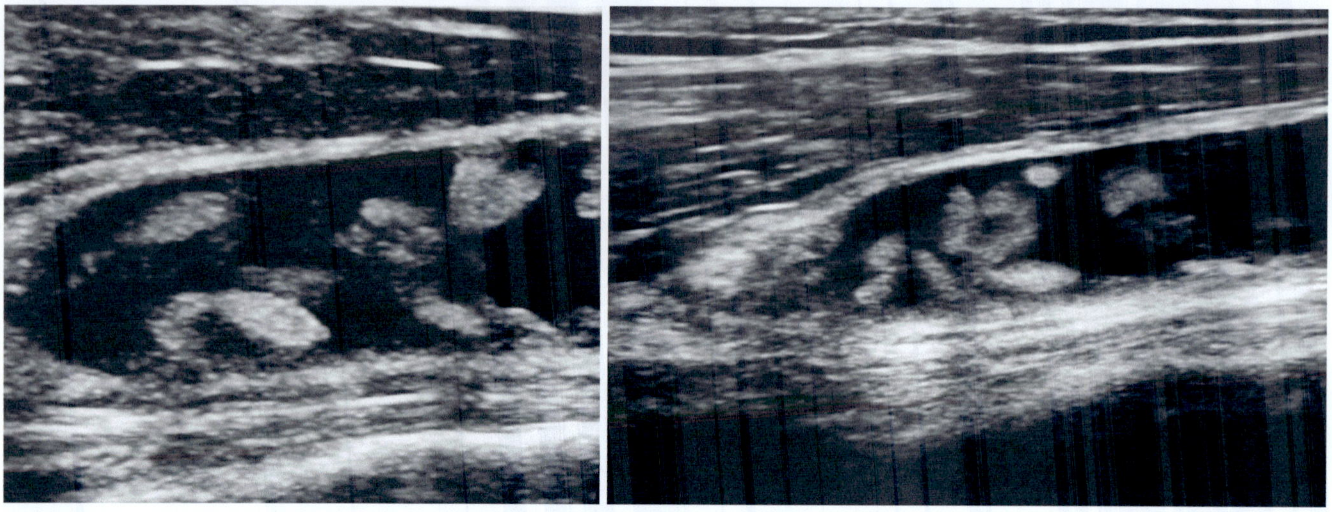

Fig. 29.2 Ultrasonography of the right shoulder joint showed subacromial and subdeltoid bursa rice body

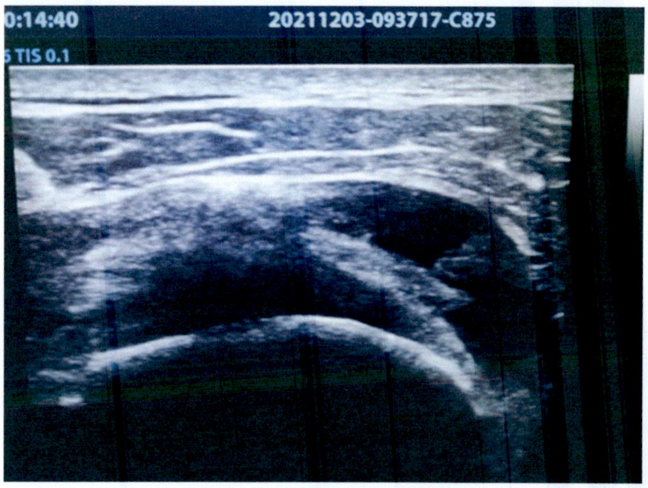

Fig. 29.3 Ultrasound of right shoulder shows rotator cuff injury

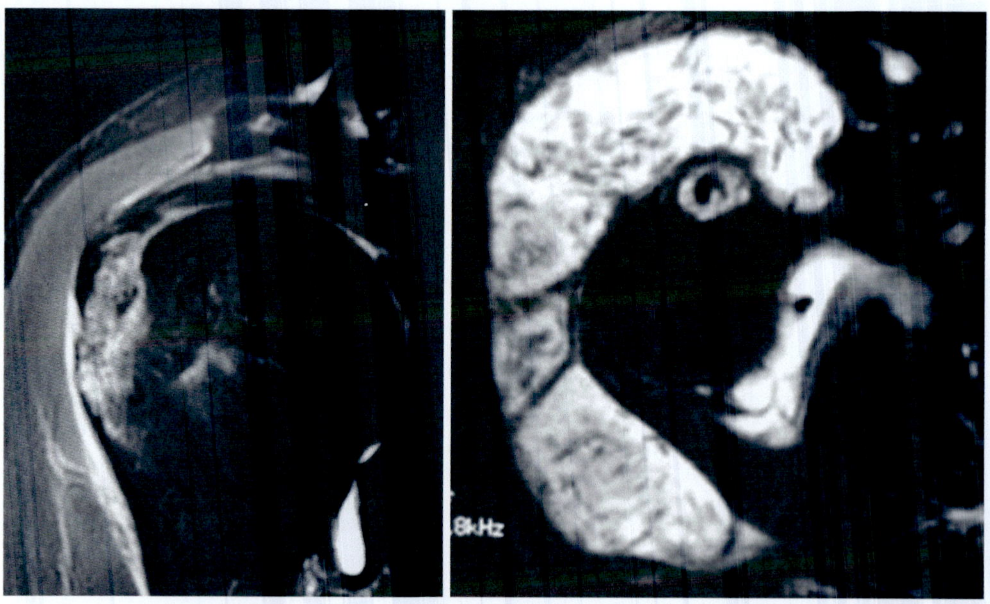

Fig. 29.4 MRI shows high signal in the subdeltoid bursa, with mixed signals

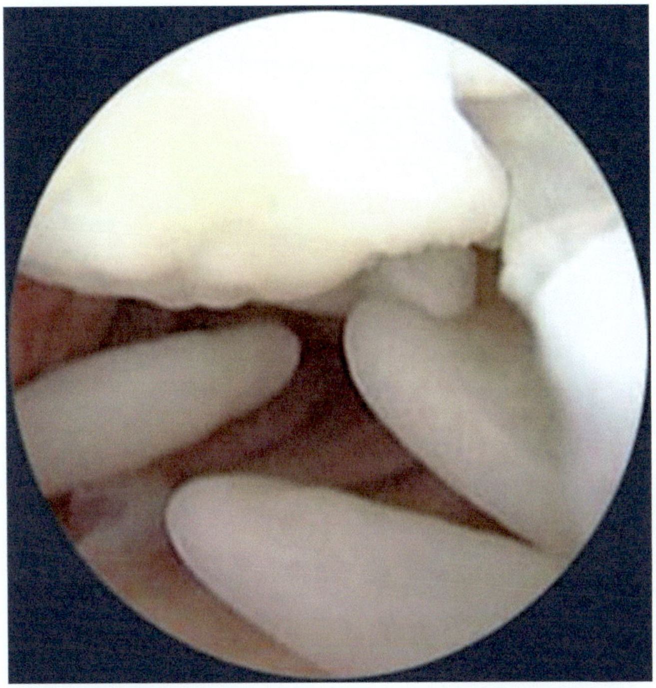

Fig. 29.5 Arthroscopy shows subacromial irregular rice-like bodies

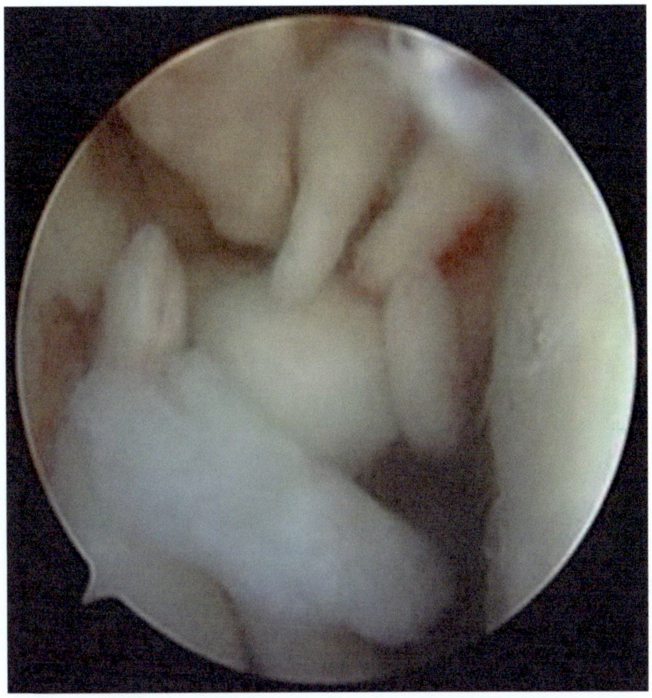

Fig. 29.6 Synovial hyperplasia in the bursa of the shoulder joint cavity with rice bodies

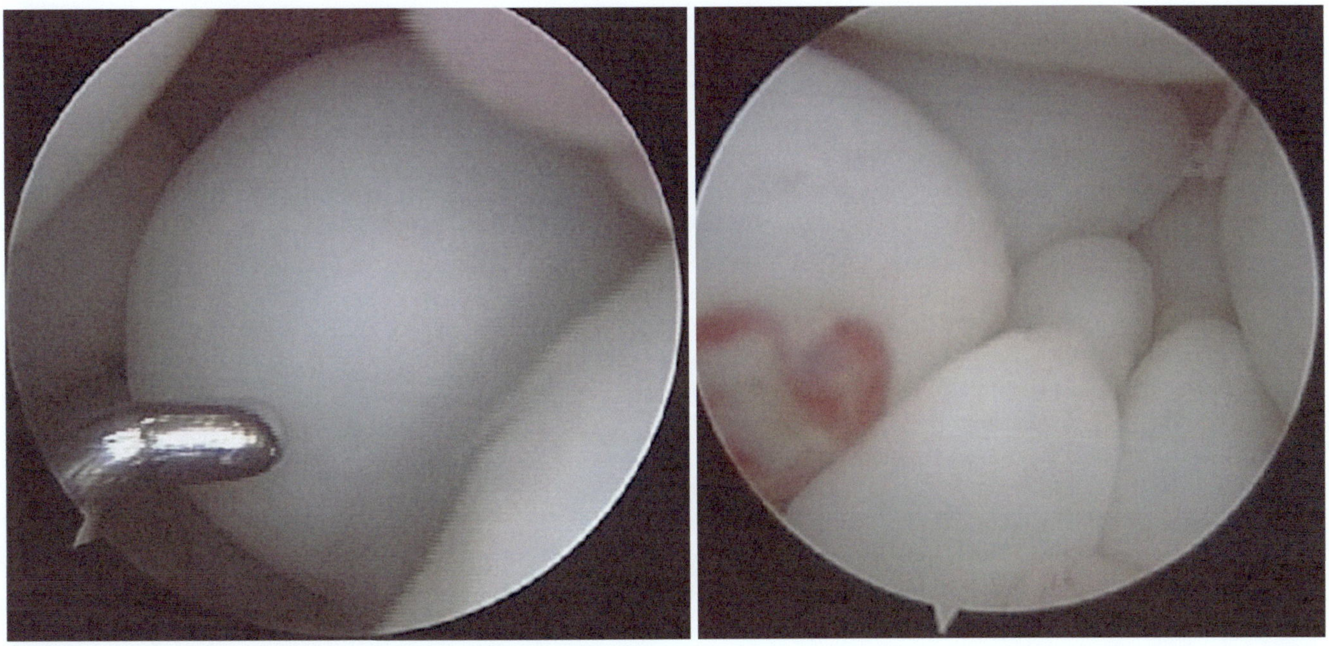

Fig. 29.7 Smooth, regular pomegranate seed–like rice bodies in the shoulder joint

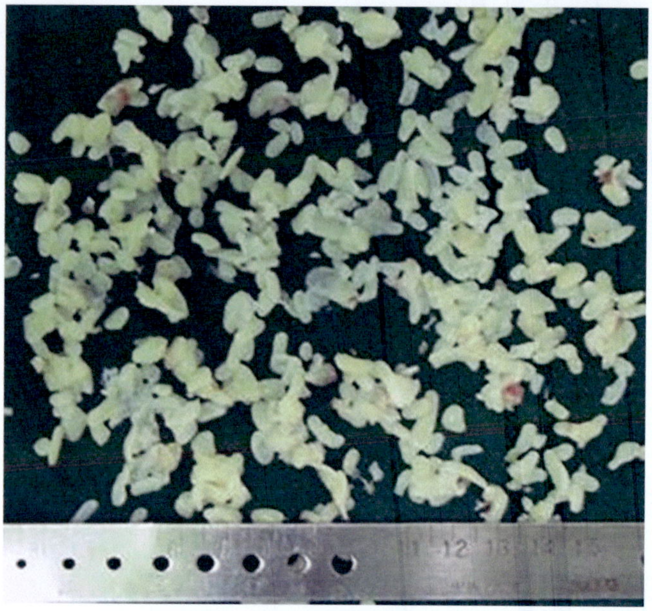

Fig. 29.8 Arthroscopic surgery to remove rice bodies

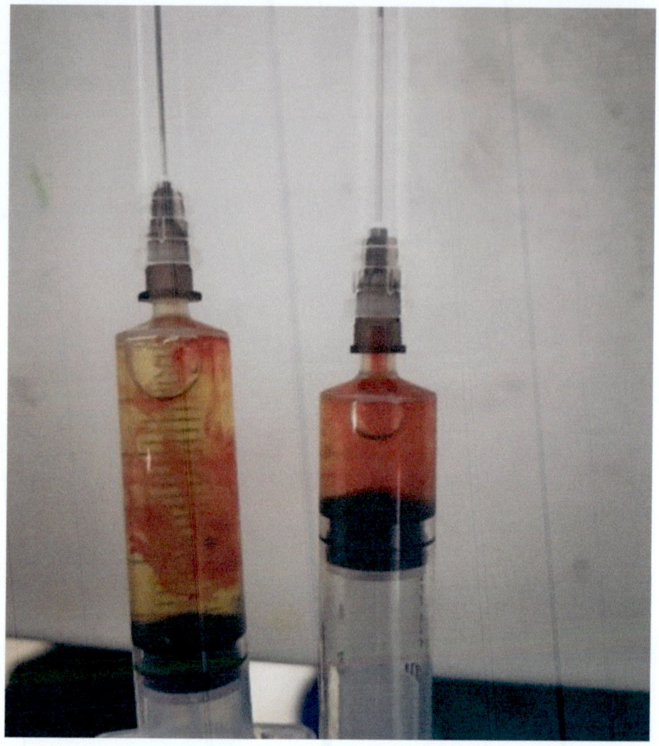

Fig. 29.9 Yellowish fluid withdrawn from a puncture of the shoulder joint with arthritis

29.2 Diagnosis

Since shoulder rice bodies can be easily misdiagnosed as tumors, tumors must be ruled out first in the case of a lump around the shoulder joint. We should figure out the benign or malignant nature of the mass, the site of its occurrence (within or outside the joint), and the origin of the tissue (bone tissue, soft tissue, or synovial tissue). Lipoma is also a common diagnosis for shoulder mass, and arthrocentesis is a valuable tool for identification and diagnosis. A soft mass with no extractable fluid is more likely to be a lipoma, while yellowish exudate on puncture fluid may indicate synovitis (Fig. 29.9). Common types include rheumatic or rheumatoid synovitis, osteoarticular traumatic synovitis, and gouty synovitis. If the fluid contains bright red blood, it is advisable to ask the patient about any history of injury, anticoagulants use (Fig. 29.10), or underlying hemophilia. Additionally, if the fluid appears coffee-colored, consideration should be given to Pigmented villonodular synovitis.

The etiology of shoulder rice bodies is associated with recurrent synovitis and exudation [1]. The exudate, which is high in protein and cartilage debris, gradually coalesces into rice-like particles resembling snowballs. These rice bodies typically range in diameter from 2 to 10 mm and may consist of fibrous proteins, collagen, reticulin, and elastin [2]. The author observed that the smoothness of rice bodies, as depicted in Fig. 29.11, may be influenced by the friction

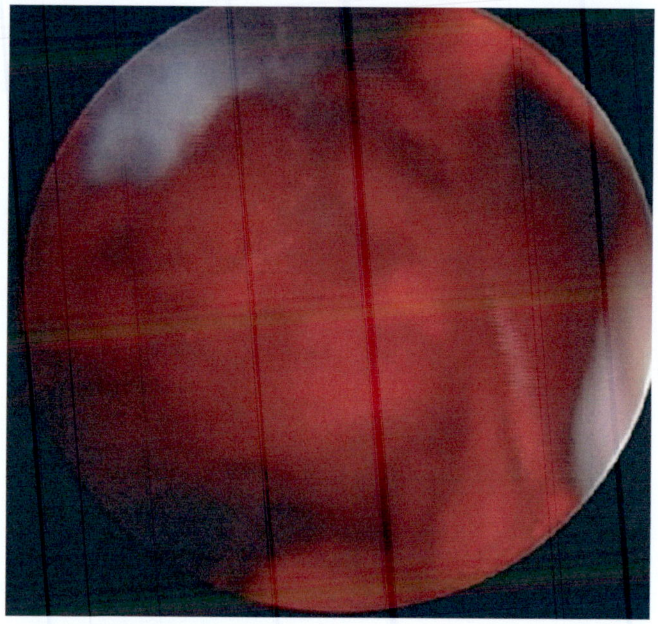

Fig. 29.10 The withdrawal of bloody fluid from the joint cavity is due to the application of anticoagulants

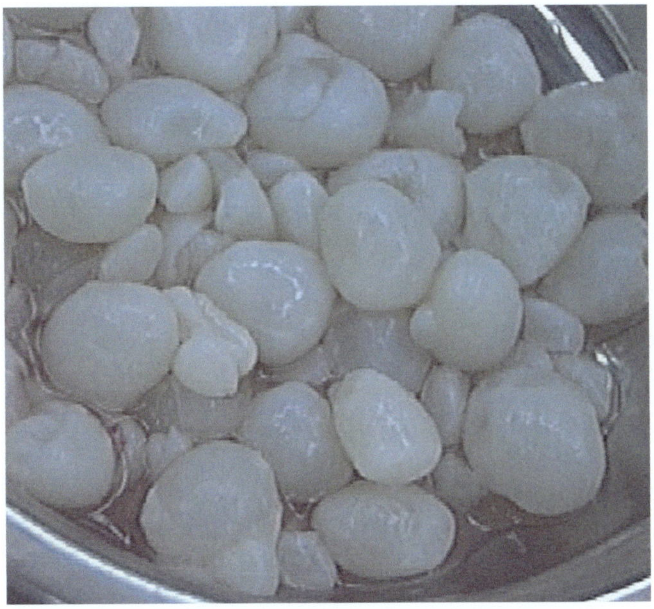

Fig. 29.11 Rice bodies in the cavity of the shoulder joint

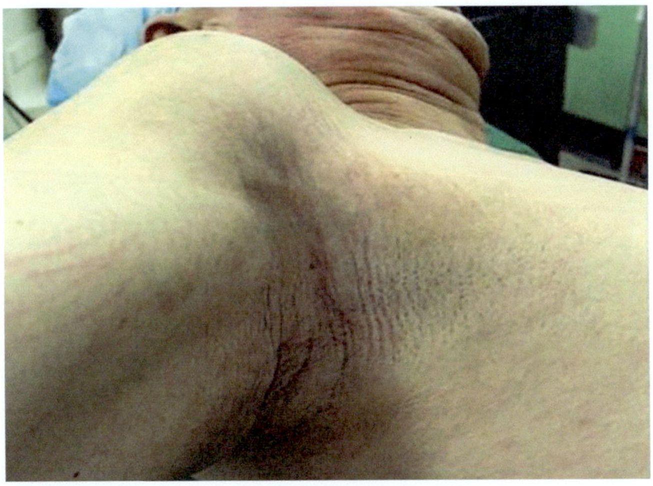

Fig. 29.12 Friction can be palpated by touching the lump formed by Synovial chondromatosis around right shoulder joint

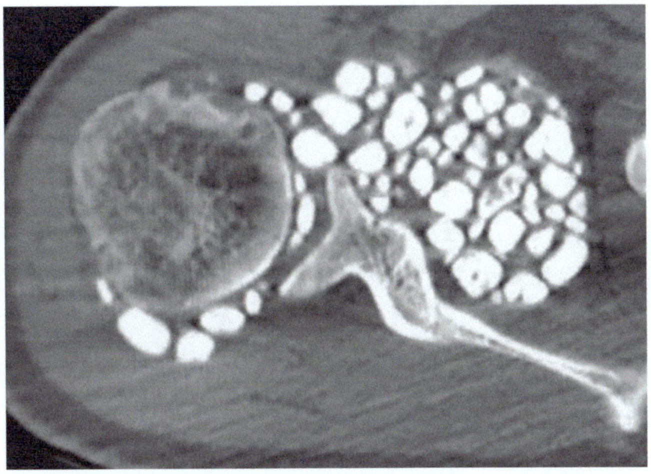

Fig. 29.13 CT scan showing loose bodies formed by Synovial chondromatosis in the shoulder joint cavity

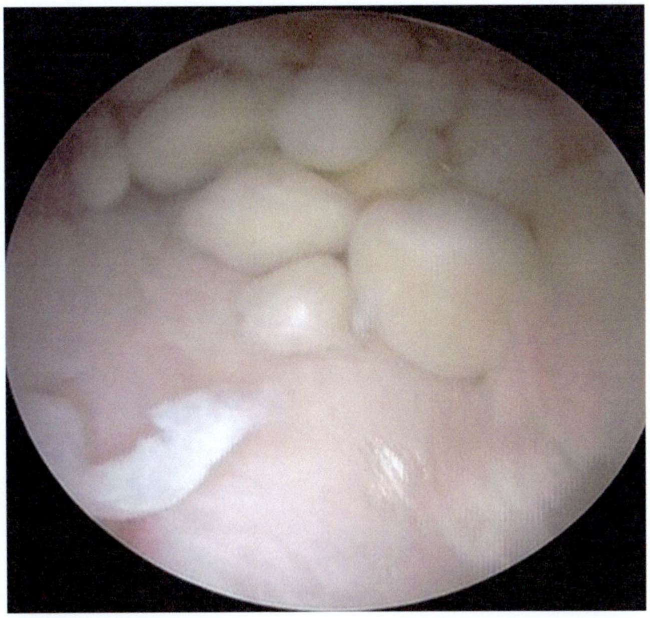

Fig. 29.14 Arthroscopy of the shoulder showing a large number of loose bodies

between the humeral head and the scapular glenoid. Due to their non-calcified nature, rice bodies cannot be seen on X-ray or CT imaging, therefore ultrasound and MRI must be used for visualization.

In addition, there are numerous similarities between synovial chondromatosis and rice body, which can be distinguished by friction sensation detected through palpation of the lump (Fig. 29.12). Radiographic imaging techniques such as X-rays and CT scans are effective in delineating the precise location and structure of the loose body associated with synovial chondromatosis (Fig. 29.13). Arthroscopic intervention allows for visualization and extraction of the loose body from the joint cavity (Figs. 29.14 and 29.15). The key strategies to minimize recurrence include arthroscopic removal of rice bodies and excision of synovium [3].

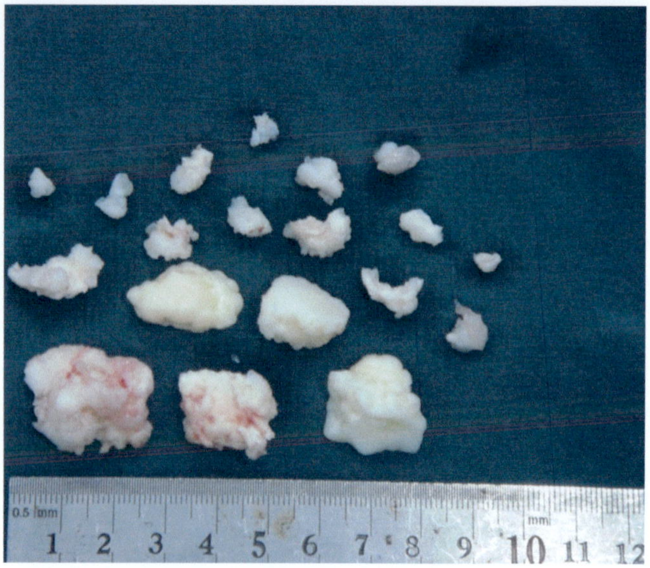

Fig. 29.15 Loose bodies from joint cavity

References

1. Edison MN, Caram A, Flores M, et al. Rice body formation within a periarticular shoulder mass. Cureus. 2016;8(8):e718.
2. Tan CHA, Rai SB, Chandy J. MRI appearances of multiple rice body formation in chronic subacromialand subdeltoid bursitis, in association with synovial chondromatosis. Clin Radiol. 2004;59(8):753–7.
3. Griffith JF, Peh WCG, Evans NS, et al. Multiple rice body formation in chronic subacromial/subdeltoid bursitis: MR appearances. Clin Radiol. 1996;51(7):511–4.

Corrections to: Misunderstandings and Countermeasures of Distal Clavicle Fracture

Chang-ming Huang, Yu-jie Liu, and Tian-hao Zhu

Correction to:
Chapter 15 in: Y.-j. Liu et al. (eds.), *Pitfalls in Diagnosis and Treatment of Shoulder Joint Diseases*, https://doi.org/10.1007/978-981-96-2472-0_15

For Fig. 15.19, we have updated the source credit line as "Source: Reprinted from the original figure."

This book was inadvertently published with an incorrect spelling of the editor's name in the front matter, which should read Chang-ming Huang instead of Changming Huang.

The updated version of this chapter can be found at
https://doi.org/10.1007/978-981-96-2472-0_15

Y. Liu et al. (eds.), *Pitfalls in Diagnosis and Treatment of Shoulder Joint Diseases*,
https://doi.org/10.1007/978-981-96-2472-0_30

MIX
Papier aus verantwortungsvollen Quellen
Paper from responsible sources
FSC® C105338

If you have any concerns about our products,
you can contact us on
ProductSafety@springernature.com

In case Publisher is established outside the EU,
the EU authorized representative is:
Springer Nature Customer Service Center GmbH
Europaplatz 3, 69115 Heidelberg, Germany

Printed by Libri Plureos GmbH
in Hamburg, Germany